BEING REDUCED

Being Reduced

New Essays on Reduction, Explanation, and Causation

Edited by
JAKOB HOHWY
JESPER KALLESTRUP

OXFORD
UNIVERSITY PRESS

OXFORD
UNIVERSITY PRESS

Great Clarendon Street, Oxford OX2 6DP

Oxford University Press is a department of the University of Oxford.
It furthers the University's objective of excellence in research, scholarship,
and education by publishing worldwide in

Oxford New York

Auckland Cape Town Dar es Salaam Hong Kong Karachi
Kuala Lumpur Madrid Melbourne Mexico City Nairobi
New Delhi Shanghai Taipei Toronto

With offices in

Argentina Austria Brazil Chile Czech Republic France Greece
Guatemala Hungary Italy Japan Poland Portugal Singapore
South Korea Switzerland Thailand Turkey Ukraine Vietnam

Oxford is a registered trade mark of Oxford University Press
in the UK and in certain other countries

Published in the United States
by Oxford University Press Inc., New York

First published 2008

British Library Cataloguing in Publication Data
Data available

Library of Congress Cataloging in Publication Data
Data available

Typeset by Laserwords Pvt. Ltd., Chennai, India
Printed in Great Britain
on acid-free paper by
Biddles Ltd., King's Lynn, Norfolk

ISBN 978–0–19–921153–1

1 3 5 7 9 10 8 6 4 2

Peter Lipton
in memoriam

Preface

To our minds, there are few more unsettling philosophical questions than this: "what happens in attempts to reduce some properties to some other more fundamental properties?" Reflection on this question inevitably touches on very deep issues about ourselves, our own interactions with the world and each other, and our very understanding of what there is and what goes on around us. If we cannot command a clear view of these deep issues, then very many other debates in contemporary philosophy seem to lose traction—think of causation, laws of nature, explanation, consciousness, personal identity, intentionality, normativity, freedom, responsibility, justice, and so on. Reduction can easily seem to unravel our world.

We asked an eminent group of philosophers to help us answer this question, and we are immensely grateful to them all for taking up the challenge—real progress is made on our question.

We wish to thank the Danish Research Council for the Humanities for funding for the research project *Naturalised Minds—Cognisant Nature* (known better as NAMICONA). This project was spearheaded by Lars Bo Gundersen whose vision for a research network on this topic proved crucial for the development and nurturing of an inspiring research milieu. We are very grateful to Lars Bo for making this possible. Thanks are also due to Jonas Christensen and Lena Frikke who assisted us all through the project; and we are grateful to Raphael Fiorese for compiling the index. Finally we should like to thank everybody at Oxford University Press for their support throughout.

Contents

List of Contributors

Louise Antony is Professor of Philosophy at the University of Massachusetts Amherst

Karen Bennett is Associate Professor of Philosophy at Cornell University

John Bickle is Professor of Philosophy at the University of Cincinnati

Tim Crane is Professor of Philosophy at University College London

Valerie Gray Hardcastle is Professor of Philosophy at University of Cincinnati

Jaegwon Kim is the William Herbert Perry Faunce Professor of Philosophy at Brown University

Peter Lipton was the Hans Rausing Professor of the History and Philosophy of Science at Cambridge University

Christian List is Professor of Political Science and Philosophy at the London School of Economics

Barry Loewer is Professor of Philosophy at Rutgers University

Peter Menzies is Professor of Philosophy at Macquarie University

David Papineau is Professor of Philosophy of Science at King's College London

Philip Pettit is the Laurance S. Rockefeller University Professor of Politics and Human Values at Princeton University

Peter Godfrey-Smith is Professor of Philosophy at Harvard University

Rosalyn Stewart is Assistant Professor of Medicine at Johns Hopkins University

Daniel Stoljar is Professor of Philosophy at the Australian National University

James Woodward is the J.O. and Juliette Koepfli Professor of Humanities at the California Institute of Technology

Introduction

1. BEING REDUCED

At least since the late 1950s reduction has been at the forefront of discussion in philosophy of mind and philosophy of science. But what is involved in the process of reduction, in something *being* reduced, or indeed in reducing a *being*? Roughly speaking, to reduce is to show that that which is reduced is nothing over and above that which it is reduced to. Reduction should thus be distinguished from a host of weaker non-causal determination relationships. For instance, to say that As do not reduce to Bs is at least prima facie compatible with saying that As are constituted by Bs. So, in the philosophy of mind, for example, rejection of reduction need not lead to outright dualism. Types of reduction can be distinguished along several dimensions. Firstly, the objects of reduction are sometimes taken to be laws, theories, explanations, concepts, or various ontological categories such as properties, kinds, or states—be they type or token. Secondly, reduction can be viewed as eliminative or conservative, for example, heat was conservatively reduced to mean molecular kinetic energy in gases, whereas caloric fluids were eliminated. Thirdly, some models of reduction assign a key role to a priori conceptual analysis, while other such models take reduction to be an entirely empirical activity. Fourthly, some hope for global reduction of for example mental states to physical states across all organisms and systems, while others settle for local species-specific reductions.

But why engage in scientific reduction? What is gained and what is lost in reducing something? Issues about reduction are typically intertwined with issues about explanation and causation. Some say that reduction facilitates reductive explanation. If we can reduce some higher-level phenomena to some lower-level phenomena, then we gain an explanation of the former in terms of the latter. For instance, if As do not reduce to Bs, how can A-type facts be explained in terms of B-type facts? Others say that reduction paves the way for mental and special science causation. For instance, if As do not reduce to Bs, how can there be any causal work left for A-type properties if B-type properties are causally sufficient for the putative effects of A-type properties? Yet others may be driven by theoretical background considerations. If we can at least in principle reduce all higher-level phenomena to physical lower-level phenomena, then we can be metaphysically satisfied that physicalism is true.

There are long-standing but relatively disjoint traditions for discussing reduction, explanation, and causation in philosophy of science and philosophy of mind. In philosophy of mind, the focus tends to be on the metaphysics of reduction, less on reductive explanation. Similarly, the discussion of mental causation has focused more on intuitive notions of causal relevance than on notions of causal inference employed in the special sciences. In philosophy of science, the focus has been more on theory reduction than reduction in terms of functionalisation and realisation. Similarly, there has been less focus on the sense in which the causes retrieved in the special sciences convey causal relevance as well as on how they cohere with what fundamental physics has to say. The papers published in this volume show very clearly that the debates on reduction, explanation, and causation will see progress by taking what is best from both philosophy of mind and philosophy of science, and that both disciplines have important lessons to learn by studying how reduction, explanation, and causation take place in such diverse empirical subjects as biology, medicine, neuroscience, and political science.

The chapters in this volume offer an astounding richness of argument and new perspectives on reduction, explanation, and causation that comfortably span the special sciences and the philosophy of mind. Below we indicate how the contributions can be situated in the wider debate, which they are likely to influence and inspire in the future. In the last section we provide brief summaries of each of the contributions.

2. REDUCTION, EXPLANATION AND CAUSATION: SITUATING THE CONTRIBUTIONS IN THE WIDER DEBATE

Nagel (1961) aimed to reduce theories by showing how the laws of the target theory could be logically derived from the laws of the reducing theory, augmented with empirical bridge laws that connect their respective kind predicates. But such laws were hard to come by, and many reductionist philosophers have instead adopted the functional model of reduction as in Lewis (1970, 1999). To reduce a target property on this model, we must first give it an a priori functional redescription in terms of its characteristic causal role. Then we a posteriori pin down the realiser in the reduction base that—uniquely or approximately—plays this role. And then finally we identify the realiser with the target property. One distinctive virtue of the functional model is that it seems to facilitate reductive explanation, at least on a deductive-nomological understanding of such explanation. In order for an explanation to be reductive, the explanatory premises of a phenomenon involving property F must not refer to any F-type properties. The first step in a functional reduction does refer to such properties, but is a definition, and definitions are not extra premises in explanatory deductions. In contrast, the classic bridge-law model of reduction cannot satisfy this constraint on reductive explanation (Kim 2005, and Chapter 5 in this volume). Crucially, functional reduction would close the explanatory gap between the physical and the phenomenal (Levine 1983, 1998): Why does pain and not something else arise from C-fibre stimulation? Why does pain arise from C-fibre stimulation and not from something else? If functional definitions of phenomenal properties are available, it looks as though a rich enough story not couched in pain-terminology could enable an a priori deduction of particular pain-facts (Chalmers and Jackson 2001).

Many believe that a priori functionalisations of phenomenal properties are not available, due to the special nature of consciousness (Tye 2002; Kim 2005). However, some philosophers are convinced that a priori functionalisations are simply not forthcoming for any properties at all (Block and Stalnaker 1999; Byrne 1999; Yablo 2000). They advance general semantic worries about analyticity, the a priori and narrow content. Instead they have adopted an identity model of reduction (Block, forthcoming), which infers identities as part of the best explanation of certain causal facts about the reduced phenomena. On their view, reductive explanation is possible without functional reduction. True, there is a sense in which appeal to identities in explanatory deductions comes for free: such identities merely rewrite the phenomena already transparently explained in a different vocabulary. But in an opaque sense such identities allow explanations we would not otherwise have. Notably, the identity model makes the explanatory gap questions illegitimate. There is no question of closing the explanatory gap, because there simply is no such gap between the *relata* of an identity.

The functionalist model of reduction and reductive explanation derives mainly from philosophy of mind and is fairly general and abstract. The question arises whether this is the pattern seen in scientific practice. Hardcastle and Stewart (Chapter 1 in this volume) argue that reduction and hence reductive explanation may be unattainable in some areas of science. For example, they report a case study where a mental illness comes quite severely apart from its commonsense causal role. And they point out that in some cases, an adequate explanation is available even if reduction for practical reasons seems out of the question. On the other hand, there is the view that science is indeed reductive but not in the abstract way normally conceived by philosophers. Bickle (Chapter 2 in this volume) uses a case study of memory research in mice to demonstrate the principles that govern the reductive process in such a scientific practice. The upshot is that reduction is much more interventionist and the reductive target much more operationalised than is normally supposed. Here, a notion of mechanism or mechanistic explanation becomes important. Some so-called new reductionists have availed themselves of this notion to ground—eliminative—reduction of special science properties without commitment to the truth of any identity statements (Gillett 2007). Godfrey-Smith (Chapter 3 in this volume) highlights this notion too, together with the importance of creating models of one's target of scientific investigation. It may be that functionalism, in its various guises, is most attractive if it involves investigating the internal architecture of the realising mechanisms. This process may involve a transition from theoretic model building to mechanistic theory.

In these discussions there is some scepticism about the discussion of reduction as it is conducted in philosophy of mind, and we can discern a trend towards a mechanistic and interventionist notion of reduction that coheres with recent trends in the debate about causation (Woodward, Chapter 12 in this volume; Menzies, Chapter 11 in this volume). Interesting issues arise in this context, since it is not clear how the functionalist model of reduction, which sees explanation as a matter of deduction, fits with the more dynamic, mechanistic model of explanation (Kim, Chapter 5 in this volume; Bickle, Chapter 2 in this volume). Part of the problem concerns the issue of levels, and how explanations may span levels or be level-bound (Lipton, Chapter 6 in this volume). Similarly, the questions arise how we can have distinct explanandum and explanans in reductive explanation, if our most clear model of reduction is identity, and conversely, how non-reductionism may be compatible with reductive explanation (Kim, Chapter 5 in this volume). Of course, the notion of supervenience is a philosophical term of art and it could well be thought that it would find no direct application in the special sciences. Yet List and Pettit (Chapter 4 in this volume) prove the opposite as they develop an example from social science of how a supervenience concept can in fact be brought in to help explain how a principled individualism can ground rational group judgements.

A predominant ontological model underlying reductionism has been to say that our world is a layered world: there is a hierarchy of distinct yet connected levels starting from the microphysical level ascending up to the chemical, biological, psychological, etc. levels. Specific to each level, there are distinct kinds of substances wholly composed of kinds from lower levels all the way down to elementary material particles. This hierarchy of levels is thus fixed by part–whole relations (Oppenheim and Putnam 1958). This model underlies much theorising in the physical sciences, e.g. trying to understand the properties of objects in terms of the properties of these objects' microconstituents. Ultimately, the world is the way the folk know it because of the microphysical way the world is.

In contrast to this reductive model stands emergentism according to which each kind has specific properties in virtue of a characteristic organisational complexity, and some of these properties have emergent causal powers. That is, emergent properties can exercise their causal power downward to affect what goes on at lower levels from which these properties somehow emerge. What is more, there are special emergent laws, neither reducible to, nor derivable from, lower-level laws, which attribute these causal powers to the types of properties in question. While emergentism may be internally coherent, and indeed, as

McLaughlin (1992) has argued, downward causation is compatible with the laws of mechanics, quantum mechanics, and relativity theory, there may be independent empirical reason for scepticism. Thus Loewer (Chapter 8 in this volume) argues that physics has accumulated much evidence that there are fundamental dynamical laws of microphysics that are complete, and no evidence that the fundamental laws can be overridden or are gappy in the way emergentism requires.

The chief worry about reductionism derives from considerations about multiple realisability. If the target property is the property that plays a certain causal role, how can this property be reduced to a particular physical property that plays that role in some organism or system, if some distinct physical property also plays that role in some other organism or system? Maybe, as Antony (Chapter 9 in this volume) suggests, the target property is identical with a not-too-heterogeneously disjunctive physical property. Alternatively, a special science property can be viewed as disjunctively realised yet not itself disjunctive. Maybe it is an ontologically distinct second-order property: the property of having a property that plays the role. Thus Fodor (1974, 1998) shares the ontological view that all items belonging to the ontologies of the special sciences are made up out of the microphysical entities that are the subject matter of fundamental physics, but he also holds that there are special science kinds and laws that are not reducible to those of physics. Basically multiple realisation shows that bridge laws are impossible, and such laws are essential to Nagel-type reduction of special science properties. Psychology and the other special sciences are thus independent of the underlying physical sciences. Fodor endorses non-reductive physicalism. This view says that although mental and special science properties are distinct from physical properties, the former are nevertheless metaphysically necessitated by the latter. Note that despite eschewing ontological reduction, Fodor maintained that special science phenomena are reductively explainable in terms of physical phenomena. Lipton (Chapter 6 in this volume) delves deeper into the status of special science laws and reductive explanation, particularly in the context of *ceteris paribus* clauses and provisos. He argues for an explanatory pluralism that allows both level-specific and reductive explanation. Such explanations seem equally affected by the perceived inadequacies of laws that contain *ceteris paribus* clauses and provisos.

It is worth dwelling on how best to characterise physicalism. Some say it is the view that everything is physical. But then we better get clear on whether this is the 'is' of strict identity, constitution, or something else. Stoljar (Chapter 13 in this volume) argues that there are a number of distinct notions of identity and distinctness in the literature that are better kept apart. For instance, what the non-reductive physicalist means by distinctness may be something modally weak and asymmetrical, while what the dualist means must be something modally much stronger and symmetrical. So, instead, physicalism is the view that everything is metaphysically necessitated by the physical. The physical is typically understood as the microphysical, but Papineau (Chapter 7 in this volume) argues that physicalists are committed to no such ranking within physics. One can consistently claim that everything is metaphysically necessitated by the physical without endorsing the microphysicalist claim that everything is metaphysically necessitated by the microphysical—if only one rejects the claim that the physical is metaphysically necessitated by the microphysical.

Another distinctive virtue of reductionism is that it sidesteps any causal competition between higher-order properties and lower-order properties. The causal exclusion argument poses the problem about the causal efficacy of the mental: how can mental properties cause physical properties if all physical effects have sufficient physical causes and no physical effect is caused twice over by distinct physical and mental causes? Strictly speaking, what the argument shows is at best that mental causation, psychophysical distinctness, completeness, and causal exclusion are incompatible. On the face of it, rejecting any one of these entails epiphenomenalism, reductionism, emergentism or overdetermination respectively. Note that the argument can presumably be generalised to the causal efficacy of special science properties. Thus Block (2003) has argued that if the reasoning is sound, then either all special science causation drains down to a bottom level of elementary particles in physics, or else all such causation drains down to a bottomless nothing! Kim's response (2003) is that identification of the competing causes at an appropriate level stops the drainage. But the problem about causal exclusion might return to haunt the reductionist. For if the relevant mental or special science properties are multiply realisable, then they are at best identical with some disjunctive physical properties. But then it looks as if mental or special science properties are causally excluded by one of the distinct physical properties out of which those disjunctive properties are constituted. Alternatively, the reductionist can opt for local reductions. This raises some further issues: what is it in virtue of which distinct species are in the same mental states? If the answer is some higher-order functional properties, then we are back to the question about their causal powers.

The non-reductive physicalist typically takes issue with the exclusion principle. Thus both Stoljar and Bennett (Chapters 13 and 14 respectively in this volume) claim that rejection of that principle is feasible if non-reductive physicalism is true, but not if dualism is true. The fact that the non-reductive physicalist believes that mental properties are metaphysically necessitated by physical properties means that mental causation isn't afflicted by vicious overdetermination; or so Bennett argues. In particular, in execution squad cases, it's non-vacuously true that if one soldier had shot, but not the other, the convict would still have died. But on this view it is not non-vacuously true that had the physical property been instantiated without the mental property, then the behavioural property would still have been instantiated. So, mental properties can cause behavioural properties that are not viciously causally overdetermined by distinct physical properties. But according to dualism, there is no metaphysically necessary connection between the mental and the physical, and so mental causation, if possible at all, is in relevant respects just like the execution squad case.

In any case, it would seem that the exclusion principle is independently implausible, at least if understood as follows: if a property is causally sufficient for some effect, then no distinct property is causally relevant to that effect. But determinable properties are not excluded from causal relevance by their determinates. Take Yablo's pigeon (1992), which is trained to peck only at red things. The redness of a triangle is causally relevant to the pecking, even though its being scarlet is causally sufficient for her pecking. But what causes the pigeon to peck when confronted with a scarlet surface? Both Menzies and Woodward (Chapters 11 and 12 respectively in this volume) follow Yablo in thinking that red is the best candidate for a cause, because it is what makes the difference. Roughly, had the triangle not been red (but some other colour), the pigeon would not have pecked, but had the triangle not been scarlet (but some other shade of red), the pigeon would still have pecked. Both Menzies' contrastivism and Woodward's interventionism falsify the exclusion principle as formulated in terms of causal sufficiency, but not as formulated in terms of causation. Their views tend to favour causal claims involving more macroscopic variables. Crane (Chapter 10 in this volume), on the other hand, thinks that scarlet is a better candidate for a cause, because sparse properties are truth-makers, and truth-makers are causes. So, what makes the statement 'the pigeon pecks when presented with this red triangle' true is that it pecks when presented with this scarlet triangle. Causes are thus always the most determinate properties. Those who accept sparse properties and their efficacy should thus give up the claim that counterfactuals track causal efficacy. If, moreover, Armstrong (1997) is right that nothing exists unless it makes a difference to the causal powers of something, then it looks as if no determinable properties exist (Gillett and Rives 2005). What scarlet and crimson have in common is merely that they fall under the determinable concept of red. Kim (Chapter 5 in this volume) defends a similar view with respect to functional properties.

3. SUMMARIES OF THE CONTRIBUTIONS

Valerie Gray Hardcastle's and Rosalyn W. Stewart's 'Reduction and Embodied Cognition: Perspectives from Medicine and Psychiatry' (Chapter 1) aims to dissociate the working cognitive sciences from various reductive strategies. Cognitive science is still a relatively young discipline and there is scope for discussion and development of its methodologies, explanatory domains, and subdisciplines. Hardcastle and Stewart advocate that cognitive science should be more inclusive in terms of what it accepts as data in developing its theories, and that it should not be wedded only to reductive strategies. They demonstrate how current cognitive science is committed to reduction in a way, moreover, that restricts the acceptable data to the brain, forgetting the role of the body for cognition. Appreciating how brains are embedded in complicated environments enlightens us about philosophical issues concerning the possibility of mind-brain reduction.

They use two fascinating case studies to support the claim that somatic states are part of our cognitive processes and, further, that as a result cognitive science cannot be reductive in the way it is normally taken to be. The case studies are on depression and somatisation, and show how there is no easy one-to-one correspondence between mental and physical phenomena. It may be that the development of mental phenomena is very sensitive to initial conditions and that as a result complete reductive stories are beyond our data-gathering capacities. This may be just a practical problem but Hardcastle and Stewart suggest that, since in both cases an explanation can be found, reduction may not be necessary for successful cognitive science.

John Bickle's 'Real Reduction in Real Neuroscience: Metascience, Not Philosophy of Science (and Certainly Not Metaphysics!)' (Chapter 2) argues that much discussion between philosophers and neuroscientists is infected by philosophical assumptions about the nature of reduction. Instead we should pursue an unbiased examination of the methods used throughout relevant areas of neuroscience. So, what is it for a scientific practice to be reductionist? In answering this question, one can either appeal to established notions of reduction from the philosophy of science (such as intertheoretic or functional reduction). Or one can appeal more directly to the details of a paradigmatic reductionist scientific practice itself. Bickle advocates the latter approach over the former and accordingly focuses on reductionist work in the neurobiological discipline of molecular and cellular cognition. The aim is to adopt a metascientific stance that will enable us to discover the scientific factors that make this research reductive, rather than see to what extent it fits with preconceived notions of reduction.

Bickle's eye-opening case study is how in mice neuronal competition for participation in a memory trace is determined by relative CREB (i.e., calcium responsive element binding protein which is a gene expression transcription enhancer) function. On the basis of this, and earlier work, he sets out two aspects of reductionist research in particular, namely that reduction is a matter of causal intervention into low level mechanisms, and tracking of the effects of these interventions through levels. When interventions provide evidence that activity in the proposed reductive mechanism co-varies reliably with activity in the target property reduction can succeed. Reduction is in these cases a matter of the lower-level mechanism being responsible for all the behavioural facts concerning the target property, in the sense that appealing to higher-level mechanisms will not add any extra explanatory power. Bickle explicitly contrasts this with functionalisation and a posteriori approaches to reduction.

Peter Godfrey-Smith's 'Reduction in Real Life' (Chapter 3) makes out a divide between the picture of reduction that philosophers of mind tend to employ and actual scientific practice in, say, psychology, biology, and neuroscience. In philosophy of mind, a certain picture of reduction holds sway. This picture, Godfrey-Smith shows, is based on less recent ideas from philosophy of science. It says among other things that scientific understanding is a matter of knowledge of forward-looking laws and it operates with a view of reduction in terms of bridge laws or supervenience. Godfrey-Smith rejects this traditional view. He argues that some of the "mid-level" special sciences are characterised by knowledge of mechanisms, of how things work, in particular he stresses the role of models in the early phases of this kind of scientific work. Reduction, on this alternative view, is a matter of explaining the properties of a whole in mechanistic terms of its parts.

Even so, as Godfrey-Smith notes, it may be that the alternative view differs in detail only from the simplified examples that philosophers of mind tend to work with. Therefore it is not given that such an alternative view would have deep consequences for metaphysical questions, for example within the philosophy of mind. However, he argues that functionalism in fact can be seen to harbour deep tensions that bear on these issues in philosophy of science. He begins by noticing how, to remain attractive, different kinds of functionalism require us to "pop the hood" and investigate the mechanism realising a given functional role. This goes against the non-reductionist aspirations of many functionalisms. Godfrey-Smith offers a novel perspective that allows us to avoid the tension between working only at higher levels and popping the hood, namely by conceiving of functionalism as moving between modelling and investigating mechanisms.

Christian List and Philip Pettit's 'Group Agency and Supervenience' (Chapter 4) argues that while group agents function in a manner that is supervenient on the contributions of individual members, this supervenience allows a surprising form of discontinuity between the individual and the collective levels. There is no mystery about how groups operate—that is the lesson of the supervenience—but this lack of mystery still leaves room for surprise.

Group agents are groups that mimic individual agents in forming more or less rational intentional states—for example, judgements of fact and value—and in acting more or less rationally on the basis of those states. List and Pettit hold by the supervenience thesis that there can be no intentional difference between two group agents without some difference in the way members think or act or relate to one another. But they show that this supervenience has to have a distinctive character. If a group agent is to be robustly rational, then the judgements it makes in favour of some propositions and against others are not guaranteed to supervene on corresponding judgements on the part of individuals.

This claim sums up some recent results in the theory of judgement-aggregation. It means, in a vivid example, that a group agent may have to form and act on a judgement that a majority of its members reject, even indeed a judgement that all of its members reject. Let a group be reliably rational and under plausible conditions it cannot be reliably responsive, proposition by proposition, to the judgements of its members. Let it be reliably responsive to those judgements, and it cannot be reliably rational. The supervenience relationship between the group level and the individual level has to be more complex than might have been expected.

Jaegwon Kim's 'Reduction and Reductive Explanation: Is One Possible Without the Other?' (Chapter 5) argues that only the functional model of reduction provides both reduction and reductive explanation. The phenomenon of multiple realisation is commonly thought to preclude type-identities, of higher properties with lower properties, and this is usually taken to show that reduction is in general not possible. Some philosophers, however, believe that in spite of this, reductive explanations are still feasible. That is, higher-level phenomena can at times be explained in terms of lower-level phenomena and mechanisms even though not reducible to them. As Kim observes, this raises many questions, among them the following: What really is a "reductive" explanation? And how are reduction and reductive explanation related to each other? Kim discusses these and related questions for the three principal types of reduction currently on the scene: bridge-law reduction, identity reduction, and functional reduction.

Kim argues that bridge-law reduction gives us neither reduction nor reductive explanation. On this model, reductive derivations assume as auxiliary premises unexplained laws connecting higher properties with properties at the lower level—that is, "bridge laws". Because of this, such derivations are incapable of generating a reductive understanding of higher phenomena in terms of lower phenomena. Moreover, higher properties remain distinct from the lower properties with which they are connected by bridge laws; hence, there is no reduction either. To avoid these and other difficulties, some philosophers have proposed that bridge laws be replaced by identities—propositions identifying higher properties with lower properties. This is identity reduction. Kim acknowledges that identity reductions do reduce. However, he argues that such reductions do not yield reductive explanations; rather, they eliminate a need for such explanations.

In contrast, functional reductions, on Kim's view, deliver reductive explanations. But do they reduce? Kim argues that if a property has been functionally reduced, its tokens can be identified with the tokens of their respective lower-level realisers. Thus, functional reductions yield token reductions. But what about the properties supposedly reduced through functionalisation? According to Kim, this question gives rise to complex metaphysical issues. After a somewhat inconclusive discussion, Kim rejects what he calls "functional property realism", settling for "functional property conceptualism", which appears to be a form of eliminativism. On this view, what the instances of a functional property have in common is that they fall under a functionally defined concept; there need be no real property had by them all.

Peter Lipton's 'CP Laws, Reduction, and Explanatory Pluralism' (Chapter 6) explores the relationships between the notions of reduction, reductive explanation, and *ceteris paribus* laws. Scientific explanations may be reductive, spanning levels, or they may be level-bound. Lipton observes that there could be a presumption in favour of reductive explanations of high-level events since lower-level laws are presumed to be strict and thus better explainers than *ceteris paribus* macro laws. He traces the *ceteris paribus* character and non-reducibility of macro laws to multiple realisability and the role of provisos and then notes that, if reduction is not possible, then it seems that there is no good explanation available at the macro levels at all. However, Lipton argues for an explanatory pluralism where what will be the best explanation depends on the explanatory question and its context.

The argument builds on distinguishing different types of reductive explanation, and Lipton sides with Fodor (1974) and Kim (Chapter 5 in this volume) in emphasising that, in Lipton's words, there can be reductive explanation without (type-identity) reduction. For example, it is possible to have reductive mechanistic explanations of macro processes; and it is possible to explain the consequent of a *ceteris paribus* macro law in terms of the antecedent of a strict micro law.

The question then remains whether such reductive explanation gets around the perceived explanatory weaknesses of *ceteris paribus* laws, in particular the worries that they cannot explain well because they are contingent (i.e., their exceptions mean the occurrence of the explanandum is not guaranteed) and that they cannot give full causes. Lipton argues that the contingency of macro laws is not avoided by appealing to micro explanations, since they too have provisos that make them contingent. Further, there is reason to think that cp laws can in fact be explanatory, and that sometimes macro explanation in terms of cp laws are better than explanations in terms of micro laws. Lipton shows how even in cases where provisos and *ceteris paribus* clauses are not satisfied, the particular contrast that a given "why"-question picks out allows a macro law to be fully explanatory.

David Papineau's 'Must a Physicalist be a Microphysicalist?' (Chapter 7) challenges the entailment from physicalism to microphysicalism—the view that all facts metaphysically supervene on the microphysical facts. Given that the conjunction of physicalism and physical microscopism—the view that all physical facts metaphysically supervene on the microphysical facts—is equivalent to microphysicalism, Papineau observes that physicalists can avoid microphysicalism by rejecting physical microscopism. So, rejecting dualism is compatible with within-physics holism: physical wholes transcend what is determined by their microphysical parts. Papineau first points out that there is no need to define 'physical' as what is microphysically determined, because the inorganically identifiable conception of 'physical' is preferable, and secondly that not every way of arguing for physicalism argues for physical microscopism too, because the causal exclusion argument does not rely on physial microscopism. All its crucial premise regarding completeness says is that all physical effects have physical, not miscophysical, causes.

Humean supervenience is a strong version of microphysicalism, and it is false if a non-Humean view of laws is true. But such a view is consistent with physicalism. A weaker form of microphysicalism adds microphysical non-Humean laws to get a broader microphysicalist supervenience base for all facts. On this view, all the laws are metaphysically determined by microphysical laws and microphysical initial conditions. In response, Papineau argues that the existence of emergent Broad-laws, i.e. macroscopic laws that are not metaphysically dependent on microphysical laws and microphysical initial conditions, is consistent with physicalism. These laws would be associated with special force fields, which would count as physical on some conceptions of the physical. So, if there were such laws, some physical facts would be microphysically emergent.

Papineau also argues that physicalists can consistently deny that facts about persisting objects, including organic and artefactual objects, metaphysically supervene on microphysical facts. For such objects supervene on their spatial parts, and if those parts are physical, then they will count as physical without any four-dimensional supervenience on time-slices. The causal exclusion argument shows that a three-dimensionalist physicalist ought to claim that organic and artefactual persisting objects supervene on their spatial parts. But this does not mean that physicalism entails that facts about persisting objects supervene on the intrinsic physical properties of (and causal and spatial relations between) their spatial parts, because quantum mechanics provide strong reason to deny this version of microphysicalism.

Barry Loewer's 'Why There *Is* Anything except Physics' (Chapter 8) deals with a tension generated by Fodor's acceptance of the following: (1) All items belonging to the ontologies of the special sciences are made up out of the microphysical entities that are the subject matter of fundamental physics, (2) The dynamical laws of microphysics are complete in the domain of microphysics, and (3) There are special science laws that are not reducible to those of physics. But it follows from (1) and (2) that special science regularities are made true by physical facts and laws, and so it looks as if those special science regularities that are lawful derive their status as laws from the fundamental laws of microphysics.

In support of (3), Fodor cites the fact that special science kinds and laws are typically multiply realised. He attempts to retain (1)–(3) by endorsing a version of emergentism according to which the laws of physics are explanatorily and modally incomplete. On his view special science counterfactuals and explanations require for their truth irreducible special science laws. So while a regularity expressed by a special science law is implied by microphysical laws and facts, its status as a law is metaphysically independent of physics. Loewer's reply is that if (1) and (2) are true, then special science counterfactuals are necessitated by fundamental physical laws and facts. So, if there are metaphysically independent special science laws then they can only overdetermine counterfactuals, and such overdetermination is puzzling.

But where does the lawfulness of special science regularities come from? Special science laws are *ceteris paribus*, temporally asymmetric, and local, whereas fundamental dynamical laws are exceptionless, temporally symmetric, and global. After examining Boltzmann's reconciliation of laws of thermodynamics with fundamental dynamical laws, Loewer proposes that the lawfulness of such regularities is grounded in the dynamical laws plus a probabilistic constraint on the initial conditions of the universe. And by adding such a constraint to the fundamental dynamical laws, it can be shown that physics misses no nomological/explanatory structure that the special sciences supply. Loewer's account is reductionist in that it denies the existence of metaphysically independent special science laws, but it does not entail that special science properties are identical to properties of fundamental physics and it allows for the multiple realisability of special science laws.

Louise Antony's 'Multiple Realization: Keeping It Real' (Chapter 9) takes Kim's causal exclusion argument to pose the following dilemma about the reality of multiple realisable properties: either they are reducible to first-order physical properties (so MR properties are not distinct from physical properties) or they are not associated with distinctive causal powers (and so are unreal). Antony detects two strands in Kim's challenge. The Incoherence Challenge is that it is incoherent to hold that one and the same set of objects or events is anomic at one level of description, but nomic at a different level of description. The Conventionality Challenge is that nomicity should depend on objective similarity, and not merely on how things are described. Antony argues that both challenges can be met, so that we can find a third way between the horns of Kim's dilemma, and vindicate multiple realisability.

Regarding the Incoherence Challenge, Antony suggests that we drop the claim that the lower-order disjunctive property is anomic. For some disjunctive predicates, e.g. 'cow-or-bull', express nomic properties. On her view, every higher-order mentalistic predicate is necessarily co-extensive with, and thus expresses the same property as, the lower-order disjunctive predicate formed by alternation of physical realisers across possible worlds. Hence, it is impossible for one of these to express a nomic property and the other not to express a nomic property. But the higher-order predicate and the lower-order disjunctive predicate can differ with respect to entrenchment, and hence with respect to their projectibility. If the best explanation of the entrenchment of the higher-order mentalistic predicate is that the property it expresses is nomic, then the unentrenched, unprojectible disjunctive predicate, no less than the entrenched higher-order predicate, expresses a nomic property.

Regarding the Conventionality Challenge, Antony argues that the practical ineliminability of mentalistic vocabulary has ontological consequences. It is not just a fact about us that such vocabulary is useful. The vocabulary would not be useful, e.g. in grounding empirical prediction, if it did not track real patterns in the world, i.e. if it did not mark out real resemblances among things. That such vocabulary is useful is an empirical fact that demands explanation, and the best explanation is that there really are laws involving the properties expressed by mentalistic terms. Antony concludes that mental properties are objective, because they are expressed by projectible predicates, and they are autonomous, because the entrenched mentalistic predicates that express them are demonstrably not co-extensive with any proprietary predicates of any lower-order science.

Tim Crane's 'Causation and Determinable Properties: On the Efficacy of Colour, Shape, and Size' (Chapter 10) is concerned with "the antinomy of determinable causation". On the one hand, there is a good argument for the thesis that determinable properties can be causes. Here Crane invokes Yablo's proportionality constraint (1992) according to which a cause must be specific enough but not too specific for its effect. Scarlet is a determinate of the determinable red. And red is more proportional to the bull's anger than scarlet, even though scarlet is causally sufficient. The counterfactual 'had the cape not been red, the bull would not have been enraged' is true, but the counterfactual 'had the cape not been scarlet, the bull would not have been enraged' is false. So, red is a better candidate to count as the cause of the bull's anger than scarlet.

On the other hand, there is a good argument for the antithesis that only the most determinate properties can be causes. Crane accepts a sparse conception of properties according to which properties may fail to correspond one–one with predicates. Crane also claims that only sparse properties are causally efficacious. Assume that causation is a relation between properties. If a causal truth has a truth-maker, it must thus relate cause and effect. The relata of the causal relation will then be truth-makers for the relata of the causal truth. But if a predication has a truth-maker, its truth-maker is a sparse property. So, these truth-makers are sparse properties. Therefore causation is a relation between sparse properties. Moreover, super-determinates are sparse; and since predications of determinables have truth-makers, then these sparse properties will be the truth-makers for these predications. It follows that only super-determinates are causally efficacious properties.

Crane opts to reject the thesis by denying any straightforward link between the truth of counterfactuals and the causal efficacy of the determinable properties mentioned in them. To predicate a determinable property of an object is to specify that it has a sparse property within some range determined by the determinable concept. To say that had the cape not been red, the bull would not have been enraged is to say that there is a determinate property, e.g. a shade of scarlet, within a range determined by the concept of red on which the effect is counterfactually dependent.

Peter Menzies' 'The Exclusion Problem, the Determination Relation, and Contrastive Causation' (Chapter 11) addresses the causal exclusion argument against non-reductive physicalism. If Yablo's proportionality constraint (1992) is imposed, then mental properties are better candidates as causes of behavioural properties than neural properties since they better meet that constraint. (Whereas determinables and determinates do not compete for causal relevance, they do compete for the role of cause.) However, Menzies rejects Yablo's objection to the causal exclusion argument on the ground that mental properties are not related to their underlying neural properties as determinables to determinates—to use Funkhouser's terminology (2006), mental and neural properties do not share determination dimensions. And the proportionality constraint applies only if mental properties are so related.

Instead Menzies proposes a contrastive account of causation, which falsifies the exclusion principle as formulated in terms of causal sufficiency, but not as formulated in terms of a double application of the concept of causation. This account is about difference-making: a cause makes a difference to its effects in that changing the value of the cause variable leads to a change in the value of the effect variable. The conditions required for a difference-making relation between mental and behavioural properties are incompatible with the conditions required for a difference-making relation between neural and behavioural properties. Nonetheless, the causal exclusion argument poses no threat to non-reductive physicalism if reformulated in terms of an exclusion principle that employs the difference-making conception of causation. A non-reductive physicalist can reject its conclusion by instead challenging the premise of the causal closure of the physical. This principle must be strengthened considerably if the argument is to be based on the viable reformulated exclusion principle: it must pertain to difference-making physical properties rather than causally sufficient physical properties. But when strengthened in the required way, it is much less plausible than it appeared in its original version. So, when there is empirical evidence that a mental property is the difference-maker of a behavioural property, there may be a physical property that is causally sufficient for the behavioural property, but it will not be a difference-making cause of that property.

James Woodward's 'Mental Causation and Neural Mechanisms' (Chapter 12) argues that many of the standard arguments for the causal inertness of the mental rest on mistaken assumptions about what it is for a relationship to be causal, and about what is involved in providing a causal explanation. These mistaken assumptions involve a conception of causation according to which a cause is simply a condition which is nomologically sufficient for its effect, and the deductive-nomological conception of explanation according to which explaining an outcome is simply a matter of exhibiting a nomologically sufficient condition for it. Given these assumptions, it is indeed hard to understand how there can be such a thing as mental causation.

However, an interventionist account of causation and causal explanation undercuts these assumptions, and allows us to reach a better understanding of what is involved in mental causation and of the real empirical issues surrounding this notion. On this difference-making account, the question of whether C causes E is identified with the question of whether E would change under some suitable experimental manipulation of C, where suitability involves the exclusion of various confounding possibilities. More precisely, X causes Y if and only if there are background circumstances such that if some intervention that changes the value of variable X were to occur in B, then variable Y would change. Woodward also holds that our practice of giving causal explanations is well founded only if the causal claims figuring in those explanations are true. Correspondingly, causal explanation consists in the exhibition of patterns of counterfactual dependency between the factors cited in the *explanans* and the *explanandum* such that changes in those factors produced by interventions are associated with changes in the outcome.

Depending on the empirical conditions and on what we are trying to explain, interventionism allows for explanations involving macroscopic variables as well as microscopic variables. So, depending on the details of the case, it can explain the causal efficacy and explanatory power of multiple realisable mental states. When it comes to the causal exclusion argument, Woodward rejects the exclusion principle according to which if an event has a sufficient cause, then no distinct event can be a cause of it, unless this is a genuine case of causal overdetermination. On his view, an event's being causally sufficient for some effect does not exclude some distinct event from causing or being causally relevant to that effect, even in the absence of overdetermination.

Daniel Stoljar's 'Distinctions in Distinction' (Chapter 13) begins with a putative puzzle between non-reductive physicalism according to which psychological properties are distinct from, yet metaphysically necessitated by, physical properties, and Hume's dictum according to which there are no necessary connections between distinct existences. However, the puzzle dissolves once care is taken to distinguish between distinct kinds of distinction. The non-reductive physicalist typically has numerical distinctness in mind, but thus construed Hume's dictum is false. For instance, being red is numerically distinct from being coloured, but being red entails being coloured. Alternatively, the non-reductive physicalist could mean that psychological properties are weakly modally distinct from physical properties, where weak modal distinctness between two properties F and G consists in the possibility of instantiating F without G or the possibility of instantiating G without F. But again determinates/determinables provide a counterexample to Hume's dictum thus understood. Stoljar considers other notions of distinctness, e.g. mereological distinctness, but it turns out in each case that either it makes no sense according to non-reductive physicalism or it is unclear whether Hume's dictum is true if pertaining to that notion.

The lesson is to take care not to conflate distinct notions of distinction. Stoljar argues that the exclusion principle is very plausible as deployed in the causal exclusion argument against the dualist according to which psychological and physical properties are strongly modally distinct, where strong modal distinctness between two properties F and G consists in the possibility of instantiating F without G and the possibility of instantiating G without F. But the causal exclusion argument against the non-reductive physicalist is very different and much less plausible. For if such properties are at most numerically or weakly modally distinct, there are counterexamples to the corresponding version of the exclusion principle. For instance, the fact that some determinate property is causally sufficient for some effect does not preclude the corresponding determinable property from being causally relevant.

Stoljar also uses distinct notions of distinction to distinguish emergentism from non-reductive physicalism. For what the former says is not that psychological properties are numerically distinct from physical properties, but rather mereologically distinct or maybe distinct in essence. Finally, Stoljar maintains that if good sense can be made of these notions of distinctness, the emergentist might also escape the exclusion problem.

Karen Bennett's 'Exclusion Again' (Chapter 14) maintains that the non-reductive physicalist's best strategy for avoiding the causal exclusion argument, as defended in her (2003), is unavailable to full-blown dualists. One strategy for denying the underlying exclusion principle is to focus on the notion of causation in play, i.e. to reject the oomphy notion of causation in favour of something along the lines of a pure counterfactual dependence notion. The other strategy focuses on the relation between the causes, i.e. in the relevant cases the causes are causally sufficient for the same effect yet are tightly related in some way that defuses the threat of overdetermination. Only the latter strategy works, but it is unavailable to the dualist.

Basically, in order to have genuine overdetermination certain counterfactuals must be non-vacuously true, and the physicalist, but not the dualist, can deny the non-vacuous truth of at least one of these counterfactuals. Unlike dualists, physicalists claim the metaphysically necessary supervenience of everything on the physical. So, in particular, it is not non-vacuously true that had the physical cause occurred without the mental cause, the effect would still have occurred. As regards the former strategy, the force of the causal exclusion argument simply does not turn upon any particular account of causation. Moving from a production to a dependence conception of causation (Hall 2004) does not alleviate the threat of overdetermination. For even counterfactual dependence accounts allow for some cases of overdetermination, and so those accounts cannot by themselves distinguish between cases of overdetermination and cases of effects with two non-overdetermining causes.

In arguing that successful denial of the exclusion principle is only open to physicalists, Bennett agrees with Stoljar in relying upon the claim that what non-reductive physicalists mean is much weaker than what dualists mean when they say that the mental is distinct from the physical. Physicalists have a clear argument for the falsity of the exclusion principle, but because dualists mean something rather different by distinctness, they wind up with no argument against that principle at all.

REFERENCES

Armstrong, D. 1997. *A World of States of Affairs.* Cambridge: Cambridge University Press.

Bennett, Karen. 2003. 'Why the Exclusion Problem Seems Intractable, and How, Just Maybe, to Tract It', *Noûs* 37, 471–97.

Block, N. 2003. 'Do Causal Powers Drain Away?' *Philosophy and Phenomenological Research* 67, 133–50.

—— forthcoming. 'Functional Reduction'.

—— and Stalnaker, R. 1999. 'Conceptual Analysis, Dualism, and the Explanatory Gap', *Philosophical Review* 108, 1–46.

Byrne, A. 1999. 'Cosmic Hermeneutics', *Philosophical Perspectives* 13, 347–83.

Chalmers, D. and Jackson, F. 2001. 'Conceptual Analysis and Reductive Explanation', *Philosophical Review* 110/3, 315–60.

Fodor, J. 1974. 'Special Sciences—or the Disunity of Science as a Working Hypothesis', *Synthese* 28, 97–115.

—— 1998. 'Special Sciences; Still Autonomous after All These Years', *Philosophical Perspectives*, 11, 149–63.

Funkhouser, E. 2006. 'The Determinable–Determinate Relation', *Noûs* 40/3, 548–69.

Gillett, C. 2007. 'Understanding the New Reductionism: The Metaphysics of Science and Compositional Reduction', *Journal of Philosophy*, 104, 193–216.

—— and Rives, B. 2005. 'The Non-Existence of Determinables: Or, a World of Absolute Determinates as Default Hypothesis', *Noûs* 39/3, 483–504.

Hall, N. 2004. 'Two Concepts of Causation', in *Causation and Counterfactuals*, (eds.) Collins, J., Hall, N., Paul, L. A., Cambridge, Mass.: MIT Press, 225–76.

Kim, Jaegwon 2003. 'Blocking Causal Drainage and Other Maintenance Chores with Mental Causation', *Philosophy and Phenomenological Research* 67, 151–76.

—— 2005. *Physicalism Or Something Near Enough*, Princeton: Princeton University Press.

Levine, J. 1983. 'Materialism and Qualia: The Explanatory Gap', *Pacific Philosophical Quarterly* 64, 354–61.

—— 1998. 'Conceivability and the Metaphysics of Mind', *Noûs* 32/4, 449–80.

Lewis, D. 1970. 'How to Define Theoretical Terms', *Journal of Philosophy*, 67, 427–46.

—— 1999. 'Reduction of Mind' in his *Papers in Metaphysics and Epistemology*, Cambridge: Cambridge University Press.

McLaughlin, B. 1992. 'The Rise and Fall of British Emergentism,' in *Emergence Or Reduction?*, (eds.) Berckermann, A., Kim, J., and Flohr, H., Berlin: De Gruyter, 49–93.

Nagel, E. 1961. *The Structure of Science: Problems in the Logic of Scientific Explanation.* London: Routledge & Kegan Paul.

Oppenheim, P. and Putnam, H. 1958. 'Unity of Science as a Working Hypothesis', in (eds.) Feigl, H., Maxwell, G., and Scriven, M., *Minnesota Studies in the Philosophy of Science*, vol. ii, Minneapolis: University of Minnesota Press, 3–36.
Tye, M. 2002. *Consciousness, Color, and Content*, Cambridge, Mass.: MIT Press.
Yablo, S. 1992. 'Mental Causation', *Philosophical Review* 101, 245–80.
—— 2000. 'Textbook Kripkeanism and the Open Texture of Concepts', *Pacific Philosophical Quarterly* 81/1, 98–122.

1

Reduction and Embodied Cognition: Perspectives from Medicine and Psychiatry

Valerie Gray Hardcastle and Rosalyn W. Stewart

Cognitive science is at an interesting stage of development. On the one hand, it is still a very new science, still feeling its way toward what its final shape will be. Exactly what it will explain, using what investigative techniques, and to what end are still very much open questions. On the other hand, cognitive science has been around long enough that we have some sense of what a complete theory in cognitive science might look like, what its component pieces should be. We know that theories in cognitive science will likely be multi-disciplinary with a distinct bias towards what Rob Wilson calls "smallism" (more on this below), a unique combination of general computational and psychological principles conjoined with underlying biological and neurological details specific to humans.

This essay aims to contribute to the discussion of what cognitive science should be when it grows up by suggesting that it should be more inclusive in what is counted as relevant data in developing its theories. It also should not be exclusively wedded to reductive methodologies. In brief, using two case studies, we suggest that somatic processing should be included as part of the domain of cognitive science and that doing so will do much to further our understanding of cognition in general. In addition, including more data from psychiatric cases will necessitate some anti-reductionistic explanations. But before we get to these suggestions, let us first spend some time summarizing the theoretical lay of the land so we have some sense of how somatic data might eventually fit into a theory of cognition and what our options for theories of cognition are.

1. INVESTIGATING COGNITION

We can divide approaches to investigating the mind and cognition into two rough categories: the top-down approach and the bottom-up approach. Each approach has its own methodologies, theoretical framework, data set, and explanatory domain, and each functions independently of the other. At the same time, both approaches result in similar reductive theories in the end. In short, both approaches produce theories that illustrate how higher-level properties are nothing more than a particular arrangement of lower-level properties.

Allow us a slight digression here to expand what we mean by a "reductive" theory, since we are using that term fairly loosely. Traditionally, philosophers of cognitive science have based their conception of reduction on Nagel's (1961) classic formulation. (See also Nagel 1949, Quine 1964, Woodger 1952.) They claim (roughly speaking) that if neuroscience reduces psychology, for example, then all the kind predicates in psychology are co-extensive with the kind predicates in neuroscience. Bridge laws (sometimes bridge principles) then express identities between predicates such that every event that falls under a psychological description or generalization will also fall under the descriptions or generalizations of neuroscience. Taken together, the bridge laws exhaust the domain of the reduced theory, in this case, psychology. Finally, the reduced theory is derivable from the union of the reducing theory and the bridge laws.

Traditional reductionists believe that the purpose behind reducing psychology is to explain psychological generalizations in terms of a more "basic" science, like neuroscience. This would show that we can think of psychological theories as special cases of neuroscientific theories. The assumption that we need to look to more basic sciences for more fundamental explanations is what Rob Wilson refers to as "smallism".

For a whole host of reasons, including that no scientific theory has actually ever been reduced according to the definition above, this version of reduction in science is untenable. However, these ideas are not without influence in cognitive science today. There remain some vestige principles of reduction that linger on. Our focus in this essay is on them.

While we think it is a mistake to outline these principles in too much detail (since they are really just guiding biases in the actual practice of cognitive scientists), some description of what these are might be useful. One of the remaining principles is that there is some sort of law-like correspondence between the objects or properties of the "reduced" and "reducing" disciplines. A second remaining principle is that this correspondence helps explain the existence of the higher-level object or property. A third principle is that even though the existence of the lower-level property might help explain the existence of the higher-level property, this fact does not make any normative comment about the relative priority of the relevant disciplines. Even if we import neuroscientific descriptions or definitions or explanations into psychology, we would not thereby expect psychology to some day disappear or that psychology somehow now loses its ability to taxonomize its own entities. While these things might happen, this looser relation of reduction does not entail it.

Our contention is that the two main approaches to theorizing in cognitive science both yield reductive theories, theories that not only connect higher-level with lower-level properties but that assume that connection tells us something important and fundamental about the higher-level property. Let us illustrate what we mean.

A top-down approach in cognitive science focuses first on decomposing mental capacities into functionally defined components (see Bechtel and Richardson 1993, Bechtel and Mundale 1999 for overviews of this strategy). This procedure falls normally within the domain of psychology, which uses reaction time and error measurements to isolate the pieces that compose our thought processes. It then matches these functional bits to underlying neural circuits or activities. This is traditionally neuroscience's domain, and neuroscientists use lesion and imagining studies to isolate the biological causal mechanisms instantiating the cognitive components.

To take a historical and well-known example, psychologists use various priming studies to differentiate implicit from explicit memory. In what is now regarded as seminal work, Endel Tulving and his research group gave a word completion task to normal (undergraduate) subjects. Subjects studied long lists of low-frequency words and were then given a yes/no recognition test and a fragment completion test one hour, one day, or one week later (Tulving, Schacter, and Stark 1982). Tulving discovered that previous exposure to a word facilitates a subject's ability to complete a fragment of it. The magnitude of this priming effect does not diminish over time, unlike recognition performance, which declined severely over the week interval.

Neurologists use that mnemonic division to explain the behavioral and neural data they gather from amnesic patients. Like normal subjects, amnesics use the prior presentation of words to complete fragments, even though the ammesics cannot recognize the words in later recognition tasks (unlike normals) (Jacoby and Witherspoon 1982, Warrington and Weiskranz 1970, 1974). Similarly, amnesics can learn skills and exhibit classical conditioning effects (Brooks and Baddeley 1976, Schacter and Graf 1986). Indeed, even though the conditioned responses of amnesics are near normal, they cannot even recognize the experimental apparatus that they had used many times before (Weiskranz and Warrington 1979). To make a long story short, neurologists involved in this research conclude that the preserved mnemonic capacities in amnesics must be due to a memory system that is neurologically distinct from the medial temporal lobes, which is what is damaged in these patients and which has been hypothesized to underwrite (at least in part) explicit memory (Squire and Zola-Morgan 1991).

Though we do not have a complete or even a fully accepted theory of explicit memory, we can see from this brief description what one should look like—at least in rough outline. We can see that a theory of explicit memory, based on experimental data such as these, would define what psychologists regard as explicit memory (the higher-level property) as some sort of activity in the medial temporal lobes or related area (the lower-level property). This theory would be reductive in the sense that it cashes out the higher-level psychological property as a lower-level neurological property and then uses this identification to reflect back on or inform our understanding of the higher-level property.

In contrast to the top-down approach, the bottom-up approach, not surprisingly, starts at the bottom. It looks for the functional pieces of cognition in the computations of neuronal interactions. Using single-cell and neurochemical studies, neuroscientists track the activity of individual neurons. They then connect these results to the cognitive processes articulated by psychology. Seeking functional mappings between neural circuits and higher-level descriptions, psychologists use double dissociation methodologies to differentiate processes relevant to previously isolated neural interactions. (Churchland 1986 appears to advocate this approach; see also McCauley 1996. Bickle 2003 and Thagard 2002 push for a slightly different version of this sort of reduction.)

For example, scientists have now isolated many molecules relevant to the mechanisms behind long-term potentiation (LTP), an activity-dependent form of synaptic plasticity many neuroscientists believe is tied to long-term memory formation. One set of these molecules in particular has been used in behavioral studies of long-term memory consolidation tasks: cyclic adenosine monophosphate response element binding proteins or CREB for short. CREB refers to a family of gene transcriptional enhancers or repressors that either turn on or turn off protein synthesis via new gene expression. Phosphorylated CREB transcriptional enhancers target, among other things, effector proteins that change the structure of active synapses, keeping those synapses potentiated for days, even weeks.

Molecular geneticists and neuroscientists have developed mice with a mutated CREB gene. These mice do not synthesize the CREB molecules required for long-lasting LTP, although they have all the molecules necessary for shorter-lasting LTP. Alcino Silva's laboratory uses these mice in a variety of mnemonic tasks, including the Morris water maze task, a fear conditioning task, and a social recognition memory task. It turns out that Silva's CREB enhancer mutant mice perform normally in short-term memory tasks but are impaired in long-term memory tasks, which is exactly what one would expect if the CREB molecules are relevant to long-term store.

At more or less the same time, psychologists developed detailed descriptions of long-term versus short-term store. (The original research for these distinctions, however, occurred in the 1970s: see especially Anderson and Bower 1973, Posner and Snyder 1975*a*, *b*, Schneider and Shiffrin 1977, Shiffrin and Schneider 1977.) In contrast to short-term processes, long-term store appears to be tied to an automated form of pattern matching. This sort of memory is massively parallel, strategy-free, with few capacity limitations, and does not require attention for processing. (While short-term retrieval is probably also a form of pattern-matching, it occurs serially and is the result of effortful and focused attention.)

Again, while we do not yet have complete theories in cognitive science of long-term store, we can see from this example how such a theory would look.

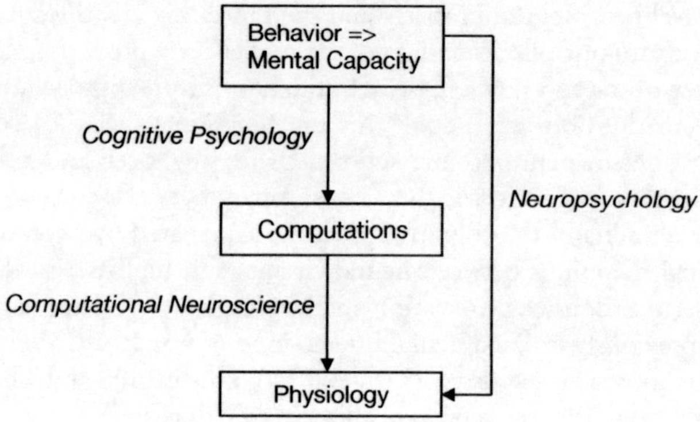

Fig. 1.1 Reductive Explanations of Mind

And, again, it would be a reductive theory, a theory that in this case would outline how something like CREB molecules and LTP underwrites what psychologists describe as long-term store, and in making this connection would explain how long-term store (the higher-level property) is nothing more than LTP and related activity (the lower-level property).

When we put both of these approaches together under the heading of cognitive science, we get the sorts of reductive explanations seen in Fig. 1.1. Cognitive psychology reduces higher-level overt behavior and its implied mental capacities to hypothesized lower-level functional computations. It reduces mnemonic behavior, for example, to hypothesized interactions of short-term and long-term store. Neuropsychology reduces essentially the same higher-level overt behavior and implied mental capacities to even lower-level underlying physiology. It reduces mnemonic behavior to a variety of long-term potentiation, perhaps. And computational neuroscience explains the hypothesized functional computations in terms of underlying physiology; following the moniker just developed, it reduces low-level properties to even lower-level properties. It explains short-term store as recurrent activity in the hippocampus and long-term store as changes in the synaptic strength in cortex. (It is important to understand that what counts as the higher- and lower-levels is relative to the inquiry at hand and its contrast class, among other things (Churchland 1986, Hardcastle 1996, Lycan 1987).)

To complicate the above rough taxonomy of reductive explanations in cognitive science (those of cognitive psychology, cognitive neuroscience, and computational neuroscience) even more, we find two additional theoretical constructs crisscrossing the divisions mentioned above: horizontal modularity and vertical modularity (originally discussed in Fodor 1983, though little remains today of the earlier characterizations). Horizontal modules refer to functional units dedicated to particular cognitive tasks across multiple input domains. Things like attention, short-term store, episodic memory are each considered a horizontal module, for each operates in the same manner over several sensory modalities. We can pay attention to visual as well as auditory inputs, for example. Or we can recall the feel of textures as well as the tastes of food. (We are deliberately leaving "in the same manner" undefined, since we really don't know how these processors operate in detail. But we can at least point to family resemblances between, e.g., olfactory memories and kinesthetic ones.)

In contrast, vertical modularity refers to domain specific tracts dedicated to processing specific inputs. The visual processing stream, a grasping reflex, audition, and so forth, represent vertical modules. In each case, we start with some particular sort of input and we can then trace that input through several computational transformations until it results in some domain-specific sort of output. The process from beginning to end is presumed to follow circuits expressly tailored for the procedures. We get a visual input of a doorknob, and then we reach to open the door. The process that takes us from that sensory input to behavioral output happens in a vertical module.

Not surprisingly, these two sorts of processing modules interact with each other on a regular basis, which is how we get complicated cognitive activity. The recent interest in so-called perception in action and conscious experience highlights the interaction between our vertical sensory processing systems and our horizontal modules for semantic/episodic memory and short-term store (Clark 1997, 2003, Gibson 1979, Noë 2006, Varela and Thompson 2001, Varela, Thompson and Rosch 1991). No matter which theoretical perspective you adopt in these matters, perception in action and conscious experience both require us to perceive (a vertical process) and to interpret those perceptions with reference to what we have experienced or done before (a horizontal one).

Similarly, meaningful behaviors require that our vertical sensory processing modules join with horizontal mnemonic modules and vertical motor ones. We can only behave meaningfully in response to our understanding of our environment, which requires that our motor responses match our interpretations of our sensory inputs. We answer the phone only when we hear the phone ringing, we understand what that ringing noise signifies, and we reach to pick up the hand piece.

The suspicion is that fully developed theories of cognition will need to address the interaction of (perhaps several) vertical and horizontal modules, with the modules and their interactions being explained either top-down or bottom-up. In short, our best theories in cognitive science are going to be very complicated affairs, replete with detailed descriptions of lots of interacting parts. And what will tie our description of these modules and their interactions together, scientists assume, will be the reductive connections made between various objects and their properties.

We can already see some progress toward this explanatory schema in recent work. For example, cognitive psychology's relatively recent move to incorporate phenomenology into cognitive science decomposes conscious experience into its component parts with the hopes of tying them to underlying sensory processing streams. As a top-down strategy, it decomposes the output of a horizontal module in the hopes of tying it to the activity of underlying vertical processors. For a second sort of top-down approach, we can look to neuropsychiatry's research into depression, which indexes alterations in neurotransmitter functionality to mood and behavior. It reduces one horizontal activity to anther type of horizontal activity. In contrast, computational neuroscience's on-going studies of things like the function of simple and complex cells in area 17 (Lehky and Sejnowski 1988) or other hypothesized computational neural processes begin at the bottom as it connects neuronal activity to the proposed computational/functional components of various higher-level cognitive processes, like shape-from-shading processes (Ramachandran 1988).

In each of these cases, we can see the interaction of horizontal and vertical modules in a reductive context. We can also see how cognitive science delimits the data relevant to cognition. These theories and theoretical approaches emphasize behavior, brains, and psychological or neural constructs and processes. They pay little attention to the bodies that house the thinking. Indeed, apart from describing inputs and outputs to our cognitive systems, theories in cognitive science generally ignore everything occurring below the neck. We believe they do so at their peril. In a moment, we shall examine two case studies that support this contention. First, though, let us explain in broad outline the challenge of being embodied for theories in cognitive science.

2. THE CHALLENGE OF EMBODIMENT

It is quite clear that somatic traits affect our mental states. Indeed, there is a whole literature that dates back to William James discussing whether our affective states are nothing more than how our minds are interpreting changes in our autonomic responses. Our favorite example comes from the mid-1970s, when Cantor, Zillman, and Bryant (1975) showed photographs of nude women to male subjects, who then ranked their own subjective sense of attraction. Some of the subjects had previously been riding an exercise bicycle to the point of autonomic arousal (flushed face, increased heart rate, panting, etc.), while others had not exerted themselves. Those who had been exercising ranked the nudes as more exciting than those who were not already aroused.

Conversely, mental functioning affects somatic traits. This direction of effect is not terribly surprising. Butterflies in your stomach are probably the quickest example of this fact. We feel nervousness in our gut, as well as other places.

These sorts of examples tell us that the body and its functioning give us clues to the functioning of the mind. This is not a controversial claim; all cognitive scientists would readily agree with it. (They would have to, else how would they be able to run their experiments?) But we wish to push a stronger line here; we believe that in many instances we need to understand the body as part of the mind itself.

This is a more controversial assertion. Many philosophers of mind who argue that perception and action are intimately tied together hold that mind and body are inextricably intertwined. However, our views are slightly different: we believe that a complete theory of our cognitive processes will include body functionality. That is, it is not just that we must recognize that minds are housed in bodies and therefore mental attributes reflect bodily needs and talents, but that what our body does—even apart from sensory transduction—is at least sometimes actually part of our cognitive processes.

We also believe that, as a result of making room for somatic functioning as part of cognitive functioning, a complete theory of the mind will not be reductive in the manner articulated above.

Let us now turn to two case studies to see why we believe such things.[1] Our first case mainly concerns the bodied mind, while the second case mainly concerns the lack of reduction.

2.1. Case Study #1: Depression

An 81-year-old Caucasian male ("Jones") arrived at his doctor's complaining of three to six months of joint pain in his shoulders and hips and worsening fatigue. Jones has a strong history of coronary heart disease, including having a pacemaker placed several years before and previous coronary artery bypass surgery, as well as at least one prior angioplasty with a stent placed in his native arteries. He reports that he had been going to cardiac rehab, but had been unable to do so for the past six months. He also used to walk daily and work out with a fitness trainer about three times a week, but over the past year and a half, he has stopped doing that as well. He's lost over twenty pounds during the past few months, but claims he has no appetite. He eats because he knows he should, not because he is hungry. He has difficulty getting into and out of bed and has difficulty standing up. He has not been able to take a bath or shower, though he does wash in a basin. It is clear that Jones had been deconditioning slowly over the past year and a half, with his condition worsening over the past six months. At the time of the exam it was hard for him to move and he was extremely lethargic.

Notice that all Jones's symptoms reflect bodily complaints: pain, fatigue, loss of appetite, problems with movement. None of his complaints are about declining cognitive capacities, or even about altered affective states. On the surface, it appears that Jones was suffering from heart failure. His medical history, coupled

[1] The two case studies recount actual patients seen at the Johns Hopkins Medical Center. Their names and some personal details have been altered to preserve patient confidentiality.

with his age, strongly suggests that his already weak circulatory system was simply giving out.

Nevertheless, Jones was diagnosed with depression, a purely mental disorder. He was prescribed anti-depressants and within a few months, he had regained his energy and appetite. His joints no longer ached; he sleeps well; he gained back the weight he lost. He is able to exercise again and can shower and dress without difficulty.

Obviously, his depression was revealing itself through physical symptoms. Depression quite often causes a loss of appetite (and hence weight loss) as well as fatigue and difficulty moving. More rarely does it cause joint pain and other similar problems. And more rarely still is depression not accompanied by the sensations of sadness, displeasure, anhedonia, irritability, hopelessness, or anger. But it does happen.

What can we learn from this case? This example tells us that there is no easy one-to-one correspondence between phenomenological experiences and underlying brain states. A putative mental disorder is identified with physical deconditioning, not to an altered mental state. We find a common explanation for multiple functional capacities (loss of balance, loss of appetite, fatigue, joint pain, muscular wasting); in particular, we find a common *mental* explanation—depression—for changes in multiple *physical* functional capacities—appetite, joint pain, etc.

Unlike our current reductive theories of depression, which link only mood and mentality to changes in neurotransmitters, Jones's depression is tied to changes in his physical performance. Though we normally understand depression as involving horizontal processing, we do not normally assume that the processing extends as widely as it did in Jones's case. Depression should refer to alterations in mood, cognitive processing, or in our somatic systems. The scope of the referent "depression" now extends beyond what we normally categorize as "mental". To explain depression—a putative mental disorder—we need to take account of not only the traditional "mind", but also the traditional "body". This theory of one corner of the mind's functioning requires the body and its functions.

At least with this example, we can see the fundamental importance of the body for explaining the mind/brain. Without Jones's bodily symptoms, not only would his depression have gone unnoticed and undiagnosed, but his bodily symptoms characterize his depression. Somatic symptoms can give us important clues regarding what is going on in the mind, if we only know how to interpret these symptoms. But, more importantly for our purposes, they can also help define, and thereby reduce, our psychological properties. This reduction, in turn, gives us a different understanding of what we previously believed was a purely mental phenomenon.

It is crucially important that we expand our notion of what counts as relevant data for explaining the mind and brain to include more than sensory input, behavioral output, and other things happening above the neck. We need to include facts about the entire body to elucidate what is going on in our "minds".

For these facts can illustrate, exemplify, or even define some of our so-called mental properties.

At the same time, we can see that the mind/brain is important for understanding the body as well. Without an in-depth appreciation of how mental disorders might affect our bodies, Jones would surely have been misdiagnosed with heart failure and sent home with a message either to live with his disability or to prepare for the worst. Appreciating the deep connections between—or the even identification of—certain aspects of mind and body allowed Jones to return to an active and happy life.

The biggest lesson from this case study, however, is that "embodied cognition" refers to more than a body moving through space (cf. Gibson 1966). Appreciating that our thoughts are tied to our being creatures who live in a three dimensional world has been an important recent advance for cognitive science. However, that sentiment does not go far enough. The fact that we move in our world and are explicitly "designed" to move does not encapsulate everything that is relevant about our bodies for cognitive science. It is not just that our minds are housed in bodies, but it is that they are inextricably part of our bodies. Our cognition is not embodied; it is bodied, full stop.

Once we recognize this fact, then we must also recognize that the scope of explanations of the mind must expand beyond brain and behavior. Our cognitive faculties are much, much richer than that and we need theories that reflect the true interconnectedness between what happens above the neck and what happens below. Complete theories of the mind will include descriptions of the body, and vice versa.

2.2. Case Study #2: Somatization

A 29-year-old Caucasian female ("Smith") reported that she had essentially been incapacitated for the past two years, unable to drive or function independently. Approximately six years ago, she developed a fatigability that has gradually gotten worse. In particular, she complained of severe sensory and emotional overload, where any extraneous sounds or sights, or any interactions with people, made her symptoms worse. Indeed, it took her several hours to dress each day and she spent most of her time sitting quietly in a chair, looking at a blank wall. Talking on the telephone, watching television, reading, walking outside—all are activities that were too much for her to endure. She counted to keep her mind active.

Smith had a history of social sensitivity, which had progressively gotten worse over time. She had always been acutely aware of people's moods, thoughts, and feelings around her. She had always had a sense of wanting to please, not wanting to disappoint others, and was a perfectionist in relationships.

At first during the exam, she had difficulty maintaining eye contact, but then she took off her glasses and was able to talk more regularly. She had shaking in her extremities, similar to the chills, and some intention tremors when she moved around. A couple of times, she became breathless and said she could not complete her sentence because it was too much.

Smith was diagnosed with a somatization, one in a spectrum of somatoform disorders, following standard DSM diagnostic procedures. "Somatization" refers to a tendency to experience psychological distress as somatic symptoms and to seek medical help for these symptoms. No diagnosed physical illness accounts for the symptoms, nor do the symptoms seem to be in proportion to what would be seen in a diagnosed illness. Somatoform disorders are not the same thing as malingering or a factitious disorder because symptoms in somatoform disorders are not intentional, voluntary, or consciously produced (though some types of somatization disorder may have elements of volition or are influenced by distress or a desire for personal gain).

Smith was treated using intensive motivational-behavioral therapy with many behavioral and cognitive interventions. She responded well to treatment, and after discharge, she was able to leave her house for short periods, talk on the phone, and spend more quality time with family members.

Just as in our previous one, this case study demonstrates that there is no easy one-to-one correspondence between mental and physical phenomena. In the first case, Jones experienced depression as joint pain and fatigue. Here, Smith experiences psychological distress as sensory overload. In neither case would we be able to predict the physical manifestation, given the mental diagnosis. How each patient responded to his or her mental ills depended on particular environmental, bodily, and historical circumstances, none of which we have adequate ways to chart.

Another way to put this same point is that it appears that at least some mental disorders exhibit extreme sensitivity to initial conditions. If we could know and follow all the relevant variables that go in to each patient's particular response to mental stress, then we could predict its symptomotology. However, charting all the relevant conditions and their interactions is beyond our data-gathering means. We simply cannot do it. As a result, we cannot predict how a mental disorder will manifest itself in any particular case.

This lack of predictability means that truly reductive theories of these disorders will be hard to construct, since it is unclear what should be included in the scope of the explanations. Instead, some of, many of, our explanations are going to be narrative descriptions of a particular constellation of environmental, bodily, and historical events that all conspire toward some particular and unique outcome. These narrative accounts will necessarily be constructed after-the-fact, since we are not able to chart the variables relevant for prediction. (Indeed, it is not clear that we even know what the relevant variables are in these cases.)

While a devoted reductionist might simply claim that all we need to do is more research, we are less sanguine about this possibility. Though we recognize that we are not presenting a deductive argument for why at least some theories of the mind will not be reductive, we take this case to highlight the difficulties inherent in such a position. While the jury is out regarding whether some day, in the distant future, and under very different circumstances, we might be able to articulate all the parameters relevant to how mental illness manifests itself, we take this case study to tell us that we do not need a reductive account to explain what has happened. A non-reductive account works just fine. Expecting reduction in this case amounts to little more than an unsupported bias toward smallism and denies the sorts of accounts doctors give every day to account for their patients' diagnoses.

What separates Smith's case from Jones's is that our best explanation and treatment for Smith's problem is at the level of cognitive capacities. Unlike Jones, we have no way to reduce Smith's difficulties down to any lower level of organization or even to isolate the relevant processing modules. Right now, the best we can do is to discuss how her thought processes affect her behavioral reactions and her sensory processing. And there is nothing on the scientific horizon that would significantly alter this sort of theoretical approach.

We fix her difficulties by talking to her about how she might think or react differently. While her thoughts clearly do have lower-level effects, we have no ways of accessing those influences other than at the level of cognition. We conclude that reduction is not the appropriate theoretical framework for all of cognition at this time.

Traditional decomposition strategies are not helpful in working with Smith or with understanding her problems. Given the restricted nature of data normally found in support of cognitive science, they are not as useful as they could be in understanding Jones's case either. It is better in both cases to take a more holistic and inclusive approach to explain the multiple symptoms and the complex and underappreciated interplay between mind and body.

In conclusion, these two case studies challenge both our assumptions regarding what counts as relevant data in explaining our minds (or how our minds break down) and our reductive strategies in explanation. While reduction may remain an admirable goal for some explanations in cognitive science, it should not be the only one. How large a processing "module" is supposed to be and how far its effects extend are issues that have not been settled. Indeed, we actually believe our examples suggest that in at least some cases modularity in processing is largely an empty expression, for what goes into the so-called module is too diverse and too diffuse throughout the organization to be any real thing, but that is a different essay. What counts as data in explaining the mind goes far beyond what cognitive scientists have traditionally demarked as the province of the mental.

Furthermore, some of our explanations—some good ones that produce positive results—are not reductive, and it is not clear how they could become reductive in the near future. We do not have minds and bodies but we have minded bodies. And some of our scientific explanations need to reflect that fact.

REFERENCES

Anderson, J., and Bower, G. 1973. *Human Associative Memory*. Washington, DC: Winston.

Bechtel, W., and Richardson, R. C. 1993. *Discovering Complexity: Decomposition and Localization as Scientific Research Strategies*. Princeton: Princeton University Press.

—— and Mundale, J. 1999. Multiple realizability revisited: Linking cognitive and neural states. *Philosophy of Science* 66: 175–207.

Bickle, J. 2003. *Philosophy and Neuroscience: A Ruthlessly Reductionistic Account*. Amsterdam: Kluwer.

Brooks, D. N., and Baddeley, A. D. 1976. What can amnesics learn? *Neuropsychologia* 14: 111–22.

Cantor, J. R., Zillman, D., and Bryant, J. 1975. Enhancement of experienced arousal in response to erotic stimuli through misattribution of unrelated residual arousal. *Journal of Personality and Social Psychology* 32: 69–75.

Chemero, A., and Heyser, C. forthcoming. Object exploration and a problem with reduction. *Synthese.*

Churchland, P. S. 1986. *Neurophilosophy: Toward a Unified Science of the Mind/Brain.* Cambridge, MA: The MIT Press.

Clark, A. 1997. *Being There*. Cambridge, MA: The MIT Press.

—— 2003. *Natural Born Cyborgs*. New York: Oxford University Press.

Fodor, J. A. 1983. *The Modularity of Mind*. Cambridge, MA: The MIT Press/Bradford Books.

Gibson, J. J. 1966. *The Senses Considered as Perceptual Systems*. Boston: Houghton Mifflin.

—— 1979. *The Ecological Approach to Visual Perception*. Boston: Houghton Mifflin.

Hardcastle, V. G. 1996. *How to Build a Theory in Cognitive Science*. Albany, NY: State University of New York Press.

Jacoby, L. L., and Witherspoon, D. 1982. Remembering without awareness. *Canadian Journal of Psychology* 36: 300–24.

Lehky, S. R., and Sejnowski, T. J. 1988. Network Model of shape-from-shading. Neural function arises from both reception and projective fields. *Nature* 333: 452–4.

Lycan, W. G. 1987. *Consciousness*. Cambridge, MA: The MIT Press.

McCauley, R. N. 1996. Explanatory pluralism and the co-evolution of theories of science. In R. N. McCauley (ed.), *The Churchlands and Their Critics*. Oxford: Blackwell.

Nagel, E. 1949. The meaning of reduction in the natural sciences. In R. Stauffer (ed.), *Science and Civilization*. Madison, WI: University of Wisconsin Press, pp. 97–135.

—— 1961. *The Structure of Science*. New York: Harcourt, Brace, and World.

Noë, A. 2006. *Action in Perception*. Cambridge, MA: The MIT Press.

Posner, M. I., and Snider, C. 1975*a*. Attention and cognitive control. In R. Solso (ed.), *Information Processing and Cognition: The Loyola Symposium*. Hillsdale, NJ: Lawrence Erlbuam Associates.

—— —— 1975*b*. Facilitation and inhibition in the processing of signals. In P. M. A. Rabbit and S. Dornic (eds.), *Attention and Performance*. New York: Academic Press.

Quine, W. V. O. 1964. Ontological reduction and the world of numbers. *Journal of Philosophy* 61: 209–216.

Ramachandran, V. 1988. Perceiving shape from shading. *Scientific American* 259: 76–83.

Schacter, D. L., and Graf, P. 1986. Preserved learning in amnesic patients: Perspectives from research on direct priming. *Journal of Clinical and Experimental Neuropsychology* 8: 727–43.

Schneider, W., and Shiffrin, R. M. 1977. Controlled and automatic human information processing: I. Detection, search, and attention. *Psychological Review* 84: 1–66.

Shiffrin, R. M., and Schneider, W. 1977. Controlled and automatic human information processing: II. Perceptual learning, automatic attending, and general theory. *Psychological Review* 84: 127–90.

Squire, L., and Zola-Morgan, S. 1991. The medial temporal lobe memory system. *Science* 253: 424–30.

Thagard, P. 2002. How molecules matter to mental computation. *Philosophy of Science* 69: 497–518.

Tulving, E., Schacter, D. L., and Stark, H. A. 1982. Priming effects in word-fragment completion are independent of recognition memory. *Journal of Experimental Psychology: Learning, Memory, and Cognition* 8: 336–42.

Varela, F., and Thompson, E. 2001. Radical embodiment: Neural dynamics and consciousness. *Trends in Cognitive Sciences* 5: 418–25.

—— —— and Rosch, E. 1991 *The Embodied Mind.* Cambridge, MA: The MIT Press.

Warrington, E. K., and Weiskranz, L. 1970. Amnesic Syndrome: Consolidation or retrieval? *Nature* 228: 629–30.

—— —— 1974. The effect of prior learning on subsequent retention in amnesic patients. *Neuropsychologia* 12: 419–28.

Weiskranz, L., and Warrington, E. K. 1979. Conditioning in amnesic patients. *Neuropsychologia* 17: 187–94.

Woodger, J. H. 1952. *Biology and Language.* Cambridge: Cambridge University Press.

2

Real Reduction in Real Neuroscience: Metascience, Not Philosophy of Science (and Certainly Not Metaphysics!)

John Bickle

PHILOSOPHICAL ACCOUNTS OF SCIENTIFIC REDUCTION

Consider what is, among philosophers, an apparently unconventional argument (at least in the sense that few seem to act upon it). Suppose we wish to understand scientific reductionism—its nature, aims, scope, and potential limits. Here's a strategy: Let us find a clear example of a "reductionistic" field of scientific inquiry, dubbed so not only by its practitioners but also by scientists working in other, related fields. Then, as unencumbered by epistemological and metaphysical assumptions as we can rend ourselves, let us investigate some paradigmatic examples of recent research from that field, with our choice of examples dictated by the field's most prominent researchers. (These choices will result from discussions with those researchers, from publication in the field's most respected journals, from decisions by prominent funding agencies, and the like.) And then let us analyze the shared practices across these examples that differentiate this field from other scientific fields investigating related phenomena, only admittedly less reductionistically. (A good analogy here might be what a historian of a science does qua historian, only we'll be working with recent and current case studies.) The resulting account should be an analysis of real reductionism in real scientific practice, as contrasted with artificial accounts of scientific reductionism that rest instead on philosophical assumptions about "what reduction has to be".

So characterized, that project strikes me as inherently reasonable. So why is it virtually non-existent in contemporary philosophy? It is virtually non-existent therein. Two accounts of "reduction" dominate the philosophical literature. One, intertheoretic reduction, has its roots in late-20th-century philosophy of science. Most detailed variations are responses to Ernest Nagel's groundbreaking work in chapter 11 of his (1961) book, *The Structure of Science.* These accounts rest on strong assumptions about the structure of scientific theories, the nature of scientific explanation, and layered hierarchical pictures of both extra-theoretic reality and the sciences themselves. Reduction of one theory to another is either syntactic derivability or some weaker notion that approximates derivability in various respects. Proponents of intertheoretic reduction often cite scientific examples from the history of physics (e.g., the 19th-century reduction of portions of classical equilibrium thermodynamics to statistical mechanics and the kinetic/corpuscular theory of gases) and genetics (e.g., the mid-20th-century reduction of Mendelian principles of inheritance to initial discoveries of molecular genetics). Many surveys of intertheoretic reductionism exist in the literature (my own is in chapters 1 and 2 of Bickle 1998). Few proponents of intertheoretic reductionism have ever worried much about whether reductionistic scientific practices remain constant, not only across distinct sciences but also across the time periods that separate current scientific practice from those of half a century (as in the case of genetics) to more than a century ago (as in the case of the gas laws and statistical mechanics).

The other currently popular account of scientific reduction among philosophers and cognitive scientists is even more philosophically loaded and removed from current scientific practice. This is "functional reduction", first championed by philosophers pursuing consciousness studies (Chalmers 1996, Levine 1993) and most recently by Jaegwon Kim (2005). According to this view, scientific reduction is a two stage process. First scientists "functionalize" the concept targeted for reduction by characterizing it exhaustively in terms of its causes and effects. Then they pursue normal empirical investigations to discover which mechanisms in the actual world play this causal role (or at least approximate playing it). The scientific examples described to illustrate this account are telling. They are not even examples from the history of real science (like the ones that intertheoretic reductionists at least appeal to). Rather, they are from *elementary school science education*—like the boiling of water near sea level due to the dynamics of H_2O molecules. One might reasonably assume that the actual practices of current reductionistic science differ substantially from those involved in the examples we use to teach children the rudiments of our scientific world view! Reductionists should also be struck by the fact that the original proponents of functional reduction are *anti-reductionists* about some features of qualitative consciousness. Here then is another methodological lesson for reductionists (that should be rather obvious): don't let your opponents define the key concept of your account.

I won't try to explain why these two accounts of reductionism have held such sway in contemporary philosophy of mind and cognitive science. That would require a long story about the extent to which armchair metaphysics and normative epistemology have re-infected "analytic" philosophy over the past three decades. My goals in this chapter are of a more positive note. I am going to sketch a metascientific analysis of real reductionism in real, current neurobiological practice and point out some of its most obvious differences from the two accounts just characterized. This account stems from a more general analysis, first articulated by neurobiologist Alcino Silva, of the conditions on sufficient evidence for establishing a cellular or molecular mechanism for a cognitive phenomenon, and further developed in collaboration between the two of us (Silva and Bickle, forthcoming). I'll provide one detailed recent case study (out of easily one hundred I could have chosen) that illustrates our analyses. And I'll do all of this without imposing any significant metaphysical or normative epistemological assumptions that are not already a part of the scientific practices I seek to articulate.

'MOLECULAR AND CELLULAR COGNITION' AS A PARADIGMATIC CURRENT REDUCTIONISTIC SCIENTIFIC FIELD

The first step of any metascientific analysis is choosing the field from which to draw paradigmatic examples of scientific research that exhibit the concept one seeks to analyze. With regard to scientific reductionism, especially as it pertains to the relationship between cognition and the brain, the relatively new field of *molecular and cellular cognition* seems an apt choice. This field began in earnest in the early 1990s with the advent of using bioengineered genetic mutations in living, behaving rodents and the use of a variety of behavioral tasks that experimental psychology had developed for investigating specific cognitive phenomena. To date, learning and memory research has provided this field's most impressive achievements, but work is now being pursued in more than 100 labs worldwide on virtually all the phenomena that comprise cognitive science. A professional society now exists, the *Molecular and Cellular Cognition Society* (or *MCCS*), whose web site (at www.molcellcog.org) states that a goal of the field is "to derive explanations of cognitive processes that integrate molecular, cellular, and behavioral mechanisms". A related goal is to "promote the study of the molecular and cellular basis of cognitive function". Molecular and cellular cognitivists set their field explicitly in contrast to cognitive neuroscience:

> Unlike Cognitive Neuroscience, which historically has focused on the connection between human brain systems and behavior, the field of Molecular and Cellular Cognition studies how molecular (ie. receptor, kinase activation), intra-cellular (i.e. dendritic processes), and inter-cellular processes (i.e. synaptic plasticity; network representations such as place fields) modulate animal models of cognitive function. (www.molcellcog.org)

Clearly, proponents of this field don't hesitate to express their reductionistic attitude.

This attitude has even reached the latest neuroscience textbooks. In the introductory chapter of the most recent (4th) edition of their *Principles of Neural Science*, Eric Kandel, James Schwartz, and Thomas Jessell write:

> This book . . . describes how neural science is attempting to link molecules to mind—how proteins responsible for the activities of individual nerve cells are related to the complexity of neural processes. Today it is possible to link the molecular dynamics of individual nerve cells to representations of perceptual and motor acts in the brain and to relate these internal mechanisms to observable behavior. (2001, 3–4)

These mind-to-molecular pathways "links" are reductions, at least in the sense that this concept is at work in actual current neuroscientific practice.

With a reductionistic scientific field in hand, our metascientific analysis next moves to finding the commonalities in scientific practices that unite investigations in this field and distinguish it from investigations of similar phenomena in less reductionistic fields. There are now hundreds of published experimental studies in molecular and cellular cognition to choose from. Space in this chapter limits me to a detailed presentation of only a single case. (I've presented others in recent publications, including Bickle 2003, chapters 2–4; 2005; 2006*a*; 2006*b*; forthcoming-*b*.) In the next section I'll present a very recent example. In light of it, I'll then present the Convergent Four principles of sufficient evidence for establishing a cellular or molecular mechanism for a cognitive phenomenon, and emphasize the two principles that constitute molecular and cellular cognition's ruthlessly reductive core. I'll then sketch the implicit account of real reductionism in really reductionistic neuroscience and contrast it with the two accounts popular in philosophy with which this chapter began.

NEURONAL COMPETITION FOR PARTICIPATION IN A MEMORY TRACE IS DETERMINED BY RELATIVE CREB FUNCTION AT THE TIME OF TRAINING

Electrophysiological studies in rodents have long suggested that only a small percentage of neurons in specific cortical regions encode a particular memory trace. For example, although roughly 80% of neurons in the lateral nucleus of the mouse amygdala receive sensory input during classical Pavlovian auditory fear conditioning, only about 20–30% display plasticity following the training phase. What factors determine which neurons are recruited to participate in a particular memory? Recent experiments by Sheena Josselyn, Alcino Silva, and their collaborators implicate as a key causal factor the functioning of gene expression transcription enhancer *cyclic adenosine monophosphate (cAMP)/calcium responsive element binding protein*, or *CREB* (especially the α and δ isoforms) in individual neurons at the time of training (Han et al. 2007).

Previous research has implicated CREB in the induction of late long-term potentiation (L-LTP), a form of activity-driven long-lasting (hours to days, even weeks) increased neurotransmission efficacy at individual chemical synapses. L-LTP requires new gene expression and protein synthesis. The multi-burst trains of activity in pre-synaptic axons necessary to induce L-LTP activate not only glutamatergic and N-methyl-D-aspartate (NMDA) receptors in the post-synaptic membrane, but also a class of dopaminergic post-synaptic receptors associated with a G-protein complex. This activity primes adenylyl and adenylate cyclase molecules in the post-synaptic terminal to convert more adenosine triphosphate (ATP) molecules into cellular energy and cAMP. cAMP then serves as a second messenger, binding to regulatory subunits of protein kinase A (PKA) molecules and freeing up enough PKA catalytic subunits to translocate back to the neuron's nucleus. There the PKA subunits phosphorylate CREB molecules, which in turn bind to cAMP responsive elements in the control region of both regulatory and effector genes, turning on new gene expression. The outcome is ultimately the synthesis of new proteins that are transported back to active synapses to restructure the cytoskeletons, keeping the synapses potentiated for hours to days (to weeks). Behaviorally, affecting these CREB-dependent mechanisms of L-LTP affects the consolidation of memories from labile, easily disrupted short-term to stable long-term form. Blocking any step in the cAMP-PKA-CREB process virtually eradicates memory consolidation, while enhancing steps can lead to faster and stronger consolidation. These basic effects have now been demonstrated experimentally for a large number of memory tasks, including hippocampus-dependent "declarative" or "explicit" memories.[1]

Building on this experimental background, Josselyn, Silva, and their collaborators first showed that only around 20% of neurons in mouse lateral amygdala (LA) displayed CREB activation after auditory fear conditioning (Han et al. 2007). CREB activity was measured using a standard immunocytochemical antibody technique for labeling the presence of phosphorylated CREB (pCREB) in individual LA neurons. Wild-type mice (with no bioengineered genetic mutations) were divided into a tone + shock group (who underwent auditory fear conditioning in a training chamber and were exposed to the conditioning tone in a novel chamber during the testing phase 24 hours later) and a number of control groups (e.g., tone alone, immediate shock, chamber alone, and home cage groups). Mice in the tone + shock group showed roughly 20% pCREB-positive neurons in LA following the testing phase. No control group showed more than 10%.

[1] See Bickle 2003, ch. 2 for a nontechnical description of the basic molecular biology of LTP and some techniques for engineering specific genetic mutations in mammals (with extensive references to the primary scientific literature). See the other references cited in the last paragraph of the previous section for nontechnical discussions of some specific experimental results using these genetically mutated mice in memory research.

This first result is consistent with CREB functioning being a key factor in neuronal recruitment to participate in specific memory traces, since the number of pCREB positive neurons following auditory fear conditioning matches up well with the number of potentiated neurons found in previous electrophysiological studies. But can CREB function be shown to be involved more directly in neuronal competition during memory training? Josselyn, Silva, and colleagues established this more direct experimental connection by microinjecting replication-deficient herpes simplex virus (HSV) vectors fused with a gene expressing green fluorescent protein (GFP) and either the wild-type CREB gene for the α and δ transcription enhancer isoforms ($CREB^{WT}$) or a gene for a dominant-negative repressor form of the CREB protein that competes with endogenous CREB for binding sites in gene control regions but inhibits gene expression ($CREB^{S133A}$, in which the serine (S) residue that occurs at site 133 in CREB α and δ isoforms has been replaced by an alanine (A) residue) (Han et al. 2007). GFP makes infected neurons easy to image and count using standard microscopy techniques; infected neurons literally synthesize a protein that distributes throughout their cytoplasms and glows green in microscopic images. The $CREB^{WT}$ insertion increases the amount of CREB α and δ molecules available and enhances CREB functioning in infected neurons over normal endogenous levels. The $CREB^{S133A}$ insertion reduces CREB transcription enhancer function. The details of this experimental work will not be familiar to philosophers and cognitive scientists, even for those who comment regularly on the scope and limits of neurobiology; but this is the sort of molecular biological knowledge and manipulation that is common in current molecular and cellular cognition.

Han et al. (2007) first manipulated CREB expression in a population of genetically mutated mice with greatly reduced levels of CREB transcription enhancers ($CREB^{\alpha\delta-}$ mice). The gene for CREB α and δ isoforms had been "knocked out" at the embryonic stem cell development phase in these mice. Previous behavioral studies have shown that these mice display significantly deficient consolidation of short-term into long-term memory on a large number of tasks. For example, in auditory fear conditioning, they only spend about 20% of testing time freezing after exposure to the conditioned tone in the testing phase 24 hours after standard one-trial tone-shock pairings, as compared to about 60% freezing time in wild-type littermate controls. (Freezing is a stereotypic rodent fear response in which the animal crouches, tucks its front paws inward beneath its chest, and ceases all movement except breathing.) Interestingly, $CREB^{\alpha\delta-}$ mutants are intact compared to wild-type littermate controls on short-term versions of this and other memory tasks, where the delays between training and test phases range from 30 minutes to 2 hours. This common result controls for motivational, perceptual, attentional, and motor confounds. The CREB expression manipulation generates a specific memory consolidation effect.

Han et al. (2007) microinjected HSV vectors containing genes for GFP and either $CREB^{WT}$ or LacZ (as a control vector) into lateral amygdala (LA) of $CREB^{\alpha\delta-}$ mutants or wild-type littermates prior to the training phase of auditory fear conditioning. Although the viral vector only infected around 18% of LA neurons in all groups (as measured by counting the number of LA neurons in confocal microscopic images displaying GFP compared to the number that did not), $CREB^{WT}$ injections completely rescued long-term auditory fear conditioning in $CREB^{\alpha\delta-}$ mutants. $CREB^{\alpha\delta-}$ mutants receiving the LacZ control vector displayed the usual failure to consolidate long-term auditory fear conditioning memories, freezing only about 20% of the time following exposure to the conditioned tone 24 hours after training, compared to the >70% freezing time in wild-types microinjected with either $CREB^{WT}$ or LacZ. Yet $CREB^{\alpha\delta-}$ mutants receiving microinjection of $CREB^{WT}$ froze about 75% of the testing time after exposure to the conditioned tone, statistically identical to wild-type performances. Furthermore, the rescued consolidation of long-term auditory fear conditioning did not result simply from the $CREB^{WT}$ injections in LA facilitating the freezing response. This was demonstrated by a supplemental study in which all groups were subjected to a hippocampus-dependent contextual fear conditioning task. In this task mice are exposed to a novel chamber, allowed to explore it briefly, and then shocked. They are placed back in the training chamber 24 hours later and measured for their freezing response. Both $CREB^{\alpha\delta-}$ mutant groups, those receiving LA injections of $CREB^{WT}$ vector and those receiving the control LacZ vector, showed the usual reduction in freezing time during re-exposure compared to both wild-type littermate control groups. This control result indicates that the LA $CREB^{WT}$ vector injections had no effect on memory consolidation deficits on hippocampus-dependent tasks and that the rescued consolidation in the auditory fear conditioning task was not due simply to facilitating the freezing response. So increasing CREB function in less than 20% of LA neurons completely rescues the consolidation of long-term auditory fear conditioning in CREB-deficient mice.

Interestingly, increasing CREB function in LA neurons of wild-type mice also enhanced auditory fear conditioning. Han et al. (2007) showed this by using low intensity shocks (0.4 mA as compared to 0.7 mA used in the earlier study) that elicit a less-than-maximal freezing (fear) response. Wild-type mice receiving the LA LacZ control vector spent about 40% of the time freezing upon tone exposure 24 hours after training. Wild-type mice receiving the LA $CREB^{WT}$ vector spent about 75% of the time freezing upon tone exposure in the testing phase. This difference reflects a statistically significant increase in tone-shock association due to increased CREB availability over normal endogenous levels.

But can one show that the specific neurons infected by the $CREB^{WT}$ vector were actually the neurons preferentially recruited into the tone-shock association memory trace? To visualize the neurons that were components of the memory trace, Han et al. (2007) took advantage of the unique time-course of the transcription of an activity-dependent gene, *activity-regulated cytoskeleton-associated protein* (*Arc*). Increased activity in a given neuron induces a rapid, transient increase in *Arc* transcription, so that Arc RNA localized in the cell nucleus 5–15 minutes after neuron activity can serve as a molecular signal of recent activity (Guzowski et al. 1999). Han et al. (2007) used a cellular imaging strategy, fluorescent *in situ* hybridization, to detect the specific LA neurons that were active (Arc+) during the testing phase of the auditory fear conditioning task. Only those neurons that were active during the testing phase, and thus part of the fear conditioning memory trace, would be Arc+. Inactive neurons during the testing phase, presumably not part of the memory trace, would be Arc−. The Arc images of LA neurons could then be merged with the GFP images to count the percentage of LA neurons that were double labeled (GFP+ and Arc+). Those neurons would be the ones that were both infected by the CREB^{WT} vector (as evidenced by their being GFP+) and hence subject to increased CREB function, and also recruited into the fear conditioning memory trace (as evidenced by their also being Arc+).

If increased CREB function at the time of training is a critical factor that influences the probability that a given LA neuron is recruited as part of a fear conditioning memory trace, then GFP+ neurons with elevated CREB function induced by the CREB^{WT} vector microinjections should have a greater likelihood of being Arc+ following the testing phase than their GFP− neighboring neurons that were not infected by the CREB^{WT} vector. What were the percentages in the various experimental groups? In wild-type mice who received the CREB^{WT} vector prior to auditory fear conditioning training, slightly more than 20% of all LA neurons were Arc+ during the testing phase (another result that coheres nicely with other measures described above about the percentage of LA neurons incorporated into a given memory trace). However, GFP+ LA neurons (which were infected with the CREB^{WT} vector and thus had higher rates of CREB function at the time of training) were roughly 3 times more likely to be Arc+ than were neighboring GFP− neurons (which had endogenous CREB function at time of training). In wild-type mice infected with the LacZ control vector coupled with GFP, once again slightly more than 20% of all LA neurons were Arc+ during the testing phase of the auditory fear conditioning task. However GTP+ neurons (and hence infected with the control LacZ vector that does not affect CREB function) and neighboring GFP-neurons were equally likely to be Arc+. This effect was even more pronounced in the CREB$^{\alpha\delta-}$ mice, who are deficient in consolidating fear conditioning memories into long-term form, but whose deficit was rescued by LA CREB^{WT} vector microinjections. In CREB$^{\alpha\delta-}$ mutants receiving the LacZ control vector, the percentage of Arc+ neurons during the testing phase was significantly lower than in any other group (less than 10% of all LA neurons), and GFP+ neurons (infected with the inactive control vector) were no more likely to be Arc+ than their nearby GFP− neighbors. However, in CREB$^{\alpha\delta-}$ mutants receiving the CREB^{WT} vector, once again nearly 20% of all LA neurons were Arc+ during the testing phase. And GTP+ neurons (infected with the $CREB^{WT}$ vector and thus with increased CREB function at time of training) were roughly *10 times more likely* to be Arc+ than their nearby GFP– neighbors. (For the quantified data, see Han et al. 2007, figure 2.) These data directly support the hypothesis that neurons with higher CREB function at the time of training are more likely to be recruited into a specific memory trace than are those with normal or low CREB function. The mechanism of this competitive recruitment process into specific memory traces has now been reduced down to particular molecular processes in individual neurons. Modifying these processes in either direction has predictable behavioral effects on memory consolidation on tasks dependent on neurons in the region of the brain whose molecular processes have been manipulated.[2]

This section has no doubt been rough sledding for many philosophers and cognitive scientists, so I'll briefly summarize the points that will be emphasized in the metascientific analysis that follows.

- Numerous previous experiments had implicated CREB functioning in individual neurons as a mechanism of long-term memory consolidation, including in lateral amygdala (LA) neurons for auditory fear conditioning.
- Intervening to block CREB functioning using molecular-genetic techniques produces mice that cannot consolidate short-term fear associative memories into long-term form.
- Intervening to increase CREB functioning at time of training in less than 20% of LA neurons (using HSV vector microinjection techniques) completely rescues long-term fear association memories in CREB-deficient mutant mice, and increases long-term fear memories in wild-type mice using a less-than-maximal aversive unconditioned stimulus.
- A fluorescent *in situ* hybridization study reveals that individual LA neurons with increased CREB functioning at time of training are statistically much more likely to be recruited into the neuronal memory trace than neighboring neurons with normal endogenous or decreased CREB functioning.

THE CONVERGENT FOUR PRINCIPLES OF MOLECULAR AND CELLULAR COGNITION

Case studies like the one described in the previous section comprise the basis on which a purely metascientific account of real reductionism in actual scientific

[2] In subsequent experiments, Josselyn, Silva, and their collaborators controlled for the possibility that neurons with increased CREB function simply have a lower threshold for inducing Arc (they don't), and that inhibiting CREB function in roughly 20% of LA neurons in wild-type mice (via HSV $CREB^{S133A}$ insertion) has no detrimental effects on memory consolidation in the auditory fear conditioning task (because enough LA neurons with relatively high CREB function remain available for recruitment into the memory trace). See Han et al. (2007) for details on these control experiments.

practice can be generated and then assessed for philosophical significance. Based on a number of such cases, neurobiologist Alcino Silva was first to sketch (in 2007 and unpublished writings) four principles that together amount to sufficient experimental evidence for establishing a cellular or molecular mechanism for a given "systems-level" cognitive phenomena, at least within the accepted practices of molecular and cellular cognition. Our recent collaborations have produced more detailed accounts of these *Convergent Four* (Silva and Bickle, forthcoming). These principles constitute metascientific fruits of a Science of Research investigation of molecular and cellular cognition—quite literally, the application of scientific practices to the study of scientific practice itself (Silva and Bickle, forthcoming). The account of real reductionism in actual reductionistic neuroscientific practice sketched in the next section derives directly from these principles.

Principle 1: *Observation.* Occurrences of the hypothesized mechanism are strongly correlated with occurrences of the behaviors used as experimental measures of the cognitive phenomenon.

Experiments in many species and neural systems have documented the *observation* that learning is accompanied by changes in synaptic plasticity in the very brain regions required for that particular form of learning. Others have documented that maintenance of these synaptic changes are correlated with memory performance. Specific forms of synaptic plasticity, like late-phase long-term potentiation (L-LTP), have been correlated experimentally with memory performance in a variety of tasks. CREB function has been observed to be correlated with L-LTP. Meeting the Observation Principle does not by itself establish that the hypothesized mechanism is part of the causal nexus generating the behavioral measures. (Molecular and cellular cognitivists aren't strict Humeans about causality!) But establishing these observations is often an early step in formulating the causal-mechanistic hypotheses that this field investigates experimentally. Before this Principle is met, investigators have no reason for pursuing the more detailed experiments required to establish sufficient evidence for a molecular mechanism for a cognitive phenomenon. In the case study discussed in the previous section, observation experiments had already long established that L-LTP followed from CREB function, that consolidation of long-term auditory fear conditioning (i.e., freezing during the testing phase) followed from L-LTP in lateral amygdala (LA) neurons, and more. (Indeed, even more than simple observation experiments already linked CREB function in LA neurons and long-term auditory fear conditioning prior to the study discussed above, as we'll see in the discussion of Principle 4 below.) In addition to these previous results, Han et al. (2007) began their investigations with an immunocytochemical antibody labeling study for pCREB that showed CREB functioning in roughly 20% of LA neurons during activation of long-term auditory fear conditioning memory (a result that matched earlier studies of plasticity in LA neurons using electrophysiological techniques). This was a straightforward example of an observation experiment.

Principle 2: Negative Alteration. Intervening directly to decrease activity of the hypothesized mechanisms must reliably decrease the behaviors used as experimental measures of the cognitive phenomenon.

Experiments that establish negative alteration are often the centerpieces of current molecular and cellular cognition investigations. For example, the engineered genetic mutation ("knock-out") that produces the $CREB^{\alpha\delta-}$ mice used in the studies reported in the previous section is a negative alteration. The mutation decreases CREB function and experimenters then track reliable decreases in behaviors that measure specific types of memory consolidation (with the appropriate controls to rule out sensory, attentional, motivational, and motor confounds).

More specific genetic interventions, with the use of either selective promoter regions on genetic insertions that limit where genes of interest are expressed or inhibited, or the use of pharmacological tools that limit the temporal dimensions of the genetic manipulation, are often used to provide evidence of negative alteration. For example, Abel et al. (1997) coupled a transgene that overexpresses regulatory subunits of PKA molecules to a promoter region that binds α-calmodulin kinase II. So while the transgene was present in every cell of the mouse's body, it was only expressed in high amounts in forebrain neurons (including hippocampus). This enabled the experimenters to demonstrate a negative alteration on hippocampus-dependent memory tasks with these mice, but no significant alteration on amygdala-dependent tasks (where the transgene was expressed in lesser amounts). A second example is the $CREB^{IR}$ mouse, developed by Silva, Mashushige, and collaborators (Kida et al. 2002), in which an inducible CREB repressor fusion protein competes with endogenous CREB for CRE binding sites, but inhibits gene expression there. The CREB repressor protein has the usual alanine-for-serine residue change at position 133, but has been fused with a ligand binding domain from a human estrogen receptor that itself has been mutated to be activated by the drug tamoxifen (TAM). Hence the CREB repressor fusion protein is only activated, and hence only inhibits CREB function, when these mice have been injected with TAM; as soon as the injected TAM has been metabolized, CREB function returns to normal endogenous levels. This creates a 6–12 hour CREB negative alteration, inducible and reversible in the same mice, and enabled experimenters to demonstrate a transient loss of memory consolidation (and reconsolidation after reactivation) in mutated animals dosed with TAM just before training (Kida et al. 2002).

Principle 3: Positive Alteration. Intervening directly to increase activity of the hypothesized mechanisms must reliably increase the behaviors used as experimental measures of the cognitive phenomenon.

Although positive alterations of learning and memory have been carried out successfully in insect studies for more than a decade, cases are still few and far between in mammal studies. That is what makes the recent studies described above especially intriguing. Both the complete rescue of long-term auditory fear conditioning in $CREB^{\alpha\delta-}$ mutants and the enhanced effect in wild-type mice using low intensity training shocks following HSV $CREB^{WT}$ microinjections into lateral amygdala (LA) are examples of positive alteration. In both cases, the inserted genetic material increased CREB function in roughly 20% of LA neurons and reliably increased the measured freezing response to tone presentation during the testing phase of auditory fear conditioning. Techniques that generate evidence of positive alteration in mammals are genuine methodological breakthroughs in current molecular and cellular cognition.

Principle 4: Integration. The hypothesis that the proposed mechanisms are key components of the causal nexus that produces the behaviors used as experimental measures of the cognitive phenomenon must be connected up with as much experimental data as is available about the hypothesized mechanism, the cognitive phenomenon, and the paths connecting them.

Principle 4 is the most abstract of these conditions on sufficient evidence, and certainly the one requiring the most extensive explication.[3] On the one hand, it serves to rule out silly objections to claimed mechanisms based on these conditions such as "removing oxygen from the animal's environment significantly alters its behavior in this memory task. Is oxygen consumption thereby a mechanism of memory?" or ". . . Does memory thereby reduce to oxygen consumption?" (These are counterexamples that philosophers sometimes raise to the Convergent Four, attempting to be cute.) Clearly, the empirical background against which serious experimental studies are performed has already ruled out such silly mechanisms or reductions.[4] Yet Principle 4 is intended to accomplish far more than just this. Data meeting it often provide the empirical reasons that motivate molecular and cellular cognitivists to attempt the specific negative and positive alteration experiments that they do, down to the particular gene expression and protein synthesis they manipulate (including the particular molecular-biological techniques they employ) and the behavioral measures they use to track the effects of their manipulations. *A lot* of information is usually

[3] Silva and Bickle (forthcoming) is a first attempt to begin this explication.

[4] Not to mention the fact that positive alterations into these silly "mechanisms" don't produce significant effects on the behavioral measures used; or if they do, then the proposed "silly" mechanisms actually are key components of the causal nexus. This fact demonstrates the independence of Principle 3 from Principle 4 and the necessity of including Principle 3 in these conditions that are jointly sufficient for establishing a molecular or cellular mechanism for a cognitive phenomenon.

known about the molecular biology and the behaviors that molecular and cellular cognitivists combine in their negative and positive alteration studies, and this goes far beyond the observational correlations that fall under Principle 1 (Observation).

Another nice feature of the study described in the previous section for our metascientific purposes in this section is the illustration it provides of Principle 4 at work. Many studies, from the behavioral down to the molecular biological, had already implicated CREB function in lateral amygdala (LA) neurons as a molecular mechanism of long-term consolidation of auditory fear conditioning. But no previous study had integrated these findings to directly implicate CREB function as the molecular mechanism for the recruitment of individual LA neurons into specific memory traces. Josselyn, Silva, and their colleagues took advantage of another recent discovery from the molecular biology of neuronal activity, the activity-dependent and temporally limited availability of Arc RNA in neuron nuclei, and an *in situ* hybridization technique for measuring this signal of recent neuronal activity. This molecular-biological insight enabled them to merge images of CREB^{WT}-infected LA neurons (GFP+), which had enhanced CREB function, with images of Arc+ neurons at the time of the testing phase of auditory fear conditioning. They were thus able to demonstrate a significantly higher probability of GFP+ LA neurons also being Arc+ than their nearby GFP− neighbors. Integrating this new molecular-biological knowledge and imaging techniques with already-available molecular and behavioral knowledge about CREB function and long-term fear conditioning consolidation provided the novel direct evidence that CREB functioning in individual LA neurons is indeed a causal mechanism of neuronal recruitment into circuits subserving specific fear memory traces.

Another interesting feature of the Integration Principle is a way that prior experimental work gets incorporated into ongoing research. In current molecular and cellular cognition research, most of the time experimental work already exists that suggests a key mechanism for the cognitive phenomenon at issue; and typically this earlier work itself already meets most of the Convergent Four principles. Often the causal interventions used in this previous work have taken place at higher "levels" of biological organization than the new experiments being pursued. This is what philosophers and cognitive scientists typically refer to as "relating different levels" of theory and explanation. In the study discussed in the previous section, earlier experiments had already established that neurons in the lateral amygdala (LA) were anatomically connected to the motor pathways that generate the behavioral measures of auditory fear conditioning, and to the sensory inputs from auditory cortex. Other work (by Joseph LeDoux, James McGaugh, and others) had established that L-LTP takes place in LA neurons during auditory fear conditioning and that CREB functioning occurs during the neuronal plasticity that resulted from the training phase of the task. These connections had already been established as more than mere observed correlations: alteration experiments had been performed successfully[5] and theoretical integration had been proposed. In fact, these connections had already been established down to the number of LA neurons that received auditory input and the number that underwent plasticity in response to the tone-shock pairing. The "higher-level" results connecting CREB to LTP, LTP to LA neuron plasticity, and LA neuron activity to long term auditory fear conditioning thus became part of the integrative theoretical background for this study described in the section above. The Han et al. (2007) study in turn established a positive alteration of CREB functioning to increase auditory fear conditioning behaviors, and CREB functioning as the mechanism for the recruitment of specific LA neurons into the circuits for particular memory traces. In this way Principle 4 captures how new results build in prior ones—where the prior ones themselves met at least some of the Convergent Four principles on their own.

The study described in the previous section is just one of at least one hundred others that could be cited as providing experimental illustrations of the Convergent Four Principles. Alcino Silva and I offer the Convergent Four as our first metascientific hypothesis from a Science of Research investigation into the scientific practices of molecular and cellular cognition (Silva and Bickle forthcoming). I'll close this essay in the final section by sketching a second metascientific hypothesis: the nature of reductionism in the actual practices of this reductionistic branch of contemporary neuroscience, drawn from the core of the Convergent Four Principles.

THE RUTHLESSLY REDUCTIVE CORE OF THE CONVERGENT FOUR

Notice that Principles 1 and 4 require "higher level" scientific investigations.[6] To establish the required observations between hypothesized mechanism and behaviors, and to integrate knowledge of molecules and behavior to establish the theoretical plausibility of the proposed mechanisms for the cognitive phenomenon in question, we need precise knowledge of what the system does under controlled experimental conditions. This means having both precise data about the system's behaviors (as grist for our lower level mechanistic explanations)

[5] With the possible exception of successful *positive* alteration experiments linking CREB function in LA neurons and auditory fear conditioning, which the Han et al. study also provided.

[6] I enclose "higher level" in scare quotes to indicate that very little hangs on its explication (here or in the previous discussion of Principle 4). I don't assume anything fancy by this term and nothing in my argument relies on any detailed account of "levels". Here I simply refer to the common assumption in neuroscientific practice that locates appeals to neural systems at a higher level than appeals to the cellular physiology of its component neurons, and the latter at a higher level than the molecular-biological processes that take place around and inside of their membranes.

and good behavioral measures for the cognitive phenomenon at issue. These are jobs for cognitive scientists and experimental psychologists, not electrophysiologists or molecular geneticists. We also need to know where to start inserting our cellular and molecular interventions. The "decomposition and localization" investigations of cognitive neuroscientists are crucial for this knowledge.[7] We also need to know what types of neuronal activity to intervene into. Action potential frequency? Action potential dynamics? Field potentials? Something else entirely? The work of neurocomputational modelers and simulators is important here. Each of these activities has distinct molecular mechanisms, and so requires different molecular-biological techniques to intervene into. Molecular and cellular cognition needs a lot of higher level cognitive science and neuroscience to accomplish its potential reductions—and it now regularly employs such scientists in order to get these details right. Molecular and cellular cognition is a reductionistic brand of current neuroscience, perhaps even "ruthlessly" so. But that in no way precludes its use of higher level cognitive science and scientists.

Yet in the end (at least at the present time), it is the experiments that illustrate Principles 2 and 3 that cinch the empirical case for a proposed lower level mechanism for a cognitive phenomena. It is certainly these experiments that typically constitute the unique contributions of molecular and cellular cognition studies. Even the case study described two sections ago, which in the previous section I argued made a significant contribution to Principle 4 for establishing the connection between CREB function and auditory fear memory consolidation, made an equally important contribution to Principle 3. That is, it established a positive alteration in CREB function to enhance the behavioral measures of auditory fear memory consolidation.

What then is the nature of the reductionism implicit in Principles 2 and 3? Unlike classic intertheoretic reduction, real reductionism in molecular and cellular cognition does not require an explicit, complete set of laws or explanatory generalizations that characterize the behaviors of reduced and reducing kinds in all contexts or circumstances. Reduction is not a logical relationship between such laws or generalizations. Unlike more recently developed and championed "functional" reduction, real reductionism does not require the reduced concepts to be characterized exhaustively in terms of their causes and effects; instead, it requires cognitive concepts to be operationalized methodologically, in terms ultimately of measures in specific behavioral protocols and paradigms, for the purposes of controlled experiments. In other words, instead of logical derivation of laws or explanatory generalizations, or functionalization of concepts, real reductionism in genuinely reductionistic neuroscientific practice is a matter of:

> *Intervening causally*, directly into processes at increasing lower levels of biological organization (cellular, intra-cellular molecular, molecular genetic)

[7] Bechtel and Richardson (1993) remains the most useful discussion of this strategy.

and then

> *Tracking* the effects of these interventions in living, behaving organisms using a variety of measures widely accepted as indicative for the cognitive phenomenon being investigated.

When these interventions generate evidence for negative and positive alterations (Principles 2 and 3 above) in light of background evidence connecting the hypothesized cellular or molecular mechanism to the behaviors serving as measures for the cognitive phenomenon, a reduction is said to have been accomplished. The cognitive phenomenon reduces to the cellular or molecular mechanisms intervened into, within the anatomical circuits leading ultimately to the motor peripheries generating the measured behaviors. Molecular and cellular cognitivists then talk explicitly about having discovered "a molecular biology of cognition" (Bailey, Bartsch, and Kandel 1996), or of "providing an experimental framework for a molecular understanding" of a specific cognitive phenomena (Abel et al. 1997).[8] Note that these are assertions made within—following Rudolph Carnap, we might say "internal to"—the practices of molecular and cellular cognition.[9] They are neither metaphysical identity claims nor normative epistemological assertions.

Meeting Principles 2 and 3 establishes experimentally that hypothesized mechanisms are actually doing the job. When Principles 2 and 3 are established experimentally (and not simply predicted to be established), our best causal-mechanistic story for the cognitive phenomenon in question now resides at the lowest level of effective interventions (in conjunction with the anatomical circuitry that gets the neuronal activity out to the motor periphery). Once again, this assertion is a part of a metascience of molecular and cellular cognition—a description of the assertive practices that take place in the research of that field. It is not offered here as a metaphysical or normative epistemological claim. It is implicit in the ways that molecular and cellular cognitivists discuss their results and develop their experimental strategies (Bickle 2003, 2005, 2006*a*, forthcoming-*a*, forthcoming-*b*; Silva and Bickle forthcoming). From the perspective of molecular and cellular cognition, when all of the Convergent Four Principles are met for a hypothesized mechanism and a cognitive phenomenon, "higher level" explanations of that phenomenon lose their status as causal-mechanistic—although such explanations still provide empirical support for two of the four principles that our currently best causal-mechanistic explanation rests upon. If you ask higher-level explanations to provide more than this,

[8] See Bickle (forthcoming-*a*) for more discussion of the differences between intertheoretic, functional, and metascientific reductionisms. Bickle (2006*a*) provides diagrams that illustrate contrasts between intertheoretic and metascientific reductionisms and a first try at distinguishing metascientific reductionism from the recent "new mechanical" philosophy of science.

[9] See Bickle (2003, chapter 1), for more on the connection between Carnap's internal/external existence question distinction and the brand of metascience advocated here.

however, after the Convergent Four principles have been met for a cellular or molecular mechanism, then you are asking for something beyond the role that the "ruthlessly reductive" practices of molecular and cellular cognition ascribe to them. That isn't necessarily a mistake. We don't yet know the explanatory scope of molecular and cellular cognition (although it already extends way beyond the range that most philosophers and cognitive scientists realize—see my publications cited below from Bickle 2003 onward). But your account thereby also isn't "neurobiologically plausible", at least in light of the practices and results of molecular and cellular cognition circa today. And that is a field of neuroscience whose practitioners increasingly populate publications in the best scientific journals, procure the largest share of external grants, and get awarded the most prestigious prizes.

REFERENCES

Abel, T., P. V. Nguyen, M. Barad, T. A. Deuel, E. R. Kandel, and R. Bourtchouladze (1997). "Genetic Demonstration of a Role for PKA in the Late Phase of LTP and in Hippocampus-Based Long-Term Memory." *Cell* 88/5: 615–26.

Bailey, C. H., D. Bartsch, and E. R. Kandel (1996). "Towards a Molecular Definition of Long-Term Memory Storage." *Proceedings of the National Academy of Sciences USA* 93/24: 13445–52.

Bechtel, W. and R. Richardson (1993). *Discovering Complexity.* Princeton: Princeton University Press.

Bickle, J. (1998). *Psychoneural Reduction: The New Wave.* Cambridge, MA: MIT Press.

—— (2003). *Philosophy and Neuroscience: A Ruthlessly Reductive Account.* Dordrecht: Kluwer.

—— (2005). "Molecular Neuroscience to My Rescue (Again): A Reply to Looren de Jong and Schouten." *Philosophical Psychology* 18/4: 487–93.

—— (2006*a*). "Reducing Mind to Molecular Pathways: Explicating the Reductionism Implicit in Current Mainstream Neuroscience." *Synthese* 152: 411–34.

—— (2006*b*). "Ruthless Reductionism in Recent Neuroscience." *IEEE Transactions on Systems, Man, and Cybernetics* 36: 134–40.

—— (forthcoming-*a*). "The Changing Faces and Scientific Bases of Mind-Brain Reductionism." In *Reti, saperi, linguaggi* (Journal of the Department of Cognitive Science, University of Messina, Italy), 2.

—— (forthcoming-*b*). "There's a New Kid in Town: Computational Cognitive Science, Meet Molecular and Cellular Cognition." In D. Dedrick and L. Trick (eds), *Cognition, Computation, and Pylyshyn.* Cambridge, MA: MIT Press.

Chalmers, D. (1996). *The Conscious Mind.* Oxford: Oxford University Press.

Guzowski J., B. McNaughton, C. Barnes, and P. Worley (1999). "Environment-Specific Expression of the Immediate Early Gene Arc in Hippocampal Neuronal Ensembles." *Nature Neuroscience* 2: 1120–4.

Han, J.-H., S. A. Kushner, A. P. Yiu, C. A. Cole, A. Matynia, R. A. Brown, R. Neve, J. F. Guzowski, A. J. Silva, and S. A. Josselyn (2007). "Neuronal Competition and Selection During Memory Formation." Science 316: 457–60.

Kandel, E. R., J. Schwartz, and T. Jessell (eds.) (2001). *Principles of Neural Science*, 4th edn. New York: McGraw-Hill.

Kida, S., S. Josselyn, S. Orliz, J. Kogan, I. Chevere, S. Masushige, and A. Silva (2002). "CREB Required for the Stability of New and Reactivated Fear Memories." *Nature Neuroscience* 5: 348–55.

Kim, J. (2005). *Physicalism, Or Something Near Enough*. Princeton: Princeton University Press.

Levine, J. (1993). "On Leaving Out What it's Like." In M. Davies and G. W. Humphreys (eds.), *Consciousness: Psychological and Philosophical Essays*. London: Blackwell, 121–36.

Nagel, E. (1961). *The Structure of Science*. New York: Harcourt, Brace, and World.

Silva, A. J. (2007). "The Science of Research: The Principles Underlying the Discovery of Cognitive and Other Biological Phenomena." *Journal of Physiology* (Paris) 101: 203–13.

—— and J. Bickle (forthcoming). "Intimology, Metascience, and the Search for Molecular Mechanisms of Cognition." In J. Bickle (ed.), *Oxford Handbook of Philosophy and Neuroscience*. Oxford: Oxford University Press.

3

Reduction in Real Life

Peter Godfrey-Smith

1. INTRODUCTION

The main message of the paper is that there is a disconnect between what many philosophers of mind think of as the scientific practice of reductive or reductionist explanation, and what the most relevant scientific work is actually like. I will sketch what I see as a better view, drawing on various ideas in recent philosophy of science. I then import these ideas into the philosophy of mind, to see what difference they make.

At the end of the paper I address a possible objection: the familiar package of ideas I reject in the philosophy of science should not be lightly discarded, because other popular views on fundamental issues depend on positions that I want to reject. I reply that those apparently attractive further ideas are not worth holding onto.

So the paper begins with issues in the philosophy of science: reduction, laws, mechanisms, and models. It then turns to philosophy of mind, and returns to broad themes in the philosophy of science at the end.

2. MECHANISMS, MODELS, AND REDUCTION

In this section I contrast two packages of views about reduction and related issues. One is a "traditional" view, the other an "alternative" view. The traditional view is not just the deliverances of older philosophy of science, however. It is a package of ideas that draws on traditional philosophy of science (especially late logical empiricism), but that has been augmented and modified by philosophers

I am indebted to those at the Aarhus conference in 2005 for helpful comments. I am grateful also to Ned Block, Carl Craver, Steven Horst, Kim Sterelny, and the editors of this collection for criticism of an earlier draft.

of mind. The "alternative" view draws on recent philosophy of science, but the position presented will be my own blend of ideas that derive from several different camps.

Here is the package of views about science that I will refer to as standard or traditional, in much philosophy of mind.

(i) Theories are essentially networks of generalizations.
(ii) The best theories feature, as central components, forward-looking causal laws. These laws treat future states and events in their domain as a function of past states.
(iii) We have theories of this kind at different "levels". The lower-level ones either reduce the higher-level ones, or are linked by a weaker explanatory relation (perhaps supervenience of facts or properties at the two levels).
(iv) Physics is at the bottom of this hierarchy of levels. Above it we find chemistry, biology, psychology, and the social sciences.
(v) There is a close link between the notions of law, natural kind, counterfactual dependence, confirmation, and explanation. In particular, not all true universal generalizations specify laws. Those that do specify laws contain predicate terms that pick out natural kinds. Laws support counterfactuals, unlike non-lawlike generalizations. Law-like generalizations, and only them, can be confirmed by their instances. Laws also have a special role in explanation.

There is plenty of debate surrounding these ideas, within mainstream thinking. But some core parts of the picture remain constant across medium-sized differences. An especially important one is the idea that genuine scientific understanding involves knowledge of laws. This package of ideas also has a fairly consistent influence on debates about the relations between "levels" in a total scientific picture. "Reduction" is associated with strong inferential relationships between levels, and the threat of the dispensability of higher-level descriptions. If reduction is possible, the coordination between levels is achieved by something like an additional set of "bridge" laws. Against this we have projects seeking more moderate options; supervenience is seen as a looser relation between levels than reduction, but one potentially preserving physicalism. Much discussion then focuses on the status of higher-level laws, which might capture patterns that cannot be seen from the point of view of a lower-level description.[1]

What is wrong with this package? The answer I offer is not intended as a description of all of science. The aim is to describe sciences that connect most directly to naturalistic philosophy of mind—roughly speaking, biology

[1] Influential versions of the view I am calling "traditional" can be found in Fodor (1974) and Kim (1993). As should be clear, what anti-reductionists sometimes call a "received" reductionist view is included with many forms of anti-reductionism within the larger category I am calling "traditional". For a detailed treatment of supervenience, see McLaughlin and Bennett (2005).

and psychology. If we focus on those areas, then the standard package is almost entirely wrong. It is false that these parts of science are organized around laws. In particular, it is false that the usual form theoretical knowledge takes is a set of forward-looking law-like causal principles that directly describe real systems. Laws appear occasionally, but they are minor players, with none of the organizing role they play in physics. I also reject the usual story about the links between laws, kinds, counterfactuals, confirmation, and explanation, and reject some popular accounts of the relations between levels.

At an earlier time in the history of science it might have been possible to think that these facts reflect badly on the biological sciences themselves. But that would be a difficult case to make now, given what biology has done and become in the last sixty years. And importantly, biology has not achieved its recent progress by moving *closer* to the traditional philosophical ideal.

I now start to present an alternative view, via three moves that draw on different parts of recent philosophy of science.

The first move is drawn (in moderated form) from John Dupré's book *The Disorder of Things* (1993). Dupré argues that when philosophers write about reductionist work in science, they imagine that what we get from such work, when it succeeds, is a low-level theory that tells us *what will happen*, in a system of a certain kind. That is, philosophers imagine science giving us a body of information that tells us how later states in a system are a function of earlier states. The "reductionist" thinks we are learning (or will one day learn) low-level accounts of this kind for the case of complex macroscopic systems like organisms and thinking agents. "Anti-reductionists" deny that this is happening, or deny that it will be possible.

For Dupré, this is a mistaken view of what actual reductionist work in many sciences looks like. He argues that in biology, and other fields in what we might call the "mid-level" part of science, we often have good reductionist theories that tell us a particular kind of thing. They tell us *how* various complex systems do what they do. But they don't tend to tell us, in any detail, *what* the systems will do. That is, we do not find low-level dynamic theories making specific predictions about how the system will change over time, what it will do next. To address such dynamic questions we tend to use a higher-level framework, even when we have a genuine reductionist understanding of the higher-level processes.

This is a useful re-orientation of the discussion. When we look at successful reductionist research programs in areas like biology, we do see an accumulation of information about how various biologically important processes occur. We now have a good understanding of processes like photosynthesis, respiration, protein synthesis, the transmission of signals in the brain, the action of muscles, the immune response, and so on. This sort of work can reasonably be, and often is, described as reductionist. We are taking a high-level process or capacity, and explaining how it works in terms of lower-level mechanisms and entities. In many of these cases, the "lower" level is the level of specific molecules or lower. (In cases like photosynthesis, for example, electrons themselves figure in the story.) But in all these cases, our theory does not take the form of a forward-looking dynamic account. The theory does not say: given this specific configuration of DNA molecules, enzymes, and other cellular mechanisms, the following processes *will* occur. Or: these processes will occur with 0.8 probability. An attempt to give a low-level story of that kind would be overwhelmed by the complexity of the system.[2] But that complexity does not overwhelm our ability to explain how things happen.

We should not go too far with Dupré, however. He would use these ideas to take us in the direction of libertarianism, and a very deflationary account of the bearing of low-level sciences on our understanding of human life. We must also be careful not to overstate the size of the separation between knowledge of how things work and knowledge of what will happen. Our knowledge of how things work includes knowledge of capacities and tendencies that can be the basis of predictions and interventions. (If this were not so, there would be acute problems in testing hypotheses.) With this knowledge we can often also formulate new generalizations, about both the characteristic behaviors of the system and how it will respond to abnormal circumstances. But these generalizations do not usually take the form of laws, and are not the central theoretical principles that organize our knowledge. Instead they appear as useful consequences and spin-offs from the growth of our knowledge of how things happen. A further qualification is that it would be a mistake to extend this picture to all of science. (I am not saying that Dupré does this.) These ideas are not intended to give a new account of the relation between thermodynamics and statistical mechanics, or even explanations of chemical reactions.[3]

The important thing is the way that Dupré's criticism re-orients the discussion for philosophy of mind. It is true, as Dupré says, that philosophers routinely picture the advance of knowledge in areas of lower-level science that are relevant to human thought and agency as the accumulation of forward-looking laws. Often, this means that the philosopher must merely *imagine* a future state of knowledge where we have such laws.[4] There is nothing wrong with imagining such a state, and imagining how this kind of knowledge might impact on us. But that state is indeed an imaginary one, and it is not a very natural near-term extrapolation from where we are now. It is not the actual form of well-developed present-day sciences that have a reductionist character. Molecular biology is, by

[2] Here I mean a direct and literal description of what will happen given a certain real-world configuration, not what would happen in an idealized model system that imagines away much of the complexity. See the discussion of models later in this section.

[3] Chemistry may be an interesting in-between case, from the perspective of this paper. For example, Stemwedel (2006) gives an account of the structure of the explanations of individual chemical reactions that includes an interesting mix of forward-looking principles explicitly christened "laws", and information that (at least to me) fits better a models-and-mechanisms framework of the kind discussed below.

[4] See, for example, Sober (1999), and commentary on that paper in Godfrey-Smith (1999).

any measure, an advanced and well-developed branch of science. Perhaps one day in the future it will be organized around a set of forward-looking laws of the kind that philosophers like to imagine. But at present, it is not organized that way at all. It is organized as knowledge of how things work, how things happen, and what structures in living cells do what.

So how might we give a better philosophical account of the content of this kind of scientific knowledge? The second idea I draw on in this section is the theory of "mechanistic explanation" recently developed by a collection of philosophers including Bechtel, Machamer, Craver, Darden, Richardson, and others. I will call these philosophers "new mechanists," and will draw especially on the summary "Thinking About Mechanisms" (2000) given by Machamer, Craver, and Darden.[5]

The aim of the new mechanists is to give a detailed account of what they take to be the predominant mode of explanation in large parts of biology, cognitive science, and some other areas. Neuroscience is often a particular focus. It would probably be appropriate to add a qualification to the analysis the new mechanists offer, and present it as an account of how these sciences work *when* they are in a reductionist mode, which they often are. (Work in different modes will be discussed briefly later in this section.)

The distinctive features of the new mechanists' account are as follows. First, they give an account of the ontology employed by these sciences, an ontology of mechanisms, activities, capacities, and processes. (I would add to their account an emphasis on structures and structural description.) Second, their account is antagonistic towards the traditional philosophical emphasis on laws, and also towards views of causation that are influenced by a focus on laws. Third, they give a very simple treatment of "levels" in these sciences. Levels are understood in terms of ordinary part–whole relations. (In the next section I discuss how a view of levels can diverge from this simple idea.)

The new mechanists take as data such scientific achievements as the explanation of protein synthesis, and the explanation of the transmission of signals across synapses between neurons. This is scientific progress, if anything is. Their argument is that there is little or no apparent role for laws in these sorts of achievements. What *does* figure essentially is a form of explanation in which complex processes are explained in terms of the capacities and organization of lower-level parts.

In mainstream philosophy of mind, the closest cousin to this picture is Cummins' discussion of functional analysis (1975), and some of his follow-up work (2000). But the new mechanists are aiming for more contentious and

[5] See also Bechtel and Richardson (1993), and Bechtel and Abrahamsen (2005). Wimsatt (1972) is an important precursor. The term "new mechanists" is one of several that seems to float around the movement. A more amusing one is Andrew Hamilton's "mechanistas". The generalizations I give here about new mechanism do have exceptions; the movement is new and quite heterogeneous.

general conclusions, as is seen in the negative treatment of laws. Their treatment of causation is also affected by these commitments. A very mild version of the mechanism-oriented view would be one that emphasized mechanisms as the currency of scientific work in these fields, but then employed a traditional regularity or nomological account of causation in the background. That is not the approach of the new mechanists. In Machamer, Craver, and Darden, in particular, the new mechanist view is associated with what we can call a "production-oriented" view of causal relations and their role in explanation. The obvious contrast is with regularity views, but we can also contrast production-oriented views with abstract difference-making accounts, that use counterfactuals and similar constructs to analyze causation (Lewis 1973; Collins, Hall, and Paul 2004). For the new mechanists, all such difference-making facts must be grounded in mechanistic facts. This last set of ideas might suggest that new mechanism is getting too close to *old* mechanism, in which a very restricted range of physical relationships are seen as scientifically legitimate. But new mechanism, properly configured, leaves it open what kinds of relations will be important in such areas as physics and physical chemistry.

The new mechanists have done a good job of giving a positive account of a kind of scientific work that had been badly misdescribed by earlier philosophy of science. They have given a fairly accurate, and philosophically informative, account of mature scientific work within the reductionist family of projects in biology and other "mid-level" sciences.

I should note that, once this picture is in place, the fate of the term "reduction" can become unclear. At a 2005 symposium on the relation between philosophy of science and philosophy of mind at Boston University, Steven Horst and William Bechtel gave talks that, on these points at least, presented fairly similar pictures of how the relevant areas of science operate, and the deficiencies of more traditional views. But Horst saw his message as anti-reductionist; his talk was titled "Beyond Reduction". Bechtel, in contrast, saw himself as describing what real reductionist work, as opposed to the philosophers' image of it, is like. In discussion, Bechtel (and Paul Churchland) argued that the term "reduction" is entirely natural for this kind of scientific work. This is work that engages in the explanation of high-level capacities in terms of lower-level ones, explanation of the big in terms of the small, and it is what most scientists themselves see as reductionist work. It is only if we tie the term "reduction" to the old philosophical picture that this kind of work could be called anti-reductionist. Terminology *per se* is not very important, of course, but I agree with Bechtel and Churchland on this point.

The third idea I will use comes from yet another camp in recent philosophy of science, that looks at the role of models and model-building in scientific theorizing.

One strand in recent philosophy of science uses the notion of a model, in roughly the logician's sense, to analyze *all* scientific theorizing. This is the "semantic view" or model-theoretic view, of theories (Suppe 1977, Van Fraassen

1980). That is not the set of ideas I will draw on; I make use of a related line of thought. This view holds that there is a particular kind of science that seeks to represent the world using models. Model-based science is a *strategy*, and often a response to a certain kind of problem.[6] In understanding this work, the logician's sense of "model" is not the right one to use. We need a different concept.

The new mechanists have not generally embraced these ideas.[7] And in the present context, there is a convenient way to approach the relation between the two. Consider the general kind of scientific work that the new mechanists discuss, but focusing on what it tends to look like in its early stages. These are stages where we do not know much about the system and its workings. Our eventual goal is an account of the structure and operation of some set of mechanisms. The goal is a list of real parts and their capacities. So in the early stages, we are dealing with hypothesized parts and their capacities. Machamer, Craver, and Darden (2000) do say a little about this stage. Their term for the products of this early work is "mechanism sketches". These are schematic mechanisms with some black-boxes that need to be filled in. In at least many areas though, the common scientific response to problems of this kind is *model-building*, in a specific sense. Model-based science features an "indirect" strategy for the representation and investigation of unknown systems. A model-builder first describes a hypothetical structure, usually a relatively simple one, and then considers similarity relations between this structure and the real-world "target" system that he is trying to understand.

A good initial sketch of this process was given by Giere (1988). Giere's aim was to describe *all* scientific theorizing, and his starting point was physics as presented in textbooks. The attempt to capture all theorizing in these terms was almost certainly over-reaching. And this paper will not try to defend any claims about physics. But Giere did succeed in giving a compact but informative sketch of one important kind of theoretical work in science, a kind that is relevant to fields impinging on philosophy of mind. This is the style of science in which a paper might begin: "Imagine an infinite population of asexual organisms . . ." "Consider a feed-forward neural network with one layer of hidden units and the following learning rule . . ." In my treatment of model-based science, I take this phenomenon at face value. What the model-builder is doing is specifying and inviting us to consider a hypothetical or fictional system (or class of systems), which he or she can describe exactly. Having done so, we can then consider ways in which the behavior of this hypothetical system might cast light on the behavior of a real system.

[6] See Godfrey-Smith (2006) and Weisberg (2006).

[7] There are exceptions to this. One is the far-seeing Wimsatt (1972). Another is Glennan (2005), but Glennan's paper could be better described as an application of some ideas from the "semantic view of theories" to the case of mechanistic description (as seen in his enthusiasm for state space descriptions of all models, whether they explicitly feature equations or not). I should also note that Horst, whose talk at Boston in 2005 is discussed above, combined a mechanistic view with an emphasis on modeling.

Model-based science gets part of its strength from a certain kind of flexibility, resulting from the indirect strategy employed. In model-based science, a lot of day-to-day discussion is about the model system—the hypothetical or imaginary system—itself. Two scientists can use the same model to help with the same target system, while having different views about the extent and character of the similarity that the model has to the target. One might see the model as a purely predictive device. The other might see it as a causal map, a good representation of a hidden dependency structure inside the target system. And there is no dichotomy between a single realist and single instrumentalist attitude here, but a spectrum or space of possible attitudes on how model and target might be related.

How does this relate to the new mechanists' account? The situation might be summarized like this: in the sciences the new mechanists are interested in, the desired *end-point* is often the sort of conceptual structure that they describe. But a different story should often be told for the early stages—the stages where people do not have a good handle on the components and their capacities. In that situation, model-building is a natural and common approach that is taken. This is not usually permanent. A description of a model can pass into a mechanistic description.

So we now have a sketch of how scientific work proceeds in the case of *early* stages of *reductionist* work on *complex* systems. In that situation, the currency of scientific work is often *models of important processes*; models of possible mechanisms, possible dependency structures, that might in time give us an account of the real mechanisms. Once we say it like this, it becomes apparent that this is what a large proportion of work in the cognitive sciences is concerned with today—models of learning, models of numerical cognition, models of the processing of syntax. And this really is quite different from the picture we would get by applying the standard philosophy of science that philosophers of mind tend to assume. Everyday work is not concerned with the assessment of hypothesized laws governing lower-level entities, with some explanatory relation to higher-level laws. Instead, models of important processes are the currency. The aim of the modeling is to eventually give an account of actual mechanisms and how they work. In the meantime, people model, with the hope that models can evolve into direct descriptions of mechanisms.

Here I have emphasized a transition from modeling to mechanistic description. I see this as specifically important for the kind of science that is relevant to philosophy of mind. But model-based science is not always a way-station. This strategy can be retained when the scientific field is mature. Idealized models may then be developed and retained for their useful generality (Levins 1966), and also for the advantages that come from simplicity. An idealized model system may be described by compact and comprehensible dynamical principles that express the future as a function of the past.

So the third and final main idea of this section is the importance and distinctiveness of modeling. Before moving on, though, I will make some further comments about generalizations and laws.

Antipathy to standard philosophical ideas about laws in science has been a theme of the paper so far. But surely it cannot be denied that scientific work of all kinds constantly deals in generalizations. Is the "alternative" view trying to deny the scientific importance of generalization itself? That would indeed be a mistake. Generalizations of various kinds are ubiquitous, and some generalizations are deeper and more important than others. Even where a science seems overtly focused on mechanisms, there is an obvious role for general statements about the systems being studied; we can often express knowledge of mechanisms in the form of generalizations. (Enzymes are made of protein. Human mitochondria are inherited maternally.) If we admit the importance of generalizations, and make distinctions among them with respect to something like "depth", is the resulting view really so different from the traditional view? It is sociologically interesting that biologists usually do not call even their deeper generalizations "laws", but might this fact be philosophically a superficial one?[8]

There is certainly space for other positions here. Sandra Mitchell (2000) has argued that plenty of generalizations in biology can reasonably be called "laws", provided that we extensively modify the usual philosophical picture of laws. She suggests that we recognize a three-dimensional space in which generalizations can be categorized by their *stability*, *strength*, and *abstractness*. The word "law" might reasonably be used in a context-sensitive way for generalizations that score highly on a relevant mix of the three dimensions, and this is applicable to all scientific fields. Mitchell has no objection to the word "law" being used broadly for "generalizations that ground and inform expectations in a variety of contexts" (p. 262). Her objections are to the usual philosophical account of what these generalizations are like.

There is a risk of the discussion becoming terminological here. But even that fact is of some interest. Mitchell, unlike me, is motivated by the fact that *some* biologists *do* want to call their claims "laws". Her examples are mostly far from the reductionist style of work that is my focus here, but I do not deny that some biologists talk this way.[9] Ecologists, in particular, worry

[8] An example of a very important generalization might be a suitably hedged version of the "Central Dogma" of molecular biology. A reasonable (though unconventional) formulation might be as follows: the linear structure of protein molecules is specified in a template process by the linear structure of nucleic acids, and this process does not occur in reverse. Note also that in this discussion of biology, I do not treat important theorems generated purely analytically from idealized mathematical models (like Fisher's fundamental theorem) as "laws".

[9] I do not agree with all her cases. One, for example, is "Mendel's law of segregation". I am always puzzled when this is called a law (except in a purely historical discussion). There are many exceptions, and these do not involve unusual breakdowns in the system. They just involve the appearance of segregation distorter alleles, which can appear easily and whose action falls squarely within the domain of ordinary biological activity (see Burt and Trivers 2006 for an extensive

more about laws more than other biologists do (Turchin 2001, Ginzburg and Colyvan 2004). So let me first emphasize my common ground with Mitchell. For Mitchell, the standard idea of a binary distinction between laws and "accidental" generalizations is mistaken. She also accepts that "laws" in biology (and elsewhere) are dependent on historical contingencies. And I think that Mitchell would probably accept the following striking difference between physics and biology. In physics, laws *matter* to the organization of knowledge. Textbooks explicitly name and discuss laws. In biology, laws rarely appear in textbooks and research articles. If no biologist ever said the word "law" again, it would make almost no difference to day-to-day work. If no physicist was allowed to say "law", the result would be wholesale reorganization of the field. The laws in physics textbooks may eventually receive unobvious and perhaps deflationary analyses by philosophers, but there is no denying their overt role in day-to-day work. The contrast with biology here is sharp. It is not the case in biology, as it is in physics, that a select group of compact, formal generalizations is installed in a central position in the theoretical structure, and used to derive and organize other information.

Having made this contrast between physics and biology, it is interesting to note the special status of some parts of psychology. If no psychologist was allowed to say "law" ever again, most of psychology would be unaffected, but a few specific sub-disciplines would be. As I understand it, psychophysics still takes laws seriously, and learning theory used to take laws seriously but does so less and less as time passes. Here it is important that the laws in question have been inherited from much earlier work. Psychophysics inherited principles known as laws from work done in the late nineteenth century, and has had reason to hang onto them. Learning theory inherited candidate laws from behaviorist work in the early to mid-twentieth century, and is showing rather less attachment to them.

In any case, when I make no attempt to defend a softened and unorthodox conception of "law" in this paper, that is because: (i) the discussion is being guided by a contrast between fields where laws matter and fields where they do not, and (ii) I think that the traditional strong connotations of "law" will seep back in to undermine revised usages like Mitchell's.

This completes my sketch of an alternative package of ideas in the philosophy of science that might be applied to philosophy of mind. The overall picture is something like this. Suppose we imagine a future science of the mind that has an organization similar to that of the reductionist parts of present-day biology. What would it look like? We would have little overt role for things called "laws". Our knowledge would be organized largely in the form of descriptions of

review). Note also that the term "law" for this and the other two main Mendelian principles was introduced by a *critic* of Mendelism, W. R. F. Weldon (1902). Counterexamples have more bite against attempts to lay down laws. However, though Mendel did not christen the three "laws" attributed to him, he did describe other principles (in particular, the 3:1 ratios in the offspring of hybrids) as laws in his 1865 paper.

mechanisms—how they are structured and how they work. High-level capacities would be explained in terms of the capacities of lower-level parts. "Levels" would be understood in terms of part–whole relations. In early stages of mechanistic investigation, in contexts where high degrees of generality are sought, and in the study of dynamics, we would see an important role for model-building, the investigation of idealized imaginary structures with complicated resemblance relations to real-world systems.

3. QUESTIONS ABOUT MODERN FUNCTIONALISM

What effect would accepting the package of ideas outlined in the previous section have on the philosophy of mind?

This is a difficult question. Late at night in the bar at the Philosophy of Science Association meetings, one might hear grumbling: "People in metaphysics and philosophy of mind have such an antiquated view of philosophy of science!" But the people in metaphysics and philosophy of mind are well within their rights to march into the bar and reply: "What *difference* does it make, to the truly foundational issues? If I fussily re-express everything in the language of the philosophy of science *du jour*, will the issues be much altered, or will they reappear more or less as before?"

In that spirit, my aim in this section is to use the preceding discussion to reexamine some issues in the philosophy of mind surrounding mainstream functionalism. I argue that there are hidden tensions within the usual picture of functionalism and functional description.[10]

My target is a position I will call "modern functionalism". Typical definitions of the view look like this: "Functionalism says that mental states are constituted by their causal relations to one another and to sensory inputs and behavioral outputs."[11] Such a view depends on the more general idea of the functional *profile*, or a total set of functional properties, of a system. A description of a system's functional profile is achieved through a certain kind of abstraction. My focus will be on the nature of these functional profiles. The argument will proceed by comparing what I see as mainstream functionalism with two slightly different views. One is "machine functionalism", an early position that has now been abandoned.[12] The other is David

[10] There is a link between the worries expressed here and some of those discussed by Ned Block (1990).

[11] This formulation from a summary given in the unpublished paper "Functionalism" on Ned Block's website, http://www.nyu.edu/gsas/dept/philo/faculty/block/papers/functionalism.pdf. Other advocates of what I call here "modern functionalism" include Fodor (1981), Stich (1983), Braddon-Mitchell and Jackson (1996), and Crane (1995).

[12] The term machine functionalism is a more recent one, coined (so far as I know) after the demise of the view.

Lewis's view about causal roles and the identification of mental states (1972, 1994).[13]

Each of these views gives a special role to a particular form of functional description. In the case of machine functionalism, this is *machine table* description. In the case of the other two views, it is something a bit different. So here is an obvious-looking question. Suppose we have a candidate functional description of a complex system. Perhaps it is a car engine, or a human agent. Which facts, described in other terms, is the functional description *answerable* to? How might it be disconfirmed? The question is asked purely in principle; we ignore all epistemic problems.

I discuss Lewis's view first. The key idea here is a distinction between *roles* and *occupants*. For Lewis, we often begin by describing a system in terms of an interlocking set of causal roles, and then we look for physical states (or maybe non-physical ones) that occupy those roles. As I understand Lewis, this process is guided by the principle that for each *bona fide* role, there should be at least an approximate occupant. And crucially, occupants have to be ordinary parts of the system, or states instantiated by ordinary parts of the system. We can employ a liberal concept here, but not a trivial one. If we find there is no *bona fide* occupant for some role that we have become accustomed to positing, then we should stop describing the system in terms of that role.[14]

So within the Lewisian style of functional description, if we have a candidate set of functional roles that might be used to describe some system, there is a straightforward way (in principle) to see if the description is OK. We "pop the hood" on the system. (For those unfamiliar with American slang, this means to lift the bonnet of a car, in order to look at the engine.) We look at its physical composition and see whether the roles we have been talking about have occupants or not. So Lewisian functional description is constrained by facts about the physical layout and organization of the system, facts we could discover by popping the hood.

I now turn to machine functionalism. In some ways this view is at the opposite end of a spectrum from the Lewisian view. Machine functionalism makes use of a special kind of analysis, in which a system is described in terms of its inputs, outputs, and a very abstract notion of inner state, or "machine state". A hypothesized functional profile for a system can be expressed in a machine table, which describes transitions between these three kinds of thing. Table 3.1 gives a

[13] Lewis's view is sometimes seen as akin to functionalism, but strictly speaking a form of the identity theory. For discussion of the subtelties here, see Braddon-Mitchell and Jackson (1996).

[14] At the Aarhus conference, Philip Pettit suggested that I am misdescribing the aims and emphasis of Lewis's work here. The aim, Pettit said, is to find ways to fit our common-sense concepts around a scientific picture of the world. The aim is not to outline a research program or a way of further developing our scientific picture. I am unsure whether this contrast captures Lewis's work well or not. If it does, then it would be more accurate to say that the "Lewisian" form of analysis discussed in this section is one that adopts Lewis-style role and occupant description, and puts it to slightly different work from that envisaged by Lewis himself.

Table 3.1. Machine table for a coke machine

Input	Current State	Next state	Output
5	1	2	
5	2	3	
5	3	1	Coke
10	1	3	
10	2	1	Coke
10	3	1	Coke + 5c

standard type of example, a simple coke machine that accepts only 5c and 10c coins, and charges 15c for a coke.[15]

We now ask the question that was asked about Lewis's view. Which facts is the machine table answerable to? In particular, when might we need to pop the hood?

This is a question about how exactly we are supposed to read machine tables, and not everyone reads them the same way. Sometimes it is said that a machine table answers only to the system's input–output profile. Two systems with same total input–output profile must have the same machine table. Then machine functionalism becomes hard to distinguish from logical behaviorism. Machine tables become a means for compact behavioral description. Indeed, without something like a machine table, describing a set of behavioral dispositions that has significant temporal structure (so that some actions occur after a specific sequence of inputs) becomes difficult.

In other discussions, however, machine table analyses are seen as making weak commitments to hypotheses about internal workings. They say something about *how* a behavioral profile is generated. This is certainly how machine tables look *prima facie*; they look as if they introduce "hidden variable" hypotheses of some kind.

What is crucial to this question is the identity conditions for machine states themselves. This is illustrated by a feature of the coke machine in Table 3.1. According to this machine table, there are two different routes by which the system can get to State 3. The coke machine can get to State 3 via receiving a 10c coin, or by receiving two 5c coins. Is there supposed to be an independent sense in which State 3 is the *same* state when reached via these two routes?[16] Could the machine table be disconfirmed if we look inside and see that there is no common physical state that these two causal paths converge on? If a machine table that is behaviorally adequate cannot ever be disconfirmed by popping the hood, then the machine table is a compact description of behavioral facts. If it

[15] Turing machines are sometimes used, instead of simple finite state automata like the coke machine, to illustrate machine functionalism, but for my purposes the coke-machine cases are much better illustrations of the key features of the view.

[16] An analogous question could be asked about the entities quantified over in Ramsey sentence formulations of functionalism.

could be disconfirmed in this way, then the machine table does make at least some commitments about how the system is structured inside.

Both interpretations of machine tables are coherent, and it turns out that different philosophers read machine tables in each of these two ways (as was clear during discussion at the Aarhus conference in 2005). Perhaps this does not matter; no one now is a machine functionalist. But I will next argue that some of the same tensions arise within current versions of functionalism as well.

I have approached modern functionalism via an indirect path because, in a sense, modern functionalism is intended to be a view lying between Lewis's view and machine functionalism. Machine table analysis treats a system as in one global inner state at a given time. So we cannot use a machine functionalist analysis to capture the idea of interaction between different inner states at a single time. We could not, for example, use machine functionalism to recognize the idea that beliefs and desires are distinct parts of the system that interact to give rise to actions (Block and Fodor 1972). In response to this problem with machine functionalism, one possibility is to move towards Lewis's view. But for some, this is moving too close to the identity theory. The Lewis position as I describe it here includes commitment to the idea that roles must have occupants that are visible from other points of view. Many want to say that functional states and properties are more "abstract" than that.[17] So modern functionalism is designed to make it possible to say two things at once:

(i) "We must capture the idea that separate components of a total psychological profile can interact causally. Beliefs have one role, and desires have another, for example. Beliefs, desires, plans, fears and memories are all functionally individuated, all separate, and all causal players in the system."

(ii) "But it is too crude to expect to be able to locate specific physical parts—distinct, localized brain structures—that realize all these functionally defined entities. That is not required."

In the 1980s, part of one's philosophical education involved learning to say both of these things at once. But the resulting position is more problematic than it initially looks, as it depends on a strong and perhaps unsustainable view about levels of description. We are apparently being asked to believe in what might be called "level-bound objects".

To isolate the place where the problem arises, suppose we have some candidate functional description. This description works well in predicting the input–output profile of the system. But suppose we then pop the hood, to see what the machinery is like. We find no simple role/occupant relations. That

[17] The sense of abstractness is not the same as that captured by saying that mental properties are "role properties" rather than "realizer properties". That issue is orthogonal here. The issue at hand concerns what sort of thing a realizer is supposed to *be*. Functionalists who think that mental properties are role properties will agree that realizers are part of the overall story.

is, we find no occupants for our roles in an inventory of the system given in independent terms. Do we then discard our initial functional description, or decide to regard it merely as a predictive device? No, we are told by the modern functionalist. The way in which we peered in when we popped the hood was too crude! The entities posited in the higher-level description are abstract, functionally defined entities. They *need not be visible* from the point of view of lower-level description. (Do not look for a "belief box". Do not look for a language of thought as if it involved inscriptions on a little blackboard.)

This seems to mean that the functionally characterized components are not just higher-level, but level-*bound*. They need not be visible at all from other points of view. But they are supposed to be real causal players in the system. We are supposed to be able to give true explanations of the system's behavior in terms of their activities and interactions.

In a discussion of this issue, Mark Johnston suggested that only careless formulations of modern functionalism give rise to these peculiar apparent consequences. If the modern functionalism was telling us to believe in higher-level *particulars* that are invisible from any other point of view, that would be odd. But modern functionalism is properly formulated as doctrine about *properties* and (hence) *states*. We should not use modern functionalism to try to treat beliefs and pains (for example) as level-bound particulars that somehow compose a thinking agent. Instead, the view gives us an account of what it is for a whole agent to have the property of believing that it is raining (or the property of being in pain). And if states are the instantiations of properties at times, then beliefs and pains are states of the whole system.

This distinction does clarify things, but I do not think it greatly ameliorates the situation for modern functionalism. A first indication that things are still awry comes from reflecting on what becomes of causal explanation within such a view.

According to this version of modern functionalism, we treat the system as a whole as having a total set of physical properties at time t_1, that give rise (non-causally) to a range of distinct higher-level properties at that time. The system may then go into a new total physical state at t_2, which gives rise to a range of new higher-level properties. It is not supposed to be the case that the various higher-level properties at t_1 are each instantiated by different physical components of the system. What then seems questionable is the idea that the higher-level states present at t_1 causally interact *with each other* such that there is a legitimate causal description of the system at the higher level, according to which its higher-level states at t_2 are consequences of interactions among its higher-level states at t_1. In the most familiar ways of thinking about causes that interact to produce an effect, the various causes are treated as distinct from each other. Here, by explicitly treating the whole system as the only relevant particular, instantiating all the various mental properties, we have "entangled" the physical bases of each of the mental states whose interactions we might have wanted to describe in causal terms. The problem can be put by saying that there seems to be no difference between this version of modern functionalism, and a version of machine functionalism that expresses its machine states as long conjunctions without positing interactions between the "components" of the total machine state.

This problem is distinct from the more standard problems about mental causation within a physicalist world view (Kim 1993, Bennett 2003). This is because the problem does not arise if the distinct mental states present at a time involve properties instantiated by different physical parts of the system. The problem only arises from the entanglement of the supposedly distinct causal players with each other at the physical level.

This argument is not intended to be decisive. It depends on difficult questions about causation, and the modern functionalist could in any case adopt a mild revisionism about causal description and explanation. But this argument has a more rigorous relative, developed by David Chalmers (1996) for different purposes.

Chalmers' argument forms part of an account of the "implementation" of computational structures by physical systems. It depends on a distinction between two kinds of computational formalisms, which are called FSA (Finite State Automaton) and CSA (Combinatorial State Automaton) descriptions. The key points in Chalmers' treatment bear generally on functionalism, however, and do not depend on linking functionalism to computationalism about the mind.[18]

In formal terms, Chalmers shows that an obvious and straightforward way of understanding what is required for a physical system to implement a CSA is far too weak. This criterion on CSA implementation turns out to require little more of a physical system than that it matches the input–output profile of the CSA. This is important because the CSA formalism is, essentially, the kind of functional specification envisaged in modern functionalism. An extra constraint on the implementation of a CSA is needed to avoid this collapse into near-triviality, and the obvious way to add such a constraint involves a move back towards (what I am calling) a Lewis-style view.

I will sketch some details briefly (though this paragraph and the next can be skipped). A pair of arguments is given. One concerns the implementation of an FSA, which is basically the sort of structure represented by a machine table. In particular, inner states of the system are treated in an atomic way, without internal structure. Surprisingly, any physical system that has the right input–output profile, has some way of recording its input history, and has a "dial" that can be set to various persisting states, implements an FSA, on a natural understanding of implementation.[19] Chalmers accepts this consequence.

[18] This is discussed in more detail in Godfrey-Smith (forthcoming).

[19] Here I only treat the case where FSAs have inputs and outputs in their specification. There are also "inputless FSAs" which are even easier to implement.

A CSA, however, is richer than an FSA. Each overall machine state is broken down into a vector (or list) of substates, and the CSA transition rule takes the system from one vector of substates (plus an input), to a new vector of substates (plus an ouput). So treating a system as a CSA seems to involve positing a number of interacting internal states present at any given time, each with its own role in the system. But suppose we say that any physical system implements a CSA if there is a mapping between the states of the physical system and those of the CSA such that causal processes in the physical system correspond to all the possible transitions in the CSA's formal specification. This simple criterion for implementation can be shown to be too weak. Any CSA can then be mapped to an FSA with a suitably large number of atomic inner states, in such a way that it inherits the weak implementation requirements of that FSA. So any system with the right input–output profile (plus an input memory and "dial") will implement the CSA. The appearance of further constraints on implementation deriving from the interactions among the substates of the CSA is illusory.

If implementing a CSA is to require more than this, some extra requirement is needed. In his discussion, Chalmers considers a simple and clearly sufficient candidate, and some weaker options that may or may not suffice. In my terms, the simple option is one that involves a move back towards the Lewisian view discussed above. This is the requirement that each CSA substate be mapped onto a *distinct spatial region* of the implementing system. Chalmers discusses the possibility that a weaker condition than this will suffice, but an extra requirement of something *like* this kind is needed. In particular, a theory of implementation must exclude a mapping in which each CSA substate is mapped holistically to a partial specification of the physical state of the entire system.

So to know whether a CSA is non-trivially implemented by some physical system, we have to work out whether the CSA substates can be mapped to something like distinct parts of the physical system. We have to pop the hood, and the aim when we do so is to see whether the roles in the CSA specification have occupants that are *bona fide* parts, or states of *bona fide* parts.

Two conclusions can be drawn. One is that the overt form of description standardly seen in modern functionalism, on its own, exerts far less constraint on the physical system being described than one might think. The other is that the obvious way (probably not the only way) to restore the lost content to functional description is to move back towards the requirement that occupants of roles have independent standing as real parts of the system.

Another moral I take from Chalmers' argument is that modern functionalism is a less worked-out and coherent doctrine than it looks. Chalmers himself does not draw this conclusion, perhaps because he sees the extra constraint that is needed on CSA implementation as being more in the spirit of standard functionalism than I do. In any case, in the remainder of this section I will put a different option on the table. This option may be a better way of making sense of the phenomena that functionalists want to capture, and a better way of describing the scientific work that is taken to support a functionalist attitude.

This alternative view distinguishes two kinds of thing that can look like "functional" description in the philosophers' sense, and that can shade into each other in some cases. Both were introduced in the previous section; they are mechanistic description, in roughly the sense of the new mechanists, and modeling. These are two real kinds of scientific work, a bit different from each other, with particular relations between them.

Scientific analysis in the style of the new mechanists is quite close to Lewisian functional description. The mechanists and Lewis use different terminologies and have different agendas, of course. Their treatments of causation are also very different. But in other ways, the two pictures are quite similar. The aim in both cases is to describe how the abstract causal analysis of a complex system works. The kind of description that results is answerable to what you see when you pop the hood. Both use a simple notion of levels of analysis, based on ordinary part–whole relations. There are no mysterious level-bound objects. In the previous section I said that the new mechanists had given a fairly good account of the explanatory style of fields like cell biology. In a considerably more qualified way, the same could be said for Lewis's framework.

As discussed in the previous section, though, when faced with complex systems that are poorly understood it can be wise to temporarily eschew the aim of direct mechanistic description. We may not have the right kind of inventory of parts; we may not know what kinds of structures to be looking for as the bearers of key causal roles. In that situation, we model. We describe possible networks of dependence relations, idealized possible machineries. We hope for similarity relations between these hypothetical structures and the real workings of the system. Modeling in this sense is different from the analysis envisaged in modern functionalism in at least two ways. First, this sort of modeling does not traffic in level-bound objects, and secondly, a crucial role is played in modeling by the complex nature of the similarity relations that may hold between model and target.

So we might consider replacing the special form of functional analysis seen in much recent philosophy of mind with two slightly different tools: mechanistic description (which is fairly close to Lewis), and modeling. This combination provides a better framework for thinking about psychological phenomena than modern functionalism does. (Indeed, it is what psychology and cognitive science have mostly been employing all along.) The important functionalist notion of multiple realizability survives intact in this view, because a given role can have physically different occupants in different cases. From this point of view, however, modern functionalism seems to be an attempt to devise a hybrid form of analysis that has some characteristics of each of two legitimate kinds of description. Sometimes it looks like abstract description of real mechanisms, and sometimes it looks like modeling, but it is supposed to be a single thing distinct from each of these. I suggest that this might be an illusion.

Here is one other way to look at the situation. Earlier I said that modern functionalism is designed to enable us to say two things at once. First, people want to treat the various components of a total psychological profile as picking out distinct things that can interact causally. Second, they do not want the useability and legitimacy of folk psychological concepts (like belief and pain) to depend on there being localized physical occupants of these roles in the brain. The suggestion I am making here enables people to say both these things, but not about the same states at the same time. Folk psychology might be something like a model, rather than a theory, of the mind.[20] As a model, it can be useable without there being a simple mapping between its structure and the machinery of the brain. But when the aim is to come up with a literally correct causal description of how mental processes work, using either folk psychological concepts or scientific ones, then we should expect and aspire to engage in the description of mechanisms.

4. LAWS, CONFIRMATION, AND KINDS

The previous section sought to export a package of ideas from philosophy of science into philosophy of mind. In this final section I return to philosophy of science. I will briefly confront a possible objection that might make people reluctant to embrace the package of ideas presented earlier. Here we leave the general topic of reduction, though, which is why this section is at the end.

The objection runs as follows. The familiar body of ideas in philosophy of science that was discarded in Section 2 is essential to the treatment of various other issues. There is a larger network of views whose viability is being questioned here.

The network of ideas I have in mind here posits a set of connections between laws, kinds, counterfactuals, and confirmation. Here I will focus on confirmation. Especially since the work of Goodman, it has been common to hold that the concept of law and the concept of confirmation are closely linked. Only law-like generalizations are confirmed by their instances; "accidental" generalizations are not. If our analysis of some part of science does not take seriously the notion of law, then, it may seem that we will not be able to understand how the confirmation of hypotheses works in that part of science. And for many philosophers, the link between law and confirmation is just one element in a rich network of ideas which it would be very costly to abandon.

My response is that the familiar network of ideas about laws, kinds, and confirmation is much overrated. We would probably be better off without it. I

[20] This idea is developed in more detail in Maibom (2003) and Godfrey-Smith (2005).

will not give a general defence of this claim in this section, but will indicate what one part of a better package of views might look like.[21]

The alleged link between laws and confirmation arises in the attempt to make sense of "instance confirmation", the support that some generalizations receive from observations of particular cases that satisfy them. Goodman's "grue" problem teaches us that not all generalizations receive support from observations of their instances (1955). Perhaps, however, instance confirmation is real when the generalization in question is law-like? Goodman linked both law-likeness and confirmation to a conception of "projectibility" based on the historical role of a predicate or category in a linguistic community, but other philosophers have generally rejected that idea while hanging onto the link between laws and confirmation.

The whole idea of "instance confirmation" is in much worse shape than even Goodman supposed. It is the creature of a particular kind of philosophical system-building, and not a genuine scientific phenomenon that needs philosophical explanation. The philosophical concept of instance confirmation is, I suggest, an unholy amalgam of two genuine inference patterns in science. One is statistical inference from samples. The other is what is usually called "inference to the best explanation" (IBE).[22] These are both real and legitimate, and each has *some* of the features that philosophers associate with confirmation by instances.

In statistical inference from samples, the *size* of sample is usually very important. Many observations are better than a few. *Randomness* of sampling is usually very important. But there is no "naturalness" constraint, of the type familiar from philosophical discussions of Goodman's problem. Roughly speaking, any predicate can be used in statistical inference from a random sample. There are problems of sample bias and confounding that have connections to Goodman's problem (Godfrey-Smith 2003*a*). But the overall status of kinds—their naturalness or lack of it—is not an issue.

In inference to the best explanation, there is no essential role for number of observations, for size of sample. Size may have some practical importance, but it is not evidentially central as it is in statistics. What is important in IBE is the specific causal and nomological structure that is relevant to the case. This is related to the "naturalness" of kinds, though it is not the same thing.

What we see in much post-Goodman thinking about confirmation, however, is a mixture of the features of these two kinds of inference. It is common to think that both the number of observations and the naturalness of kinds are important, while randomness of sampling is rarely discussed. This category is a philosophical fiction. And the idea that positive instances confirm law-like

[21] A more detailed discussion is found in Godfrey-Smith (2003*a*), especially the final section.

[22] In Godfrey-Smith (2003*b*) I preferred the modified term "explanatory inference" because I think IBE suggests the wrong kind of link to an independent notion of goodness of explanation (in the sense discussed in the Hempel, Salmon, Van Fraassen (etc.) literature on explanation). Here I will use the more common term.

generalizations, and only them, is not a feature of either statistical inference or IBE.[23]

This last section has traveled some distance from the topic of reduction. But these points do play a role in the earlier discussion. It seemed for some time that philosophy of science had generated a tightly-knit and plausible package of ideas about laws, confirmation, and kinds. When someone argues, as I did earlier, that there is no important role for laws in some part of science, the appeal of the larger package of ideas linking laws and confirmation (etc.) is one motivation for attempts to find a *hidden* role for laws, lurking in work that is ostensibly quite different in organization. But at least in the scientific fields that border on philosophy of mind, the lawless nature of reduction in real life is something we can, and should, take at face value.

REFERENCES

Bechtel, W. and A. Abrahamsen (2005). "Explanation: A Mechanistic Alternative." *Studies in History of Philosophy of the Biological and Biomedical Sciences* 36: 421–41.

—— and R. Richardson (1993). *Discovering Complexity*. Princeton: Princeton University Press.

Bennett, K. (2003). "Why the Exclusion Problem Seems so Intractable, and How, Just Maybe, to Tract it." *Noûs* 37: 471–97.

Block, N. (1990). "Can the Mind Change the World?" In G. Boolos (ed.), *Meaning and Method: Essays in Honor of Hilary Putnam*: Cambridge: Cambridge University Press, 137–70.

—— and J. A. Fodor (1972). "What Psychological States are Not." *Philosophical Review* 83: 159–81.

Braddon-Mitchell, D. and F. Jackson (1996). *The Philosophy of Mind and Cognition*. Oxford: Blackwell.

Burt, A. and R. Trivers (2006). *Genes in Conflict: The Biology of Selfish Genetic Elements*. Cambridge MA: Harvard University Press.

Chalmers, D. J. (1996). "Does a Rock Implement Every Finite-State Automaton?" *Synthese* 108: 309–33.

Collins, J., N. Hall, and L. Paul (eds.) (2004). *Causation and Counterfactuals*. Cambridge MA: MIT Press.

Crane, T. (1995). *The Mechanical Mind: A Philosophical Introduction to Minds, Machines and Mental Representation*. London: Routledge.

Cummins, R. (1975). "Functional Analysis." *Journal of Philosophy* 72: 741–65.

—— (2000). "'How Does it Work?' vs. 'What are the Laws?' Two Conceptions of Psychological Explanation." In F. Keil and R. Wilson (eds.), *Explanation and Cognition*. Cambridge MA: MIT Press, 117–45.

[23] The argument in this paragraph is structurally similar to an argument from the preceding section. In each case (confirmation, functional analysis) the recent philosophical tradition has drawn on two real phenomena and combined their elements in the wrong way.

Dupré, J. (1993). *The Disorder of Things*. Cambridge MA: Harvard University Pres.

Fodor, J. A. (1974). "Special Sciences." *Synthese* 28: 97–115.

—— (1981). *Representations*. Cambridge MA: MIT Press.

Giere, R. (1988). *Explaining Science: A Cognitive Approach*. Chicago: Chicago University Press.

—— (1999). "Using Models to Represent Reality." In L. Magnani, N. J. Nersessian, and P. Thagard (eds.), *Model-Based Reasoning in Scientific Discovery*. New York: Kluwer/Plenum, 1999, 41–57.

Ginzburg, L. and M. Colyvan (2004). *Ecological Orbits: How Planets Move and Populations Grow*. Oxford: Oxford University Press.

Glennan, S. (2005). "Modeling Mechanisms." *Studies in the History and Philosophy of the Biomedical Sciences* 36: 443–64.

Godfrey-Smith, P. (1999). "Procrustes Probably: Comments on Sober's Physicalism from a Probabilistic Point of View." *Philosophical Studies* 95: 175–81.

—— (2003*a*). "Goodman's Problem and Scientific Methodology." *Journal of Philosophy* 100: 573–90.

—— (2003*b*). *Theory and Reality: An Introduction to the Philosophy of Science*. Chicago: Chicago University Press.

—— (2005). "Folk Psychology as Model." *Philosopher's Imprint* 5/6: 1–16.

—— (2006). The Strategy of Model-Based Science. *Biology and Philosophy* 21: 725–40.

—— (forthcoming). "Triviality Arguments Against Functionalism." *Philosophical Studies*.

Goodman, N. (1955). *Fact, Fiction, and Forecast*. Cambridge MA: Harvard University Press.

Harman, G. (1965). "The Inference to the Best Explanation." *Philosophical Review* 74: 88–95.

Horst, S. (unpublished). "Beyond Reduction: What Can Philosophy of Mind Learn from Post-Reductionist Philosophy of Science?" Presented at Boston Colloquium in the Philosophy of Science, 2005.

Kim, J. (1993). *Supervenience and Mind: Selected Philosophical Essays*, Cambridge: Cambridge University Press.

Levins, R. (1966). "The Strategy of Model-Building in Population Biology." *American Scientist* 54: 421–31.

Lewis, D. (1972). "Psychophysical and Theoretical Identifications." *Australasian Journal of Philosophy* 50: 249–58.

—— (1973). "Causation." *Journal of Philosophy* 70: 556–67.

—— (1994). "Reduction of Mind." In S. Guttenplan (ed.), *A Companion to the Philosophy of Mind*, Oxford: Blackwell, 413–31.

Machamer, P., C. Craver, and L. Darden (2000). "Thinking About Mechanisms." *Philosophy of Science* 67: 1–25.

McLaughlin, B. and K. Bennett (2005). "Supervenience." *Stanford Encyclopedia of Philosophy*. http://plato.stanford.edu/entries/supervenience/

Maibom, H. (2003). "The Mindreader and the Scientist." *Mind and Language* 18: 296–315.

Mitchell, Sandra D. (2000). "Dimensions of Scientific Law." *Philosophy of Science* 67: 242–65.

Sober, E. (1999). "Physicalism from a Probabilistic Point of View." Philosophical Studies 95: 135–74.

Stemwedel, J. (2006). "Getting More with Less: Experimental Constraints and Stringent Tests of Model Mechanisms of Chemical Oscillators." *Philosophy of Science* 73: 743–54.

Stich, S. (1983). *From Folk Psychology to Cognitive Science: The Case Against Belief.* Cambridge MA: MIT Press.

Suppe, F. (ed.) (1977). *The Structure of Scientific Theories*. 2nd edition. Urbana: University of Illinois Press.

Turchin, P. (2001). "Does Population Ecology have General Laws?" *Oikos* 94: 17–26.

Van Fraassen, Bas C. 1980. *The Scientific Image.* Oxford: Oxford University Press.

Weisberg, M. (2006). "Who is a Modeler?" *British Journal for the Philosophy of Science* 58: 207–33.

Weldon, W. (1902). "Mendel's Laws of Alternative Inheritance in Peas." *Biometrika* 1: 228–54.

Wimsatt, W. (1972). "Teleology and the Logical Structure of Function Statements." *Studies in the History and Philosophy of Science*, 3: 1–80.

4

Group Agency and Supervenience

Christian List and Philip Pettit

1. INTRODUCTION

In this paper, we sketch an account of group agency. We take groups, whether agents or not, to be sets of individuals who are networked with each other in a way that matters to them or others, and that affects their behavior or that of others. The networking may matter because it marks members off in their own perceptions or those of others, or in their capacities or disabilities relative to others; the possibilities are various. Those of a certain religious or ethnic background may form a group on this account, as may those in a particular profession or those with distinctive skills. But those who live at a certain latitude on earth do not form a group, nor do those who are of the same unexceptionable height or hair colour.

What distinguishes group agents from other groups, then? We argue that it is their capacity to mimic the more or less rational way in which individual agents act. Examples of groups constituting agents include committees and commissions, partnerships and companies, expert panels and joint authorships, governments and courts. These groups are not just networked collections of individuals. They are networked collections whose performance parallels that of individual agents. They can take on tasks, commit themselves to goals, enter into contractual relationships, and be held responsible for what they do. They are entities that may have the status of legal persons.

Where does the capacity for group agency spring from? Does it emerge mysteriously, without a clear basis at the level of individuals, as some traditions

Originally published in *Southern Journal of Philosophy*, vol. 44 (Spindel Supplement) (2006), 85–105. Earlier versions of this chapter were presented at the NAMICONA Conference on Reductive Explanation, University of Aarhus, May 2005, and at the 2005 Spindel Conference on Social Epistemology, University of Memphis, Sept. 2005. We thank the participants at both occasions for helpful comments and suggestions.

have suggested (Runciman 1997)? Or does it appear in virtue of how things are organized among individual members? Is it consistent with an underlying individualistic ontology? We explore and defend an individualistic account of group agency here.

If a group is to be a rational agent, under any plausible form of individualism, then it must be constituted in such a way that certain 'inputs' by the group members—for example, their actions, judgments or dispositions—give rise to suitable 'outputs' at the group level: to outputs that manifest the group's standing as an agent. The rational agency of the group must 'supervene' on the group members' individual contributions—in analogy to the way in which, on standard accounts, the rational agency of an individual human being supervenes on certain physical processes in this human being's brain and body. But what exactly is the nature of this supervenience relation? We address this question here.

We argue that the relation required is more complex than might have been expected. Focusing on group judgments in particular, we show that a group's judgment on a particular proposition cannot generally be a function of the group members' individual judgments on that proposition. Rather, it must be a function of the group members' inputs in their entirety. The upshot is that knowing what the group members individually think about some proposition does not generally tell us how the group as a whole adjudicates that proposition. While our account preserves the individualistic view that group agency is nothing mysterious, it also supports the interesting possibility that a group may hold judgments that are not directly continuous with the group members' corresponding individual judgments.

Our discussion is structured as follows. We suggest general conditions of agency in section 2 and introduce the supervenience account of group agency in section 3. Drawing on the emerging theory of judgment aggregation (e.g. List and Pettit 2002; Pauly and van Hees 2003; Dietrich 2006), we then present some impossibility results in section 4 which show that group agency is not generally consistent with the requirement of 'proposition-wise supervenience'. We explore the possibility of group agency under the less restrictive requirement of 'set-wise supervenience' in section 5. In section 6 we draw some conclusions. The crucial notions of proposition-wise supervenience and set-wise supervenience will be defined below.

2. CONDITIONS OF AGENCY

When does a system, natural or artificial, individual or social, count as an agent? We think that four conditions are individually necessary and at least close to being jointly sufficient. We state the conditions here but do not provide a full-scale defence of them, if only because they reflect a broad consensus in psychology, economics and the philosophy of mind. The conditions are the following:

- First, the system forms representational and goal-seeking states; for example, beliefs and desires, or judgments and plans.
- Second, in forming and revising these representational and goal-seeking states, the system satisfies appropriate conditions of (theoretical) rationality. We will give attention to three such conditions in particular: completeness, consistency and deductive closure, as defined below.[1]
- Third, the system acts or intervenes in the world on the basis of its representational and goal-seeking states, as conditions of (practical) rationality require; it acts so as to realize its goals, under the guidance of its representations.
- Fourth, the system exhibits these properties not just accidentally or contingently, but robustly—that is, not just in actual conditions, but also in a class of relevant possible conditions.

These conditions should be readily intelligible. Consider a human being, a simple animal, or perhaps a swarm of bees. In each case we can discern a pattern of behavior that invites us to adopt the 'intentional stance', as Daniel Dennett (1987) calls it. Once we adopt this stance towards a system, we cannot help but take the conditions above to be fulfilled. We recognize a complexity in the interaction between the system and its environment that leads us to analyze it as a system that more or less rationally espouses representations and goals; it acts rationally in accordance with its representations and goals; and it displays these properties more or less robustly, not as a product of fortuitous chance or occasion.

The conditions of agency are formulated in a somewhat abstract way, so as not to engage with unnecessary questions of detail. They say nothing on what internal organization a system must have to count as a rational agent. We may want to stipulate that the system must be wholly present in the spatial boundaries it represents; that it must not be controlled from outer space, for example (Peacocke 1983). We may also want to stipulate that it must generate its responses on the basis of causal connections between successive, evolving states, not on the basis of clever pre-emptive rigging (Block 1980). Both of these qualifications answer to ordinary intuitions (Jackson and Pettit 1990). But beyond those general stipulations, we need to say nothing further on how an agent must be internally constructed. For all we suppose, the architecture of agency may be otherwise unconstrained.

Just as we do not suppose anything specific on this organizational question, so we make no demanding assumptions about how far agents must engage with matters of value. We take it that agents form goals (thereby instantiating states such as plans, desires, preferences, or utilities); agency requires intervention, after

[1] One might also add certain conditions of truth-tracking.

all, not just representation. But we can be neutral on the source of those goals. We can preserve our picture of agency, regardless of whether or not we assume that the system's goals are supported by underlying representations to the effect that something is inherently or instrumentally desirable or plan-worthy. Details of our picture may change with changes in our account of these goals, but we need not commit ourselves to any particular account here.

In the following discussion we shall be concerned with how group agents meet one particular necessary condition for agency: that the system robustly satisfy constraints of theoretical rationality, such as the constraint of consistency, in the formation of representational states. More particularly still, we shall be concerned with how group agents can meet this condition with respect to those representational states we describe as 'judgments'. We use the notion of 'judgment' in a broad sense, to include both judgments of fact, bearing on what is to be believed, and judgments of value, bearing on what is to be desired. While 'beliefs' (and 'desires') come in degrees of strength, 'judgments' are categorical. I may believe to this or that degree that *P* but I will judge that *P*, period, or I will not judge that *P*, period. Under what may be a regimentation of common usage, there is no room for holding a judgment more or less strongly. This is not a great restriction, as there is still room for judging that it is more or less probable (or more or less desirable) that *P*.

We focus on judgments because in the case of those group agents we are especially interested in here—such as committees, expert panels, governments, courts, co-authorships—judgments are particularly important representational states. But why focus on judgments rather than plans? Plans are also on–off states, after all, and they also engage constraints like consistency.

We are influenced by the following consideration. Whereas rationality constraints on plans will track corresponding rationality constraints on judgments—judgments of value as to what should be done or brought about—the converse does not hold. We achieve a greater simplicity by focusing on judgments, and we do so without any great loss of generality.

3. THE SUPERVENIENCE ACCOUNT OF GROUP AGENCY

Under an individualistic ontology, a group's agency cannot emerge mysteriously without a clear basis at the level of the group members. The 'outputs' at the level of the group—here the group's judgments—must 'supervene' on certain 'inputs' at the level of the group members. And given the conditions of agency discussed in the last section, the supervenience relationship must guarantee the rationality of the group judgments formed.

We say that one set of facts, B, 'supervenes' on another set of facts, A, if and only if, necessarily, fixing the A-facts also fixes the B-facts. There is no variation possible in the B-domain without a variation in the A-domain. An individualistic

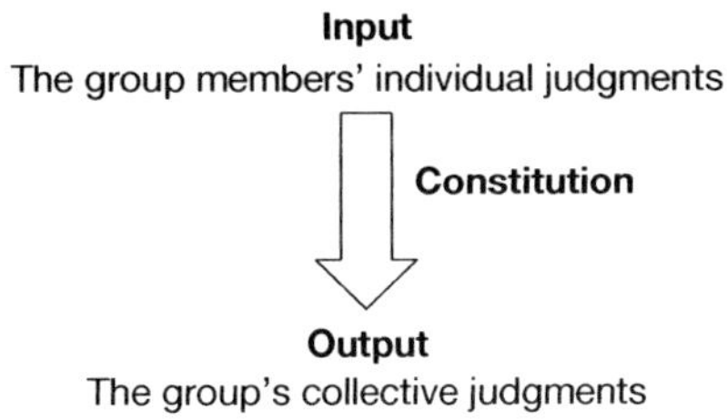

Fig. 4.1 A Constitution

ontology commits us to the view that a group's judgments supervene on the contributions of individuals: say, on what the individuals judge and do. More precisely, a group's judgments supervene on these individual contributions once the group's 'constitution' is put in place. As illustrated in Fig. 4.1, a 'constitution' is a set of rules, formal or informal, for determining how the inputs of individuals are to be put together to generate group judgments as outputs (see also List 2005). A simple example of a constitution is the rule that a group judges any given proposition to be true whenever a majority of group members individually judge this proposition to be true.

In the absence of any constitution, it hardly makes sense to ascribe judgments to a group. The group members' individual contributions are integrated into a group judgment only when an appropriate constitution is explicitly or implicitly in place. Take the people who happen to be in the same subway train at the same time. Clearly there is no formal or informal constitution in place among them, and so it does not make much sense to talk of the group judgments that they hold. By contrast, many groups in public life—such as committees, judiciaries, organizations, companies, expert panels—are organized by appropriate formal or informal rules. And so, at least in principle, they are capable of generating group judgments from individual contributions.

Does the need for a constitution in any plausible supervenience account of group agency compromise the hope for an individualistic ontology? We do not think so. That a constitution is in place among a collection of people merely means that they share certain interpersonally connected dispositions: the dispositions to follow or license certain procedures in the derivation of group judgments from individual contributions. We might think of the constitution, therefore, as yet another individual contribution on the part of the members: a contribution that consists in their possession of the appropriate dispositions. For convenience, however, we shall treat the constitution as a framework within which individual contributions—paradigmatically, judgments and actions—are made and a framework in virtue of which the group-level judgments are formed.

We can now present our main results. If an individualistic account of group agency is to be vindicated, then it must be possible to find a constitution such that the group judgments generated by it from individual contributions are robustly rational. It must be possible to identify a supervenience relation that is capable of securing this result. We turn now to some results in the recently developed theory of judgment aggregation and explore their significance for this inquiry.

4. IMPOSSIBILITY RESULTS: THE INCONSISTENCY OF ROBUST GROUP RATIONALITY WITH 'PROPOSITION-WISE' SUPERVENIENCE

Consider a group of two or more individuals faced with the task of making judgments on some interconnected propositions. In a paradigmatic and much discussed example (Kornhauser and Sager 1986), the group is a multi-member court making judgments on the following propositions:

P: The defendant did action X.

Q: The defendant had a contractual obligation not to do action X.

R: The defendant is liable for a breach of contract.

The propositions are interconnected by the constraint that proposition *R* (the 'conclusion') is true if and only if propositions *P* and *Q* (the 'premises') are both true: more formally, '*R* if and only if (*P* and *Q*)'. More generally, there might be more than two premises; or, in other cases, the disjunction rather than conjunction of the premises might be taken to be necessary and sufficient for the conclusion.

The set of propositions considered by the group—including the logical constraint '*R* if and only if (*P* and *Q*)'—is called the 'agenda'. Throughout this paper, we assume for simplicity that the agenda is as in the multi-member court example or one of its generalizations, but many other kinds of agendas have been investigated in the literature on judgment aggregation.[2] We also assume that, whenever a proposition is included in the agenda, then so is its negation; this enables the group to accept as true either the proposition or its negation or neither.

Each group member forms judgments on (some or all of) the propositions in the agenda. We say than an individual's judgments are:

- 'complete' if, for every proposition in the agenda, the individual judges either the proposition or its negation to be true;

[2] While we here state all formal results just for the agenda of the court example, they can be shown to hold for larger classes of agendas. Proposition 1 holds for all agendas that have a minimal inconsistent subset of three or more propositions; Proposition 2 holds for all so-called 'minimally connected' agendas; and Proposition 3 holds for all so-called 'strongly connected' agendas. For technical details, see Dietrich and List (2005).

- 'consistent' if, for every proposition in the agenda, the individual does not judge the proposition and its negation to be true;
- 'deductively closed' if, whenever the propositions in the agenda judged true by the individual logically entail another proposition included in the agenda, then the individual also judges that other proposition to be true.

Now, given our earlier definition, the group's 'constitution' is a set of rules by which the group members' individual contributions determine the group's judgments on the propositions in the agenda.[3] We assume in our formal discussion that the group members' contributions are their relevant individual judgments, but in our conclusion below we also consider other possible individual contributions. Moreover, we here assume that the constitution has the 'universal domain': it accepts as admissible input all possible combinations of complete, consistent and deductively closed individual judgments. If that domain is further enlarged so as to include combinations of individual judgments that are not fully rational, our results essentially continue to hold.[4]

What does it mean for the multi-member court in our example to be a group agent? In terms of our necessary condition for agency, the court must form judgments on the propositions in the agenda that satisfy certain rationality conditions.[5] We can capture this by the following condition, which applies the individual rationality requirements defined above to a group as a whole.

> **Robust group rationality.** The group's judgments (generated through the constitution) are robustly (by which we mean: for all admissible combinations of individual judgments) complete, consistent and deductively closed.

Robust group rationality might seem rather strong: especially completeness and deductive closure seem to be demanding requirements. But notice that completeness and deductive closure are required only for the propositions in the agenda, that is, the propositions on which the group is supposed to make judgments; no such requirements are made for propositions outside the agenda, whose resolution may not be required.

Can the group be constituted in such a way as to meet the condition of robust group rationality? And, if it is, how exactly do the group's judgments supervene on the group members' inputs? A simple and initially plausible thesis about how the group's judgments supervene on these inputs is the majoritarian supervenience thesis.

[3] Formally, a constitution is a function that maps each admissible combination of individual judgments on the propositions in the agenda to corresponding group judgments on these propositions. As noted above, a simple example of a constitution is the rule that the group judges a proposition to be true whenever a majority of the group members judge that proposition to be true.

[4] Some technical refinements may be needed in this more general case.

[5] Perhaps additional conditions are required for group agency, but we here consider just a simple necessary condition.

Table 4.1.

	P	*Q*	*R*	*R* if and only if (*P* and *Q*)
Individual 1	True	True	True	True
Individual 2	True	False	False	True
Individual 3	False	True	False	True
Majority	True	True	False	True

Majoritarian supervenience. The group judgment on each proposition in the agenda is robustly the majority judgment on that proposition.

But if this is the way in which group judgments supervene on individual inputs, then group agency, in the sense defined above, is not generally possible, as the following result shows.

Proposition 1. For a constitution with universal domain, robust group rationality is inconsistent with majoritarian supervenience.

This result is a slightly generalized version of the much discussed 'discursive dilemma' (e.g. Pettit 2001, ch. 5); for a proof of the present version, see List (2006). To sketch the argument, assume, for a contradiction, that a group of two or more individuals is constituted in such a way that robust group rationality and majoritarian supervenience are both met. By robust group rationality, the group's judgments are complete, consistent and deductively closed for all combinations of individual judgments in the domain of the constitution. In particular, in the special case of a three-member group, consider the individual judgments in Table 4.1, where the agenda is the one from the court example. This combination of judgments is clearly admissible under the universal domain assumption; similar examples can be constructed for different group sizes and different agendas of propositions.

By majoritarian supervenience, the group's judgment on each proposition is the majority judgment on that proposition. But the majority judgments resulting from the individual judgments in Table 4.1 violate deductive closure: propositions *P* and *Q* and the logical constraint '*R* if and only if (*P* and *Q*)' are each judged to be true by a majority, and these propositions jointly entail proposition *R*; yet *R* is judged to be false by a majority. This contradicts robust group rationality. Notice that this rationality violation occurs despite the fact that the judgments of all group members are individually rational here, in the sense of being complete, consistent and deductively closed.[6]

For a group to be an agent, then, the relation between the group judgments and those of the group members cannot be that of majoritarian supervenience.

[6] So the inconsistency between robust group rationality and majoritarian supervenience does not depend on any irrationality on the part of the group members.

Could the relation be something similar to majoritarian supervenience? After all, it seems plausible to assume that the group's judgment on a proposition supervenes *in some way* on the group members' judgments on that proposition, albeit not necessarily in a majoritarian way. Consider the following supervenience thesis, which is weaker than majoritarian supervenience.

> **Uniform proposition-wise supervenience.** The group judgment on each proposition in the agenda is robustly a function of the individual judgments on that proposition, where the function depends on more than one individual's judgment and is the same for all propositions.

While the majoritarian supervenience thesis permits only one such function—namely the majoritarian one—the present supervenience thesis permits a large class of functions; it only rules out functions according to which group judgments depend only on the judgments of a single fixed individual. But even if majoritarian supervenience is weakened to uniform proposition-wise supervenience, group agency, in the sense defined above, is not generally possible.

> **Proposition 2.** For a constitution with universal domain, robust group rationality is inconsistent with uniform proposition-wise supervenience.

This result is a strengthened version of an impossibility result in List and Pettit (2002), proved in this strengthened form by Pauly and van Hees (2003). As the proof is more technical than that of Proposition 1 above, we omit it here. But the result shows that the problem illustrated in the sketch proof of Proposition 1 persists even if the group judgment on each proposition is not determined by the majority judgment on that proposition, but by another, more general function of the individual judgments. Again, the result does not depend on any irrationality on the part of the individuals; it is true despite the favorable assumption that individual judgments are rational.

So, for a group to be an agent, the relation between the group judgments and those of the group members cannot be that of uniform proposition-wise supervenience either. Let us relax our supervenience thesis further. Perhaps the problem lies in the 'uniformity' of the supervenience relation, that is, the fact that the functional dependence between individual judgments and group judgments is the same for all propositions. Consider the following weakened proposition-wise supervenience thesis.

> **Proposition-wise supervenience.** The group judgment on each proposition in the agenda is robustly a function of the individual judgments on that proposition, where the function depends on more than one individual's judgment and in addition respects unanimous individual judgments,[7] but may differ from proposition to proposition.

[7] This means that, whenever the individuals unanimously agree on some proposition, this agreement is respected by the group judgment.

Proposition-wise supervenience would permit, for example, that on some propositions the group judgment is the majority judgment, while on others it is a different function of the individual judgments. Each such function must only have the specified minimal properties (that is, it must depend on more than one individual's judgment and respect unanimous individual judgments). But even if we assume proposition-wise supervenience alone, dropping the 'majoritarian' and 'uniformity' requirements, we are still faced with an impossibility result.

> **Proposition 3.** For a constitution with universal domain, robust group rationality is inconsistent with proposition-wise supervenience.

Extending an earlier impossibility result by Pauly and van Hees (2003), this result was proved by Dietrich and List (2005); again, we omit the proof. In summary, for a group to be an agent, the relation between the group judgments and those of the group members cannot be that of proposition-wise supervenience. Although this does not refute the supervenience account of group agency, we can already conclude that the supervenience relation cannot be as simple as one might have thought. The group's judgment on a particular proposition cannot generally be a function of the group members' individual judgments on that proposition. So if the group is constituted in such a way as to form an agent, the group members' individual judgments on a proposition are not generally sufficient to determine the group's judgment on that proposition. The supervenience relation must be more complex.

5. POSSIBILITY RESULTS: THE CONSISTENCY OF ROBUST GROUP RATIONALITY WITH 'SET-WISE' SUPERVENIENCE

The core idea of the supervenience account of group agency is that the rational agency of a group—if indeed the group is an agent in its own right—supervenes on the group members' individual contributions, here specifically on their individual judgments. In our conclusion, we briefly consider the possibility that the group's judgments supervene on other, non-judgmental contributions by the group members.

Is group agency ever possible according to this core idea, given that group judgments cannot generally supervene on individual judgments in a proposition-wise way? The following supervenience thesis preserves the core idea of the supervenience account, while giving up the requirement of proposition-wise supervenience.

> **Set-wise supervenience.** The *set* of group judgments on all the propositions in the agenda is robustly a function of the individual *sets* of judgments on (some or all of) these propositions.

We now show that there are possible group constitutions under which a group satisfies both robust group rationality and set-wise supervenience. This finding supports our claim that, at least in principle, group agency is possible under the supervenience account.

Again, consider the multi-member court example. In that example, the group has to make judgments on the propositions *P*, *Q*, *R*, and '*R* if and only if (*P* and *Q*)' (and their negations). Can it do so in a way that meets both robust group rationality and set-wise supervenience? Consider the following constitution.

> **The premise-based procedure.** The group first makes a group judgment on each premise (here *P*, *Q*) by taking a majority vote on that premise (with some constitutional provision for breaking majority ties). The group also accepts the appropriate logical constraint (here '*R* if and only if (*P* and *Q*)') and then derives its group judgment on the conclusion (here *R*) from these group judgments on the premises, using that logical constraint.

In our example, the premise-based procedure would require the court first to take separate votes on whether the defendant did action X and on whether he or she had a contractual obligation not to do X, and then to derive its judgment on the defendant's liability from the outcomes of these votes, using the appropriate logical constraint.

> **Proposition 4.** A group using the premise-based procedure as its constitution satisfies both robust group rationality and set-wise supervenience, but not proposition-wise supervenience.

It is easy to see why this possibility result holds (Pettit 2001, ch. 5). First, the premise-based procedure is guaranteed to generate group judgments that are complete, consistent and deductively closed, regardless of the group members' individual judgments: under the premise-based procedure (i) propositions are always decisively adjudicated; (ii) it is impossible for a proposition and its negation to be judged true simultaneously; and (iii) the adherence to the appropriate logical constraint ensures the satisfaction of deductive closure. For example, if the individual judgments are as in the 'problematic' case of Table 4.1 above, then the premises *P* and *Q* are each accepted by a majority vote, the logical constraint '*R* if and only if (*P* and *Q*)' is accepted by default, and the conclusion *R* is accepted by logical implication, an overall rational set of judgments.

Second, under the premise-based procedure, the set of group judgments on the propositions in the agenda is a function of the individual sets of judgments on those propositions: once the individual judgments on all propositions are fixed, the group's judgments are also fixed.

Third, to prove that a group using the premise-based procedure as its constitution violates proposition-wise supervenience, consider proposition *R* in our example (the conclusion) and notice that the group judgment on *R* is not determined by the individual judgments on *R* alone. In particular, there exist two possible situations in which all individuals hold the same judgments on *R*, and

Table 4.2.

	P	Q	R	R if and only if (P and Q)
Individual 1	True	True	True	True
Individual 2	False	False	False	True
Individual 3	False	False	False	True
Majority	False	False	False	True

yet the group judgment on R differs between the cases. Compare, for example, the cases of Table 4.1 and Table 4.2 (above). The individual judgments on proposition R are the same in these two cases (the column corresponding to R is the same in both cases). Yet, if the group uses the premise-based procedure as its constitution, the group judges proposition R to be true in the case of Table 4.1 but not in the case of Table 4.2.

It is worth noting that the supervenience relation here has not only a set-wise character (as opposed to a proposition-wise one), but also a further property (Pettit 2003). Under the premise-based procedure, the individual judgments on the premises alone are sufficient for determining the group judgments on all the propositions. So the group judgments are non-continuous with the group members' individual judgments in two senses. The individual judgments on the conclusion are not only insufficient for determining the group judgments on the conclusion (a weak discontinuity), but also unnecessary (a strong discontinuity).

The premise-based procedure can be generalized to more than two premises and to other logical constraints (for example, disjunctive rather than conjunctive ones). Moreover, neither the classification of certain propositions as 'premises' and 'conclusions' nor the choice of the logical constraint need to be built into the group's constitution. A generalization of the premise-based procedure to other agendas of propositions is the following (List 2004, 2006; for informal versions, see Pettit 2001, ch. 5; 2003).

> **A sequential priority procedure.** First, an order of priority among the propositions in the agenda is specified. Earlier propositions are interpreted as 'prior to' later ones: they may serve as 'premises' in relation to later ones. Second, the group considers the propositions in the given order. For each proposition thus considered, if that proposition is not logically constrained by earlier propositions judged to be true, then the group takes a majority vote on the new proposition; but if the new proposition is logically constrained by those earlier propositions (such as a 'conclusion' that is constrained by 'premises' judged to be true earlier), then the group derives its judgment on the new proposition from its judgments on those earlier propositions.

It is easy to see that Proposition 4 continues to hold if the premise-based procedure is generalized to a sequential priority procedure. A group using either of these two procedures as its constitution satisfies both robust group rationality and set-wise supervenience, but violates proposition-wise supervenience. Like the premise-based procedure, the sequential priority procedure may give rise to discontinuities between group judgments and corresponding individual judgments.

The premise-based and sequential priority procedures are both constitutions under which all group members contribute to the group judgments in exactly the same way. In particular, if we permute the group members' contributions, the group judgments are unaffected. For example, if we permute the rows in 4.1 and 4.2, the resulting group judgments under the premise-based procedure remain the same in each case. Formally, we say that the supervenience relation between individual judgments and group judgments has a 'homogeneous supervenience base'.

> **Homogeneity of the supervenience base.** The set of group judgments on the propositions in the agenda is invariant under permutations of the group members' individual sets of judgments on those propositions.

By contrast, we say that the supervenience relation between individual judgments and group judgments has a 'heterogeneous supervenience base' if this condition is violated. Are there any interesting constitutions under which the group judgments supervene on the group members' individual judgments in a heterogeneous way and where these group judgments are robustly rational? Consider the following constitution (List 2005).

> **The distributed premise-based procedure.** The group is subdivided into multiple subgroups, one for each premise (e.g. one for *P* and one for *Q*). Each subgroup 'specializes' on precisely one premise and takes a majority vote on that premise only (e.g. one subgroup specializes and votes on *P*, another on *Q*). Now the outcomes of these majority votes are taken as the overall group judgments on the premises. Again, the group also accepts the appropriate logical constraint (e.g. '*R* if and only if (*P* and *Q*)') and derives its group judgment on the conclusion (e.g. *R*) from its group judgments on the premises, using that constraint.

In the court example, the distributed premise-based procedure would require subdividing the court into two subgroups, where the members of one subgroup would 'specialize' on the question of whether the defendant did action X and vote only on this first issue, and the members of another subgroup would 'specialize' on the question of whether the defendant had a contractual obligation not to do action X and vote only on this second issue. The members would not necessarily have to form individual judgments on whether the defendant is liable. Rather, the court's overall judgment on the liability issue would be derived at the group level from the judgments reached by the relevant subgroups on the two premises.

In the case of a court, this is an unfamiliar (and perhaps implausible) constitution. However, large committees, and particularly legislatures, are often subdivided into several subcommittees that play exactly the role assigned to subgroups by the distributed premise-based procedure.

> **Proposition 5.** A group using the distributed premise-based procedure as its constitution satisfies both robust group rationality and set-wise supervenience, but not proposition-wise supervenience.

For technical details, see List (2005). The judgments of a group using the distributed premise-based procedure as its constitution are non-continuous with the group members' individual judgments in several senses. First, for each premise, the judgments of a subset of the individuals are sufficient for determining the group judgment on that premise, whereas the judgments of other individuals are unnecessary; there are different such subsets for different premises. Second, to determine the group judgments on all the propositions in the agenda, each individual needs to contribute only a single judgment on a single proposition, namely on the premise on which that individual 'specializes'; no contribution on any of the other propositions is necessary. And, third, no individual judgments on the conclusion are necessary for determining the group judgment on the conclusion.

The distributed premise-based procedure is an example of a constitution that allows a group to perform as a unified rational agent based on an internal division of labor.

6. CONCLUSION

In our formal discussion, we have focused on the question of how the judgments of a group must supervene on those of its members for the group to be rational. A supervenience relation can be proposition-wise or set-wise. Among proposition-wise supervenience relations, we have further distinguished between uniform ones and others, and among uniform proposition-wise supervenience relations between majoritarian ones and others. Among set-wise supervenience relations, we have distinguished between cases where the supervenience base is homogeneous and ones where it is heterogeneous. Fig. 4.2 summarizes the different supervenience relations we have considered and our formal results.

We have begun with the observation—drawn from the 'discursive dilemma'—that a majoritarian supervenience relationship is inconsistent with robust group rationality. But a majoritarian supervenience relation is a highly special one, as it is a special case not only of a proposition-wise supervenience relation, but also of a uniform one. We have seen that even if the restrictions of majoritarianism and uniformity are dropped, proposition-wise supervenience remains inconsistent with robust group rationality.[8] By contrast, set-wise supervenience is consistent

[8] It is, of course, possible to identify some special conditions under which (some version of) robust group agency *is* consistent with (some version of) proposition-wise supervenience. With

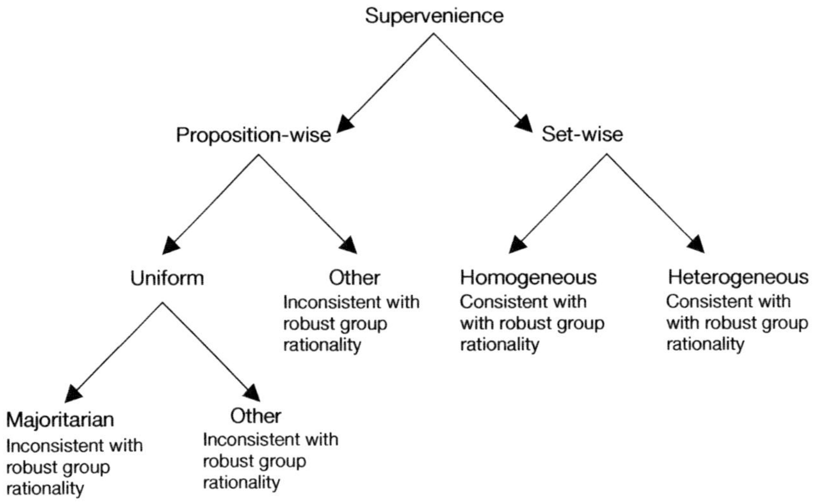

Fig. 4.2

with robust group rationality. The premise-based and distributed premise-based procedures are examples of group constitutions under which group judgments are both robustly rational and set-wise supervenient on individual judgments. Here the supervenience base is homogeneous in the case of the regular premise-based procedure and heterogeneous in the case of the distributed one.

The possibility results are meant to be indicative of how group agency is possible, not exhaustive of the different ways in which it may be achieved. There are a variety of possibilities open, as should be fairly clear. They include informal procedures in which members of the group are invited to think explicitly about the requirements for group consistency, and adjust in the light of these; there is no reason to exclude that possibility (pace McMahon 2005). An example of such a procedure might be the following: individuals take a straw vote on each proposition that comes up, determine whether the straw judgment is inconsistent with existing judgments on other propositions, and then seek to

respect to robust group agency, we might relax the robustness requirement of agency, for example by restricting the domain of the constitution. Or we might relax the rationality requirement of agency, for example by relaxing the requirements of completeness or deductive closure. With respect to proposition-wise supervenience, we might permit a trivial proposition-wise supervenience relation whereby the group judgments depend only on a single 'dictatorial' individual. Or we might relax the 'respect for unanimity' requirement in 'proposition-wise supervenience' and permit a trivial proposition-wise supervenience relation whereby the group judgments are held constant across all possible combinations of individual judgments. Finally, we might shrink the agenda of propositions on which collective judgments are to be formed. These possibilities correspond to various escape-routes from the impossibility results on judgment aggregation. See List and Pettit (2002) and List (2005, 2006).

resolve any inconsistency by eliciting a second round of voting on which of the conflicting judgments to revise (List and Pettit 2005; Pettit 2006).

We said above that we would not make any particular assumptions about the internal make-up of agents. The idea was that so long as a system behaves like an agent, it should generally count as an agent. The most that might be required in addition, we suggested, was that the system's responses were not generated from a distant center and that they were not pre-empted by prior rigging. In effect, what we proposed was that function rather than structure is what matters for agency.

We have illustrated in the later sections of the paper ways in which a group's structure or constitution may vary while group agency is preserved: in particular, while the rationality of the group agent's judgments is preserved. But the question that naturally arises, in conclusion, is whether we have pointed at the further reaches of possibility in this domain. Does our approach make room for all the possible ways in which individuals might cooperate with one another to constitute a group agent?

In rounding off this discussion we have to admit that we may have been too conservative in one respect. Especially in our examples of possible group agents, we have implicitly assumed that the individuals who constitute a group agent do so in a knowing and willing manner. They do so, if they do it in full-dress form, on the basis of certain 'joint intentions' (Tuomela 1995; Bratman 1999; Gilbert 2001). Each member intends that together members sustain the group agent in operation; members will at least acquiesce in the more or less salient fact that how they act together secures that result. And, regimenting their attitudes in full dress, each member intends to do his or her bit; believes that others will do their bit; intends to do his or her bit because of this belief; where all of this is above board, as a matter of shared awareness (Pettit and Schweikard 2006).

Might individuals ever constitute a group agent without anything, however implicit, approximating this condition? The question can be sharpened with an example from non-human animals. It is often said that a swarm of insects can behave as if it were a single, organized agent, even though each individual insect presumably responds in a more or less rote way to chemical signals from its neighbors or environment (Seeley 1989). The swarm, we may suppose, behaves like a proper agent, the individual bees with the inflexibility of automatons, and so without any awareness of the swarm-level behavior. Can we imagine human beings constituting a group agent on a similar basis: on a basis that does not require any one of them to have the conception of what they as a group are doing?

Some of Tolstoy's discussions in *War and Peace* suggest that he thought of populations having this sort of emergent agency, without individuals really understanding what was going on. But we remain skeptical about the possibility. The requirements for such emergent agency look, on the face of it, to be implausibly strong. The individuals who contribute to the group in action will presumably do so, at least in some part, by acting in their own right. But if they act without a conception of their contribution to the group, then their reasons for action must be unrelated to the group's performance. And in that case it is not easy to see what sort of organization, what sort of unrecognized constitution, could guarantee that group agency would be secured. How could any constitution ensure that no matter what people's personal reasons for acting, they will always act as is required for the group as a whole to be robustly rational (Pettit 1993, ch. 3)?

It is hard to see how a constitution could do this, unless the whole enterprise was directed centrally and members deferred to the director. Take Ned Block's China-body system (Block 1980, pp. 276–7). In this imaginary scenario each of the billion members of the Chinese population takes charge of a particular task in the Turing-machine replication of someone's mental life. Without individuals understanding what they are doing, their electronic connections with one another and with the artificial body through which they act ensure that the body manifests agency. Does this mean that the members of the population constitute a group agent? Perhaps, but the presence of central direction, and the widespread deference to the director, would mean that we have a special sort of joint intention here: an intention on the part of each that they together follow what the director enjoins.

If standard social and economic theory is to be believed, then the individually rational inputs of individuals can generate, as by an invisible hand, a pattern of collectively rational results. The question is whether a group agent might emerge in the same way. And it is not clear to us how, empirically, it could. Collectively rational results—say, a pattern of competitive pricing—are stable across many variations in context. But the outputs that would have to be generated for the emergence of a group agent will have to be tailored to different circumstances of action. No existing theory makes sense of how this could happen.

Donald Davidson once said that the secret in exploring a philosophical thesis is to maintain the excitement while increasing the intelligibility. We have explored the thesis that rational group agency supervenes, but not in a straightforward way, on the contributions of individual members. The most exciting version of that thesis is certainly the doctrine of emergent agency that Tolstoy supports. But at this margin of excitement, alas, the intelligibility runs out. We have to settle for less.

REFERENCES

Block, N. (1980). "Troubles with Functionalism?" In *Readings in Philosophy of Psychology*, vol i. London: Methuen.

Bratman, M. (1999). *Faces of Intention: Selected Essays on Intention and Agency*. Cambridge: Cambridge University Press.

Dennett, D. (1987). *The Intentional Stance*. Cambridge MA: MIT Press.

Dietrich, F. (2006). "Judgment Aggregation: (Im)possibility Theorems." *Journal of Economic Theory* 126/1: 286–98.

—— and C. List (2005). "Arrow's Theorem in Judgment Aggregation." Working paper, University of Konstanz.

Gilbert, M. (2001). "Collective Preferences, Obligations, and Rational Choice." *Economics and Philosophy* 17: 109–20.

Jackson, F. and P. Pettit (1990). "In Defence of Folk Psychology." *Philosophical Studies* 57: 7–30; repr. in F. Jackson, P. Pettit and M. Smith, *Mind, Morality and Explanation.* Oxford, Oxford University Press (2004).

Kornhauser, L. A. and L. G. Sager (1986). "Unpacking the Court." *Yale Law Journal* 96/1: 82–117.

List, C. (2004). "A Model of Path-Dependence in Decisions over Multiple Propositions." *American Political Science Review* 98: 495–513.

—— (2005). "Group Knowledge and Group Rationality: A Judgment Aggregation Perspective." *Episteme: A Journal of Social Epistemology* 2/1: 25–38.

—— (2006). "The Discursive Dilemma and Public Reason." *Ethics* 116/2: 362–402.

—— and P. Pettit (2002). "Aggregating Sets of Judgments: An Impossibility Result." *Economics and Philosophy* 18/1: 89–110.

—— —— (2005). "On the Many as One." *Philosophy and Public Affairs* 33/4: 377–90.

McMahon, C. (2005). "Pettit on Collectivizing Reason." *Social Theory and Practice* 31/3: 431–50.

Pauly, M. and M. van Hees (2003). "Logical Constraints on Judgment Aggregation." *Journal of Philosophical Logic*, 35(6): 569–85.

Peacocke, C. (1983). *Sense and Content.* Oxford: Oxford University Press.

Pettit, P. (1993). *The Common Mind.* New York: Oxford University Press.

—— (2001). *A Theory of Freedom: From the Psychology to the Politics of Agency.* Cambridge and New York: Polity and Oxford University Press.

—— (2003). "Groups with Minds of their Own." In F. Schmitt (ed.), *Socializing Metaphysics.* New York: Rowan and Littlefield: 167–93.

—— (2006). "Participation, Deliberation and We-thinking." In D. O'Neill, M. Shanley and I. Young (eds.), *The Illusion of Consent: Essays in Honor of Carole Pateman.* Philadelphia: Pennsylvania State University Press.

—— and D. Schweikard. (2006). "Joint Action and Group Agency." *Philosophy of the Social Sciences* 36: 18–39

Runciman, D. (1997). *Pluralism and the Personality of the State.* Cambridge: Cambridge University Press.

Seeley, T. D. (1989). "The hone bee colony as a superorganism." *American Scientist* 77: 546–53.

Tuomela, R. (1995). *The Importance of Us.* Stanford CA: Stanford University Press.

5

Reduction and Reductive Explanation: Is One Possible Without the Other?

Jaegwon Kim

I

A certain picture seems widespread and influential in recent discussions of issues that involve reduction and reductive explanation—especially, in connection with the mind-body problem. The same picture is also influential in the way many think about the relationship between the "higher-level" special sciences and "basic" sciences. What I have in mind is the idea that *reducing* something is one thing and *reductively explaining* it is quite another. Thus, there supposedly is a vital difference, from both the scientific and philosophical point of view, between reducing psychological phenomena to biological/physical phenomena and reductively explaining the former in terms of the latter. The significance of the difference, on this line of thought, derives from the purported fact that reductive explanation is often an achievable scientific goal whereas reduction is an overreaching metaphysical aspiration that is seldom, if ever, realized.

To see what this picture is and appreciate its appeal, consider two domains (or "levels", if you like) of phenomena, M and P. (For concreteness, we may think of M as "mental" and P as "physical".) To reduce M to P, we must show, to use J. J. C. Smart's suggestive expression, that the M-phenomena are "nothing over and above" the P-phenomena (Smart 1959). It may be that a proposed reduction is "eliminative"—that is, it consists in the claim that there really are no such things as M-phenomena ("there really are no such things as caloric fluids; there is only molecular motion"). If so, there trivially are no M-phenomena over and above P-phenomena. Whether eliminative reduction is a serious form of reduction can be debated, but we should keep in mind that "reduction" is a term of art and there need be no harm in the idea of eliminative reduction. A more central form of reduction is "conservative" (or "preservative", "retentive") reduction whereby the reduced phenomena survive as legitimate entities of the world. It's only that they now turn up as entities in the base domain. Heat was conservatively reduced—it survives as molecular kinetic energy—whereas caloric fluids were eliminated. Genes were conservatively reduced; vital forces and entelechies were eliminated. If M-phenomena are to be conservatively reduced to P-phenomena, they must be shown to be "nothing over and above" the P-phenomena, and it is hard to see how this could be done unless each M-phenomenon is claimed, and shown, to be identical with a P-phenomenon. That is, reduction appears prima facie to require the identification of M-phenomena with P-phenomena, and this means that M is turned into a subdomain of P. This is no surprise: reduction must reduce, and if M is reduced to P, M-phenomena no longer exist as something *extra*, something *in addition to* P-phenomena.

In contrast, when we think about reductive explanation—that is, explaining M-phenomena on the basis of P-phenomena (including P-laws), what seems like a natural train of thoughts leads us to a considerably different picture. Suppose we explain an M-phenomenon in terms of P-phenomena. We now understand why, and how, this M-phenomenon arises from certain P-phenomena: it is because these particular P-phenomena constitute an underlying mechanism whose operations yield phenomena of kind M. Prima facie, this doesn't seem to undermine, or weaken, the ontological status of the M-phenomenon vis-à-vis P-phenomena. It apparently remains an entity with a legitimate, independent standing in its own right; it's only that its existence and character has been made intelligible in light of the underlying phenomena and mechanisms. There seems no reason to think a reductive explanation of an M-phenomenon carries any commitment, explicit or implicit, to the claim that it is "nothing over and above" the P-phenomena; nor does it imply, or suggest, that the M-phenomenon must be identified with a P-phenomenon. (As an analogy, think about causal explanation: we do not think that a causal explanation of an event adversely affects its status as an independent entity.) If something like this is right, reductive explanation should be possible even where there is no reduction. Or so it seems at first blush.

Conversely, it is difficult to see why we should expect reduction to yield reductive explanation: M-phenomena may be nothing over and above P-phenomena, but that in itself says nothing about explanation, something that has essential epistemic dimensions. If an M-phenomenon is identical with a P-phenomenon, there seems no specifically M-phenomenon that needs to be, or can be, reductively explained. The M-phenomenon *is* a P-phenomenon after all, and it is prima facie a bit incoherent to talk of "reductively" explaining a P-phenomenon in terms of other P-phenomena. It almost seems as though reduction might actually preclude reductive explanation. It is clear in any case that there are issues about reduction and reductive explanation that need to be sorted out and clarified.

Jerry Fodor's "Special Sciences" (Fodor 1974) was the canonical source of the antireductionist arguments in the latter half of the 20th century. As is widely known, Fodor's antireductionist argument, based on the so-called multiple realizability of psychological and other special-science properties, played a pivotal role in creating what Ned Block has aptly dubbed "the antireductionist consensus" (Block 1997). The consensus has perhaps lost some of its pervasive hold, but it is still a widely shared orthodoxy with considerable reach and influence. However, few commentators seem to have noticed the following surprising paragraph in Fodor's paper:

> It seems to me (to put the point quite generally) that the classical construal of the unity of science has really badly misconstrued the *goal* of scientific reduction. The point of reduction is *not* primarily to find some natural kind predicate of physics coextensive with each kind predicate of a special science. *It is, rather, to explicate the physical mechanisms whereby events conform to the laws of the special sciences* [emphasis added]. I have been arguing that there is no logical or epistemological reason why success in the second of these projects should require success in the first, and that the two are likely to come apart *in fact* wherever the physical mechanisms whereby events conform to a law of the special sciences are heterogeneous. (Fodor 1974, p. 107)

Here, Fodor is saying that although the "bridge laws" required for Nagelian reduction (more on bridge laws below) are unavailable (since, as he says, special science predicates in general have no coextensive physical predicates) and so reduction is impossible, this does not preclude reductive explanations of special-science laws in terms of "physical mechanisms" at the lower levels. In fact, he is suggesting something bold and revolutionary, namely that the idea of reduction be reconstrued as, or be discarded in favor of, reductive explanation. So, for Fodor, reduction is not possible anywhere; yet, reductive explanation is a legitimate scientific procedure which presumably is often successfully executed. Unfortunately, Fodor drops the matter here and says nothing further about how he conceives reductive explanation, or why explanation in terms of "physical mechanisms" is an appropriate replacement for reduction as traditionally conceived.

The idea that reductive explanation can thrive even where reduction fails appears to reflect a natural way of thinking about the interlevel relations in the sciences, and it reappears, more than twenty years later, in the following remarks by David Chalmers:

> A reductive explanation of a phenomenon need not require a *reduction* of that phenomenon . . . In a certain sense, phenomena that can be realized in many different physical substrates—learning, for example—might not be reducible in that we cannot *identify* learning with any specific lower-level phenomena. But this multiple realizability does not stand in the way of reductively *explaining* any instance of learning in terms of lower-level phenomena. (Chalmers 1996, p. 43)

Chalmers has evidently bought into the Putnam-Fodor multiple realization argument against reduction, or type-identity reduction, but he claims that this in no way affects the possibility of reductively explaining higher-level phenomena in terms of phenomena and mechanisms at lower levels.

But how is that possible? Chalmers doesn't address this question directly, but the following thought seems implicit and it is not an implausible one. Reduction requires type identities, which are excluded by the phenomenon of multiple realization; however, reductive explanation can target individual instances instead of types: any instance of a higher-level phenomenon occurs by being realized by a lower-level phenomenon, and it can therefore be explained in terms of its underlying realizer. This means that two instances of the same higher-level phenomenon (as a type) may receive two distinct reductive explanations, each in terms of its own realizer. This is the initial thought; we will explore below how it might be fleshed out.

A related thought is that physicalism itself can, and perhaps should, be understood in a new way. In order to secure physicalism, we do not need a reduction of all phenomena to a physical base; all that is required is the reductive physical explainability of all phenomena other than fundamental physical phenomena. If all mental phenomena are shown to be explainable on the basis of physical phenomena and physical laws, why isn't that physicalism enough? For that would mean that physical phenomena suffice for the understanding of everything about mentality—why the phenomena of the mind occur in the way they do, why they interrelate among themselves and relate to physical phenomena as they do, and all the rest. It is perhaps no accident that what many regard as the most important obstacle to physicalism is called the problem of "explanatory gap" (Levine 1983). The problem, as everyone knows, is that of explaining—presumably, reductively explaining—phenomenal consciousness, or qualia, in terms of physical/biological phenomena. The idea is that once such an explanation is achieved, or shown to be achievable, the gap is closed and physicalism is home free. Conversely, if the gap resists closure, that should defeat physicalism.

But can we separate reduction and reductive explanation so easily and neatly? Is it really possible to reductively explain a mental phenomenon, say pain, in neural terms and for this phenomenon to remain "over and above" neural phenomena, as a distinct and separate entity? Conversely, if mental phenomenon M has been shown to be "nothing over and above" a physical/biological phenomenon P, will that give us a reductive explanation of M in terms of P? In this paper, I consider these and related questions in regard to three models of reduction currently on the scene—bridge-law reduction, identity reduction, and functional reduction. As will be seen, answers to our question vary depending on the kind of reduction involved. Bridge-law reduction, I will argue, is an oxymoron: it yields neither reduction nor reductive explanation. In contrast, identity reduction gives us reduction but no reductive explanation. Finally, functional reduction can be seen to yield reductive explanation and, arguably but not unproblematically, reduction as well.

II

Bridge-law reduction was developed by Ernest Nagel in the 1950s and 60s (Nagel 1961) as an account of inter-theoretic reduction in science. The model as it has been generally understood in the debate over reduction and reductionism in the decades that followed is a somewhat simplified version of the model actually stated by Nagel (Nagel 1961, 1970), and here we will use this simpler and more familiar version. Let T_1 and T_2 be two theories where theories are construed as sets of laws, with some laws designated as "basic" and the rest being logically derivable from them. According to the bridge-law model:

> T_2 is reducible to T_1 = def. (1) [the bridge-law condition] for each primitive predicate F of T_2 there is a T_1-predicate G such that a "bridge law" of the biconditional form "$Fx \leftrightarrow Gx$" holds, and (2) [the derivability condition] each law of T_2 is logically derivable from the laws of T_1, with the bridge laws taken as auxiliary premises.

On this mode, then, the reduction of one theory to another amounts to a deductive absorption of the former into the latter augmented with the bridge laws. Since the proprietary vocabularies of the two theories must be expected to be disjoint, or at least not to completely overlap (for example, thermodynamics and statistical mechanics, classical and molecular genetics), Nagel thought that principles connecting, or "bridging", the two vocabularies are needed to enable the derivation, and that these would typically be empirical scientific laws correlating phenomena of the two domains involved.[1]

It is easy to appreciate the centrality of bridge laws to reductions of this form. For we can quickly see that if the bridge-law requirement (1) is met, the derivability condition (2) is automatically met as well—with a small caveat. Let L be any law of T_2, the theory being reduced, and assume that the bridge-law condition has been satisfied. We can now use these biconditional laws as definitions and rewrite L entirely in the vocabulary of T_1, the base theory. Let L^* be this T_1-rewrite of L. Either L^* is derivable from T_1-laws or it is not. If it is, then L can be derived from the T_1-laws (derive L^* first and then derive

[1] Nagel's final formulation of his model (Nagel 1961) does not require the bridge laws to be biconditionals in form; however, in discussions of reduction they are standardly taken to be biconditionals; see, e.g., Fodor's talk, in his quotation above, of classical reduction requiring "some natural kind predicate of physics *coextensive* with each kind predicate of a special science"(added emphasis), and we follow this practice here. In any case, this is one reason to call the model as presented here "bridge-law reduction", not "Nagel reduction" (the second, and more important, reason is the centrality of bridge laws to the model as will shortly be discussed). Also, condition (1) is simplified in that it only refers to monadic predicates.

L from L* using the bridge laws) and the derivability condition is met. If L* is not derivable from T_1-laws, add L* to T_1 as an additional basic law. This is permissible because in missing L*, T_1 is missing an important truth, a lawlike truth, in its domain (here we are assuming T_2 and the bridge laws to be true). In this case, L is derivable from this augmented base theory $T_1 + L^*$, again with the help of the bridge laws. In either case, therefore, the derivability requirement is met, either in regard to T_1 or with respect to an augmented version of T_1 stated in the same theoretical vocabulary.[2]

There is another way to see the importance of bridge laws. Checking the derivability condition in any given case requires us to look at whole theories. For this to have real significance, the theories we examine must be completed theories, or nearly completed ones. This makes it difficult to discuss, say, whether psychology is reducible to neuroscience because we have nothing like a completed psychology—or a completed science of the brain. However, the question whether or not we can expect to find bridge laws connecting psychological states with neural/physiological states has seemed more amenable to discussion—even at the present state of knowledge. Many well-known antireductionist arguments about psychology aim at showing that there can be no such psychoneural laws, quite independently of what completed psychology or neuroscience will look like. The Putnam-Fodor multiple realization argument (Putnam 1967; Fodor 1974) is one such example; Donald Davidson's anomalist argument is another (Davidson 1970). These arguments are largely independent of the current state of the psychological or neural sciences, and simply bypass consideration of the derivability requirement.

Suppose that we have a theory about pain and that this theory includes the following law:

(L) Pain causes distress.

Suppose further that this pain theory has been bridge-law reduced to neurophysiology, with the help of psychoneural bridge laws, including these:

Pain occurs to $x \leftrightarrow$ neural state N_1 occurs in x.
Distress occurs to $x \leftrightarrow$ neural state N_2 occurs in x

If (L) has been derived from neurophysiological laws with these bridge laws as extra premises, neurophysiology must include the following law:

(L*) N_1 causes N_2.

By carrying out this bridge-law reduction, have we reduced pain? Do we have a reductive explanation of pain? And do we have a reduction, or reductive explanation, of psychological law (L)?

I believe the answer is no to each of these questions. On the standard conception of bridge-law reduction, bridge laws are a posteriori and contingent,

[2] Note: if T_1 is physics, so is $T_1 + L^*$; if T_1 is biology, so is $T_1 + L^*$.

and this means that the properties or states connected in a bridge law remain distinct entities. The bridge law connecting pain with N_1 does not entitle us to say: pain is "nothing over and above" neural state N_1. We do not think that nomological equivalence or coextensiveness guarantees identity, or warrants "nothing over and above" or "nothing but" talk. We might say that N_1 is the neural correlate, or substrate, of pain, and that's all the bridge law entitles us to say. Does our bridge-law reduction of pain give us a reductive explanation of pain in neural terms—more specifically, in terms of N_1? The answer, again, is no. The reduction takes the pain–N_1 correlation as an unexplained, underived, premise in the derivation of the pain theory from neurophysiology. That is, it takes the correlation law as something brute and fundamental. The "explanatory" gap between pain and N_1 remains untouched. In fact, what creates the explanatory gap is exactly the pain–N_1 correlation. The gap arises because we are apt, or perhaps fated, to ask questions like the following: why does pain correlate with N_1 rather than another neural state?; why doesn't itch correlate with N_1?; why does any qualitative experience correlate with N_1?; and so on. Clearly, what is in need of explanation—reductive explanation—is why the bridge law correlating pain with N_1 holds—what it is about the physical nature of N_1 that explains why it correlates with a conscious state with the phenomenal character constitutive of pain. Finally, do we get from this bridge-law reduction an explanation of the psychological law (L)—that is, why pain causes distress? Again, the answer is no. All we can conclude from (L*) and the two bridge laws is that pain correlates with a neural state which causes the neural state with which distress is correlated.[3] That doesn't come anywhere near an explanation of why pain causes distress.

The conclusion is unavoidable: Bridge-law reduction gives us neither reduction nor reductive explanation. At least in this case, reduction and reductive explanation go together—by both being absent.

III

A natural step to take at this point is to consider upgrading bridge laws into something more robust and stronger, something that could support reductive claims and perhaps also handle the explanatory issues. And it didn't escape philosophers' attention that identities might be just the replacements we needed for the bridge laws. The idea goes back to the early mind-body identity theorists like Herbert Feigl and J. J. C. Smart. Feigl famously called these psychoneural bridge laws "dangling" laws (Feigl 1958), and Smart's explicit aim in promoting psychoneural identity theory was to eliminate these "nomological danglers" and

[3] To mimic an admirably felicitous sentence from Block and Stalnaker (1999).

replace them with psychoneural identities (Smart 1959).[4] So instead of the likes of:

Pain occurs $\leftrightarrow$ N_1 occurs

we would now have identities like:

Pain = N_1.

These identities are stronger than the corresponding correlations and can do their work in inferential contexts. So theory reduction construed, à la Nagel, as logical derivation of the reduced theory from the reducer can be based on identities as well as correlations (Sklar 1967, Causey 1972).[5]

Early psychoneural identity theorists considered these identities contingent and a posteriori. Things have changed in our post-Kripkean modal paradise: the identities are generally taken to be necessary truths (if true), though they are allowed to retain their a posteriori character. Their epistemic and theoretical status, according to some influential latter-day identity theorists (for example, Hill 1991, Block and Stalnaker 1999, McLaughlin 2001), is supposed to be the same as, or at least similar to, that of scientific identities like "water = H_2O", "heat = molecular kinetic energy", and "genes = DNA molecules". So it isn't surprising that some have claimed psychoneural identities to be justifiable by the same sort of evidence and consideration that warrant acceptance of these familiar scientific identities (Block and Stalnaker 1999).[6]

We may call this mode of reduction "identity reduction": reduction is accomplished by identifying phenomena and properties being reduced with appropriate items in the base domain. The return of psychoneural type identity theory, during the 1990s, is one of the more interesting developments in the recent debate on the mind-body problem.[7]

There is no question about the reductive import of identity reduction. If pain = N_1, there is no pain over and above N_1; and if mental states are identical with brain states, there are no mental states over and above brain states. This is an open-and-shut affair if anything in philosophy ever is: Identities do reduce. For reduction nothing works as magically as identities, and it may well be that identities of some sort are required for any genuine reduction.

[4] It should be noted that Feigl didn't see eye to eye with Smart on this issue; see Feigl (1967, pp. 136 ff). Here my discussion focuses on Smart's views.

[5] Nagel himself later recognized identities as a form of bridge laws (his examples include "water = H_2O" and "light waves are electromagnetic waves" (Nagel 1970). But he never seems to have considered the issue of *property* identities; for Nagel, bridge laws involving properties seem to have remained empirical correlations.

[6] This suggestion would seem to turn the mind-body problem into a scientific problem, one that can be resolved by scientific research. We should keep Smart's remark to the effect that while the choice between the brain-state theory and the kidney-state theory is an empirical scientific issue, the choice between the brain-state theory and epiphenomenalism is not (Smart 1959). I believe that Block and Stalnaker's argument for their proposal is seriously flawed (Kim 2005).

[7] How does the multiple realizability argument affect the new identity theory? This question has not been extensively explored. For some useful discussion see Hill (1991, 101 ff) and Block (1997).

It is of course an independent question where we can get these identities, in particular psychoneural identities. We must earn our entitlement to them; it is not acceptable to argue that the identities are warranted because they would give us psychoneural reduction. I believe this is the biggest remaining hurdle for identity reduction; I do not myself believe it can be overcome.

But does identity reduction yield reductive explanation? Does the identity "pain = N_1" help close the supposed explanatory gap between pain and N_1? If the identity holds, there is here only one thing, not two, and, to push the "gap" metaphor a bit, at least two distinct items are needed to create a gap. If psychoneural identities hold, there isn't any mind-brain gap to be closed and there never was. If we stay with the correlation "pain occurs $\leftrightarrow$ N_1 occurs", we face explanatory challenges of the sort the emergentists have raised: Why does pain, not itch or tickle, correlate with N_1? Why doesn't pain correlate with a different neural state? And so on. As I believe Ned Block remarked somewhere, the problem of the explanatory gap is to answer the question "Why do phenomenal states correlate with the neural states with which they correlate?" On behalf of the identity theory, Block and Stalnaker deliver a decisive dismissal for such explanatory requests (Block and Stalnaker 1999, 24):

> If we believe that heat is correlated with but not identical to molecular kinetic energy, we should regard as legitimate the question of why the correlation exists and what its mechanism is. But once we realize that heat *is* molecular kinetic energy, questions like this can be seen as wrongheaded.

In general, there are two ways of responding to an explanatory request "why *p*?" The first is to provide a correct answer to the question, by offering an explanation of why *p*. The second is to show that the presupposition of the request, namely that there is here something to be explained, is incorrect, and that in consequence no explanation is needed, or even possible. When *p* is false, the question "why *p*?" obviously has no correct answer (consider "Why does oil dissolve in water?") In the present case, we could say either that the identity of pain with neural state N_1 shows that there is here no correlation between the two states, and that this makes the presupposition of the question "Why does pain correlate with N_1?" false, or we could say that the identity trivializes the question into "Why does pain correlate with pain?" or "Why does N_1 correlate with N_1?" In either case, there is nothing to be explained here, and there is no gap to be closed.[8]

That, however, is not the end of the story. There is an important further point that has to hold if psychoneural identities are to resolve the explanatory

[8] We should take note of a different take on the issue of identities and the explanatory problem. According to Hill (1991) and McLaughlin (2001), psychoneural identities provide explanations for psychoneural correlations—that is, "Why does pain correlate with N_1?" is correctly answered, and explained, by saying that "pain = N_1". I do not think this view is correct; for discussion see Kim (2005, chapter 5). In any case, I don't believe that either Hill or McLaughlin would claim that identities deliver "reductive" explanations of the correlations.

gap problem, and it is this: Identities like "heat = mke" and "pain = N_1" are immune to further explanatory challenges. It isn't enough that, as Block and Stalnaker say, "heat = mke" renders the question "Why does heat *correlate with* mke?" wrongheaded; it must also be the case that the question "Why is heat *identical with* mke?" is also a wrongheaded question. If this is a legitimate question requiring an answer—a "correct" answer—then, a "gap" or no "gap", the identities like "pain = N_1" will fail to free us from the burden of explaining psychoneural relations, and the emergentists' explanatory challenges cannot be stopped. In order to put an end to them, we must assume that identities are terminal points of regressive explanatory challenges "Why *p*? Because *q*. Why *q*? Because *r*. Why *r*? . . ." When we are finally able to come up with an answer in the form of an identity "Because $x = y$", that will, it is hoped, stop the why-questions in their tracks. The reason, as the thought runs, is that it makes no sense to ask for an explanation of why $x = y$—namely that identities are not proper explananda. But is this correct?

Prima facie, there seem to be any number of identities for which we can sensibly ask for explanations—and find them if we are clever or lucky. Consider:

Michael Jordan = the most valuable player of the Chicago Bulls
32° F. = the freezing point of water
Black = the color of my true love's hair

It surely makes sense to ask why Michael Jordan is the most valuable player of his team, why 32° F. is the freezing point of water, and so on, and receive informative answers that explain the facts in question. However, we also notice that, unlike "Cicero = Tully" and "water = H_2O", these identities don't seem to be genuine identities—they are easily paraphrased into equivalent predicative statements like "Michael Jordan is a more valuable player than anyone else on the team", "Water freezes at 32° F.", and "My true love's hair is black". It surely makes sense to ask why Jordan is a more valuable player than any of his teammates, why water freezes at 32° F., and so on. Further, these identities are all contingent, each with a nonrigid designator flanking the identity sign.

In contrast, identities like "heat = mke" and "pain = N_1" are taken, in this context, to be necessary truths. What does the contingency or necessity of an identity have to do with the question whether it is a fit object of explanation? If *p* is a contingent truth, we can always ask the question "What is it about this world that makes it the case that *p*?"—that is, "Why is this world one in which *p* is true rather than one in which *p* is false?" If *p* is a necessary truth, *p* is true everywhere and the question "What is it about this world that makes it the case that *p*?" either receives a put-down answer "Nothing special—*p* holds in every world", or can be charged with having a wrong presupposition, to the effect that there are certain special features of this world, not present in every world, which are responsible for *p*'s holding here. In either case, the question "why *p*?", where

p is a necessary truth, does not receive a "correct" answer; rather, the response it elicits dissipates the point of the question.[9]

What we have just said applies to all necessary truth, not just necessary identities. Is there anything specific to be said contra identities as possible explananda? There is this train of thought: If necessarily $x = y$, saying that $x = y$ says no more, and no less, than that $x = x$, or that $y = y$. Therefore, asking "why $x = y$?" makes no more sense than asking "why $x = x$?" One might protest: saying that Cicero = Tully *is* saying more than that Cicero = Cicero, or that Tully = Tully. We can grant that. "Cicero = Tully" carries information that "Cicero = Cicero" does not. What could this information be? As far as I can tell, it is the fact that the names "Cicero" and "Tully" name the same object. And of course *this* fact can be a proper explanandum. But "Cicero = Tully" is not a statement about the names "Cicero" and "Tully", and it does not report a fact other than the fact (if there is a fact here) reported by "Cicero = Cicero". It is difficult to see any fact here that can be a suitable object of explanation. In contrast, if it is only contingent that $x = y$ (e.g., Benjamin Franklin = the inventor of bifocals), we can no longer say that "$x = y$" says nothing more than "$x = x$" or "$y = y$", and there can be an explanation of the fact that Benjamin Franklin = the inventor of bifocals.

I am not certain exactly what these considerations add up to show; I cannot say I find them, singly or together, wholly compelling or satisfying, though not entirely vacuous or irrelevant either. There undoubtedly is more, probably much more, to be said on the role of identities in explanations, either as elements in an explanans or as possible explananda. This is a large and complex topic in its own right, and what I have said is pretty much all that I have to say.[10] In any case, we can safely conclude that identity reduction does reduce but yields no reductive explanations. Rather, it deals with the explanatory questions of the sort the emergentists raised in a different way: it asserts that there is something seriously defective about the presuppositions of those questions, and that this renders these explanatory requests improper and misguided. If this is right, we have a case in which reduction and reductive explanation do not go hand in hand—identity reduction does reduce but generates no reductive explanations.

IV

We now turn to the last of the three models of reduction. Functional reduction proceeds in three steps. Suppose that property M is to be so reduced:

9 One pertinent issue here concerns the possibility of explanations of mathematical truths. One could argue, it seems, that proofs, especially constructive proofs, explain why the theorems are true. I have nothing interesting or informative to say about this, but it seems to me that mathematical explanations, if there are such things, must be radically diverse in kind from explanations of natural events, facts, laws, and the like.

10 I discuss the role of identities as part of an explanans in Kim (2005, chapter 5).

Step 1. Functionalize M by providing a functional definition/characterization of the following form:

> For *x* to have M (or to be an M) = for *x* to have some property or mechanism P such that C(P), where C(P) states a causal specification that P must meet.

Step 2. Identify—that is, ascertain—the P, or Ps, that meet the causal specification C in the system, or a population of systems, of interest in a given research program. Such Ps are called the "realizers" of M.

Step 3. Develop a theory that explains how these realizers of M perform the causal task specified by C in the systems in question.

Steps 2 and 3 are likely to go concurrently, hand in hand. As a simplified schematic example, consider this:

(i) For *x* to be a gene = for *x* to have, or be, a mechanism that encodes and transmits genetic information.

(ii) DNA molecules are the mechanisms that perform the task of encoding and transmitting genetic information (in biological organisms of interest to us).

(iii) Molecular biology explains how DNA molecules perform this task.

When all this is in, we may say that genes have been reduced—functionally reduced—to DNA molecules in the population of interest to us, presumably various sorts of terrestrial organisms.

Philosophically, step 1 is the critical step. Steps 2 and 3 are obviously matters of scientific research. The question whether M can be defined functionally is a conceptual issue, though not necessarily a wholly a priori or philosophical one—in particular, just how a functional definition for a given M is to be formulated is likely to have to be informed by empirical findings and theoretical needs. The philosophical interest and importance of the issue of functionalizability stems from the fact that once M has been functionalized (or shown to be functionalizable), we know that M is functionally reducible—whether, and how, M is going to be reduced, that is, whether and how steps 2 and 3 will be carried out, is an empirical scientific issue. Given that M is a functional property, if anything has M, it logically follows that it has one or another of the realizers of M, though we may not have a lower-level description of the realizer involved. Further, we will argue that any particular instance of M is reducible and reductively explainable in terms of M's realizer on this occasion.

Let us first take up the issue of reductive explanation. Suppose that pain has been given the following functional definition—along the lines indicated by early functionalists:

> For *x* to be in pain = for *x* to be in some state P such that tissue damage is apt to cause P and P is apt to cause winces, groans, and aversive behavior.

(This is for illustrative purposes only; I am not suggesting that pain can be functionally defined or reduced—on the contrary, I believe pain is not functionally definable.) Supposing neural state N_1 to be the realizer of pain in humans, let us consider explanatory questions like these:

Why is Jones in pain at *t*?
Why did Jones experience pain when he stepped on a thumbtack?
Why is neural state N_1 invariably accompanied by pain (in humans)?

Can we formulate explanations as responses to these questions, explanations in terms of neural laws and neural facts about Jones? I believe the following is a possible neural explanation of why Jones is in pain at *t*:

Jones is in neural state N_1 at *t*.
Tissue damage is apt to cause N_1 in Jones, and N_1 is apt to cause Jones to wince, groan, and engage in aversive behavior.
Being in pain = being in a state apt to be caused by tissue damage and apt for causing winces, groans, and aversive behavior.
Therefore, Jones is in pain at *t*.

The argument is clearly valid, and it derives a pain fact from neural/physical facts alone. If anything could count as closing the explanatory gap between pain and its neural correlate, this explanation should. Please note that the third sentence is a definition; it is not a "fact" about pain's correlation with any neural/physical fact; if it is about any fact, it is about a semantic/conceptual fact about the term "pain". Definitions don't count as premises in a proof; they come free. Notice one more thing: at the second sentence, the argument invokes a nomological fact. The argument is an empirical lawful regularity that this particular neural state, N_1, has the specified causal role in Jones and creatures like him. It has the form of a Hempelian deductive-nomological explanation.

We now turn to formulating a reductive explanation in answer to the second explanatory question "Why was Jones in pain when he stepped on a thumbtack?":

Jones stepped on a thumbtack.
This caused tissue damage in Jones.
This in turn caused neural state N1.
N_1 is apt to be caused in Jones (and like individuals) by tissue damage and is apt to cause Jones to wince, groan, etc.
Being in pain = being in a state apt to be caused by tissue damage and apt for causing winces, groans, etc.
Therefore, Jones was in pain.

We may assume that the second and third sentences are derivable from the first sentence from physiological laws; or they can be taken as independent premises. I believe the argument again is a plausible reductive explanation of why stepping on a thumbtack in the way Jones did caused Jones pain. Again, a pain fact is derived from premises concerning neural/physical facts alone. A reductive explanation can be formulated, on a similar pattern, as a reply to the third explanatory request above.

Plausibly, then, functional reduction delivers reductive explanations. But does it reduce? Take a given instance of a functionally reduced property, M—that is, something *x*'s having M at *t*. If *x* has M at *t*, it follows that *x* instantiates at *t* a realizer of M, say P_k. I believe that the identification of this instance of M, *x*'s having M at *t*, with the instance of the realizer involved on this occasion, *x*'s having P_k at *t*, is all but compelling. This is for at least two reasons. First, the definition of M says that for *x* to have M at *t is* for *x* to instantiate, at *t*, a property that plays causal role C (for *x*); and P_k is exactly the property that *x* has at *t* which plays causal role C. There is no further fact about *x*'s having M at *t* than the fact that *x* has P_k at *t*. Second, there are causal considerations: What are the causal powers of this instance of M? The only reasonable answer seems to be that they are identical with the causal powers of this instance of P_k. (This is what I have called elsewhere the causal inheritance principle (Kim 1992).) These considerations point to a form of token identity thesis: this instance of M is identical with the instance of the realizer of M on this occasion. In general, then, if mental properties are functionally reducible, instances of mental properties are identical with the instances of their physical realizers. That, at any rate, is the proposal. We may call it token reductionism.

Let us first deal with a possible objection. It might be argued that token reductionism of this form doesn't sit well with the earlier claim that functional reduction yields reductive explanation. Consider the first of the two displayed derivations above. As may be recalled, the claim was that it is an explanation of why Jones has pain at a time on the basis of why Jones is in neural state N_1 at that time. In this example, N_1 is the realizer of pain on that occasion, so on the token reduction thesis, Jones's having pain at $t =$ Jones's in neural state N_1 at *t*. If so, this would turn supposed explanation into one in which something is explained in terms of itself—a self-explanation. But the very idea of explaining something by simply re-invoking it under another name seems foolish and incoherent.[11] There may be a general lesson here: there is a prima facie incompatibility between reducing something *x* to *y* and reductively explaining *x* in terms of *y*—a point noted at the outset of this paper. Once *x* has been reduced to $y, x = y$, and any attempt to explain *x* in terms of *y* would only result in an absurd self-explanation. Since the derivations that were claimed to be reductive explanations do seem to be explanatory, one might argue, the upshot is that we must reject the identity claim for pain-instances and N_1-instances and, more generally, reject token reductionism. This is the objection to be considered.

I believe that we can make good sense of the explanatory claim in a way that is consistent with the token identity thesis. Let us begin by reminding ourselves that

[11] Compare: Why is Cicero wise? Because Tully is wise and Cicero = Tully!

the relationship between x's having pain at t and x's being in neural state N_1 at t is contingent, not necessary. This stems from the contingency of the realization relation: that N_1 is a realizer of pain in x and like systems is contingent, not necessary. N_1 realizes pain in this population in virtue of satisfying the causal specification definitive of pain. That these particular causal relations hold for state N_1 in systems like x is a contingent fact, a fact that depends on what laws prevail in our world. In worlds in which different laws hold (we are assuming that laws, or causal laws, are contingent), different causal relations will hold, and N_1 might no longer meet the causal specification associated with pain. In some such worlds, N_1 will fail to realize pain. Thus, the identity "x's having pain at $t = x$'s having N_1 at t" is contingent. In some worlds where x has pain at t, it might be that x's having pain at $t = x$'s having Q at t ($Q \neq N_1$), where Q realizes pain in x in that world. The contingency of these token identities is the key to seeing how "self-explanations" apparently involved in our reductive explanation can be perfectly harmless. By providing a reductive explanation of the sort displayed above, we show how the description "x is in pain at t" applies to something as a causal-nomological consequence of the fact that the description "x is in neural state N_1 at t" applies to it. Or think of it this way: the identity "x's being in pain at $t = x$'s having M at t" is contingent, so it makes sense to ask: What is it about this world that makes it so? Why is it that in this world this identity holds whereas in those other worlds it does not? The answer: It is because in this world these laws hold, enabling N_1 to fill the causal role that defines pain, whereas different laws hold in those other worlds and these laws do not confer similar causal powers on N_1. This is what the suggested reductive explanation does; it invokes laws holding in this world and shows that N_1 has the causal powers required to realize M.

We now turn to another question: Might the contingency of the identity "x's having M at $t = x$'s having P_k at t" undermine its reductive import? I don't see why it should. The reductive claim is this: x's having M at t reduces, in this world, to its having P_k at t—that is, in this world, x's having M at t is "nothing over and above" its having P_k at t. In another world, x's having M may reduce to x's having P_j (where $k \neq j$), and so on. Moreover, given that M is a functional property, in every world in which something has M at t, there is a realizer of M such that the object's having M at t reduces to its having that realizer at t. So then, there is no world in which something's having M is "over and above" its having some physical realizer of M. That is, in no world are there instances of M that are unidentified with instances of M's physical realizers. Once you have all actual and possible instances of M's realizers, you've got all instances of M, actual and possible; M-instances add nothing ontologically to the instances of its realizers. This seems reduction enough for all instances, or tokens, of M, actual or possible. The contingency of the token identities, therefore, appears to be consistent with the efficacy of these identities as vehicles of reduction; necessary identities are not necessary for reduction.

So token reductionism takes care of pain instances. But what of pain itself? That is, once a functional reduction of pain has been achieved, what happens to the type, or property or kind, *being in pain*? Is this property reduced and if so, to what? If not, aren't we still stuck with an unreduced, and irreducible, nonphysical property? These are the questions we must now face.[12]

Let P_1, P_2, . . . be all the realizers of M at this world; this means that for something to have M in this world, it must have one of the Ps, and if something has one of the Ps in this world, it has M. Consider the (possibly infinite) disjunction P_1 v P_2 v. . . (or UP for short). Then anything has M at this world if and only if it has UP. So can we say that M = UP? Is this a way of physically reducing M? In considering this question, we must first recognize the proposed type identity as a contingent truth, as in the case of token identities: the identity holds at this world, and worlds like this one in respect of causal laws but in worlds in which different laws and causal relations obtain, M may have a different, perhaps a wholly disjoint, set of realizers, say Q_1, Q_2, . . ., and M = UQ at those worlds. Thus, "M", or "having M", is not a rigid designator; it refers to different properties in different worlds—to UP in this one, to UQ in certain other worlds, to UR in still others, and so on. To give a property designator a functional definition in terms of a causal specification is to make it nonrigid. M so defined is no longer a unitary property that can be tracked from world to world; "M" can designate one property in this world and a different property in another, and perhaps nothing at all in some worlds.

So should we go with M = UP? Accepting this identity would commit us to the token identity "*x*'s having M at *t* = *x*'s having UP at *t*". This contrasts with our earlier recommended token identity "*x*'s having M at *t* = *x*'s having P_k at *t*". Thus, the identification of M with the disjunction of its realizers at a world yields a competing token identity thesis, an alternative form of token reductionism. Which of these two token identity claims is preferable? We should remember that UP is, or can be, an extremely heterogeneous and unmanageably huge disjunction; this makes it unclear what causal-nomological import UP can have. Consider two properties, each with a specific set of causal powers, say having a temperature of 100° C. and having a mass of one kilogram. What causal powers are to be associated with the disjunctive property of *having a temperature of 100° C. or having a mass of one kilogram*? What causal powers does an object have in virtue of having this disjunctive property? It isn't clear what we should say. All we can say appears to be that if an object has this disjunctive property—that is, if it either has a temperature of 100° C. or has a mass of one kilogram—then it either has the causal powers associated with the temperature or those associated with the mass. The last "or" in the preceding sentence is sentence disjunction, not a special operator designating some kind of "disjunction" operation on properties.

[12] I have discussed this question elsewhere, in particular in Kim (1998). What I am going to say here is similar to what I have said before but not exactly identical.

That is, to say that something has causal powers C_1 or causal powers C_2 is to say only that either it has C_1 or it has C_2; there is no need to posit a disjunction of C_1 and C_2, which one might denote as $[C_1 \vee C_2]$, and say that the thing has this disjunctive causal power $[C_1 \vee C_2]$. If such disjunctions are to be posited, we will need an explanation of what the disjunctions stand for in terms of what each of their disjuncts stands for. But such an explanation is exactly something we don't have. In consequence, we are without an understanding of what causal powers are to be associated with disjunctive properties, or with their instances.

What this means is that if we identify *x*'s having M with *x*'s having UP, we are putting the causal status of *x*'s having M in jeopardy—or at least in a limbo; it seems that we can say nothing clear and motivated about what causal powers this token event should be credited with. In contrast, P_k is, by assumption, a specific causal-nomic property, and identifying *x*'s having M with its having P_k gives the M-instance robust causal reality and a specific causal profile. It seems to me that this is a sufficient reason for rejecting the proposal that we identify M with UP.

One might suggest that if something has the disjunctive property $[P_1 \vee P_2]$ in virtue of having P_1 (that is, the truthmaker of "*x* has $[P_1 \vee P_2]$" is "*x* has P_1"), we identify the causal power of *x*'s having $[P_1 \vee P_2]$ with the causal power of *x*'s having P_1. And likewise if *x* has $[P_1 \vee P_2]$ in virtue of having P_2. So, in the case of M, supposing that *x* has UP in virtue of having P_k, the suggestion is that we identify the causal powers of this instance of M with the causal powers associated with P_k. This means that if another thing *y* (this could be *x* at another time) has UP, *y*'s having UP may have causal powers quite diverse from those of *x*'s having UP. In consequence, UP fails to represent a uniform set of causal powers, and it seems to drop out of the picture in favor of its realizers. I think we might as well be straightforward and identify *x*'s having M at *t* with *x*'s having P_k at t, bypassing unwieldy disjunctions like UP.

For these reasons, we may set aside the possibility of identifying a functionally reduced property with the disjunction of its realizers. What then? I believe there are two other options to consider: what we may call *functional property realism* and *functional property conceptualism*. Let us begin with functional property realism (it corresponds to what some have called *role functionalism*). On this approach, if M is a functional property, with the kind of functional characterization as indicated earlier, M is a robust property in its own right with a clear identity as a unitary property from world to world. Take pain: being in pain is the property of being in some state with such-and-such input and such-and-such output conditions. This property has diverse realizers from world to world, from species to species, from an individual at one time to the same individual at another time, and so on. But it is a single, unitary property with its own integrity as a property; it's just that this one property has different realizers along various dimensions. The important thing to remember is that, on this view, the functional property only "has" realizers, and that it remains ontologically distinct from them, individually, taken in disjunctions, or whatever. Whence the name functional property *realism*.

Those who hold this view will reject the claim that functional reduction in our sense gives us reduction, since there is no physical property with which M can be identified. One mark of this is the fact that, on this view, "M" is a rigid designator which tracks the same nonphysical property world to world; in this way, the view contrasts with the disjunction approach (M = UP) earlier considered which makes "M" nonrigid. The position is strongly antireductionist with regard to psychological properties; its proponents include those, like the original functionalists such as Putnam and Fodor, who took functionalism as an essentially antireductionist and antiphysicalist view.[13]

I believe there are two plausible arguments against functional property realism, both of them based on causal considerations. The first argument goes like this: token reductionism we earlier recommended is highly plausible, but if token reductionism is true, functional property realism has little to recommend itself. We have already argued why token reductionism, of the sort we urged, should be accepted. So assume token reductionism. Functional property realism asserts that a functionally characterized property M is a real property in its own right. If so, it must represent a specific set of causal powers; in each world, M must confer on each and every object that has M some specific and uniform set of causal powers. (On some views, these causal powers go toward defining M; that is, they are constitutive of the very identity of M as a property.) If, as token reductionism claims, all actual and possible instances of M are instances of M's realizers, M cannot have causal powers that go beyond the causal powers of its diverse realizers; there are no new causal powers that M brings to the world other than those contributed by its realizers. This seriously undermines the claim that M is a genuine property in its own right, distinct from its physical realizers. At best, M's causal powers are going to be very diverse and heterogeneous—as diverse and heterogeneous as the causal powers of its many diverse realizers—whereas we would expect genuine properties to show at least a certain degree of nomological and causal unity.[14] M cannot be the kind of property in terms of which productive scientific theorizing could be conducted; M's causal profile is too heterogeneous and fragmented for it to be a projectible nomic property, the kind of property that can be considered a causally efficacious property on its own (Kim 1992; for replies see Block 1997, Fodor 1997). When M is invoked in a causal claim or explanation, this should be understood in terms of a tacit reference to a realizer of M which is doing the causal work.[15]

[13] Ross and Spurrett (forthcoming) are recent advocates of this version of functionalism; there are others, including Ned Block (I believe; see Block 1997). Also see McLaughlin (2006).

[14] I realize that I am here touching on some general issues about properties, causality, realization, and other related topics. They obviously require more extended discussion and consideration than what I can do here.

[15] That is, when we say "*x*'s having M caused E", we should be understood as saying something like "there is a realizer P of M such that *x* had M on this occasion in virtue of having P, and *x*'s having P caused E".

Invoking M rather than one of its realizers masks either our ignorance of the details of the situation or our laziness. Psychological properties on this view seem to form a badly gerrymandered taxonomy overlaid on the underlying domain of physical/biological properties.

The second causal argument against functional property realism is the familiar exclusion argument: if *x*'s having M at $t \neq$ *x*'s having P_k at *t*, where P_k is M's realizer on this occasion, the M-instance's causal role is threatened with preemption by the P_k-instance, or else we would have a case of spurious causal overdetermination (Kim 1998; see also McLaughlin 2006 for recent discussion). To insist on M as a real property only to have its causal status undermined and usurped by its realizers, anywhere and everywhere it is instantiated, should strike as an empty and futile gesture. Since the basic considerations on the exclusion argument are well known, there is no need to rehearse them here. I believe that all these considerations should convince us that functional property realism is untenable, or at least highly problematic.

We now turn to functional property conceptualism, our final option on the status of functional properties. The proposal is that we should take the causal and nomological disunity of the functionalized M seriously and abandon M as a genuine, unitary property. Ned Block once asked what all pains have in common in virtue of which they are instances of pain (Block 1980). If pain is a functional property definable in terms of physical inputs and behavioral outputs and realized in many diverse neural/biological/physical structures, then what all pain instances have in common is merely the fact that they all fall under the *concept* of pain as given by its functional characterization—no more and no less. That is to say, pains are pains because they conform to the definition of pain, not because they all share some hidden essence, like C-fiber stimulation or a pain quale. So there is the concept of pain, a concept given by its functional definition, but no property of pain, or being pain, that all pain instances have in common. There simply is no property in the world with causal and nomological unity required of genuine properties which answers to our concept of pain, and which is shared by all instances of pain (pains in humans, pains in reptiles, pains in Martians, and the rest). More generally, psychological functionalism may be characterized as the view that *psychological kinds have no real essences, only nominal essences.* (If you feel that this doesn't do full justice to pain, and that there obviously is a genuine property there—well, all pains hurt!—you would reject the functionalization of pain. Remember our question is this: What happens to pain, as a kind or property, if it has been functionally reduced?)

This option may sound like a form of eliminativism, and perhaps rightly so. M as a property is gone; it has been eliminated. It remains true that, in Smart's idiom, M as a property is nothing "over and above" its realizing properties for the trivial reason that M *is* nothing. If mental properties are functionally reduced, we may well have to live with mental eliminativism and irrealism.[16] But note a couple of things. First, M as a concept stays, and individual instances falling under M are perfectly legitimate entities with causal-explanatory efficacy. The situation with the mental eliminativism of the sort advocated by Paul Churchland (1981) is quite different: as I take it, Churchland's eliminative materialism discards psychological concepts—the concepts of propositional attitudes, like those of belief, desire, and intention—as well as psychological states and properties. The concept of belief suffers the same fate that befell the concepts of phlogiston and caloric fluid. Second, we should remember that functionalism about the mind as originally formulated by Hilary Putnam (1967) was a thesis not about mental states or properties but about psychological predicates and concepts. Putnam's seminal 1967 paper, which first introduced psychological functionalism, carried the title "Psychological Predicates", which later took an ontological turn and became "The Nature of Mental States". It shouldn't surprise us that functional reduction of the mental, at least on one reading, ends up not as a reduction of mental properties but as a thesis about mental concepts.

We have reviewed three ways of dealing with psychological properties in functional reduction, the disjunction approach, functional property realism, and functional property conceptualism. I believe that reasons for rejecting the first are quite compelling, and that there are nearly as compelling reasons for rejecting the second. The third smacks of psychological antirealism and, for that reason, is not very appealing. But it seems to me that it is the best of the unappetizing lot, the only one that is free of major philosophical difficulties. I am willing to admit that this whole scene may well be worth revisiting and reconsidering.

V

To conclude, I have argued three main points. First, bridge-law reductions deliver neither reductions nor reductive explanations. The source of the trouble is the use of bridge laws, construed as empirical and contingent, as unexplained, unreduced auxiliary premises of reductive derivations. Second, identity reductions, in which bridge laws are replaced by identities, give us reductions but no reductive explanations. Rather, such reductions eliminate the need for—indeed, the possibility of—such explanations. Instead of "closing" the explanatory gap, reductions of this type imply that no such gaps exist in the first place. That is a perfectly effective way of dealing with the supposed explanatory gap problem. Finally, I argued that functional reductions give us reductive explanations of the sort we expect and help close the gap, and that it arguably gives us reductions as well, though there remains room for further debate as to the exact nature of the reductions involved.

[16] Terry Horgan, I believe, was the first to remind me of this possible implication of functional reduction.

What our discussion makes clear is that as far as reduction goes, nothing beats identities. That appropriate identities achieve reduction is intuitively obvious and beyond any philosophical second thoughts. That, unsurprisingly, is the chief attraction of the psychoneural identity theory as a form of reductionist physicalism. Unsurprisingly again, the main issue about the reductive significance of functional reduction comes down to the question whether and how functional reduction can yield appropriate identities, for psychological properties/kinds and their instances. All this goes toward reconfirming the point, perhaps an obvious one when we think about it, that identities are absolutely central to reduction.[17] Finally, we should note that in this paper we have not touched on the important question whether or not reductionism of either form can be plausibly held—that is, the question whether and how we may earn our entitlement to psychoneural identities or to the functional definability of mental kinds and properties.[18]

REFERENCES

Block, Ned (1980). "Introduction: What is Functionalism?" in *Readings in Philosophy of Psychology*, vol. i, ed. Ned Block, Cambridge, Mass.: Harvard University Press.

—— (1997). "Antireductionism Slaps Back", *Philosophical Perspectives* 11: 107–32.

—— (forthcoming). "Functional Reduction".

—— and Robert Stalnaker (1999). "Conceptual Analysis, Dualism, and the Explanatory Gap", *Philosophical Review* 108: 1–46.

Causey, Robert (1972). "Attribute Identities in Microreductions", *Journal of Philosophy* 69: 407–22.

Chalmers, David J. (1996). *The Conscious Mind*, Oxford: Oxford University Press.

Churchland, Paul M. (1981). "Eliminative Materialism and the Propositional Attitudes", *Journal of Philosophy* 78: 67–90.

Davdison, Donald (1970). "Mental Events", repr. in Davidson, *Essays on Actions and Events*, Oxford: Oxford University Press, 1980.

Feigl, Herbert (1958). "The 'Mental' and the 'Physical'", *Minnesota Studies in the Philosophy of Science* 2, 370–497.

—— (1967). "Postscript after Ten Years", in Herbert Feigl, *The "Mental" and the "Physical": The Essay and a Postscript*, Minneapolis: University of Minnesota Press.

Fodor, Jerry A. (1974). "Special Sciences—the Disunity of Science as a Working Hypothesis", *Synthese* 28: 97–115.

—— (1997) "Special Sciences: Still Autonomous after All These Years", *Philosophical Perspectives* 11: 149–63.

Gillett, Carl (forthcoming). "Understanding the New Reductionism: The Metaphysics of Science and Compositional Reduction", *Journal of Philosophy*.

Hill, Christopher (1991). *Sensations*, Cambridge: Cambridge University Press.

[17] Carl Gillett defends the view that compositional relations, rather than identities, are fundamental to much scientific reduction (Gillett, forthcoming).

[18] For further discussion see Block and Stalnaker (1999), Kim (2005), and Block (forthcoming).

Horgan, Terence (1996). "Kim on the Mind-Body Problem", *British Journal for the Philosophy of Science* 47: 579–607.

Kim, Jaegwon (1972). "Phenomenal Properties, Psychophysical Laws, and the Identity Theory", *The Monist* 56: 177–92. Excerpted in *Readings in Philosophy of Psychology*, vol. i, ed. Ned Block, Cambridge, Mass.: Harvard University Press, 1980.

—— (1992). "Multiple Realization and the Metaphysics of Reduction", repr. in Kim, *Supervenience and Mind*, Cambridge: Cambridge University Press, 1993.

—— (1998). *Mind in a Physical World*, Cambridge, Mass.: MIT Press.

—— (2005). *Physicalism, or Something Near Enough*, Princeton: Princeton University Press.

Levine, Joseph (1983). "Materialism and Qualia: the Explanatory Gap", *Pacific Philosophical Quarterly* 64: 354–61.

Lewis, David (1980). "Mad Pains and Martian Pains", *Readings in Philosophy of Psychology*, vol. i, ed. Ned Block, Cambridge, Mass.: Harvard University Press.

McLaughlin, Brian (2001). "In Defense of New-Wave Materialism", in *Physicalism and Its Discontents*, ed. Carl Gillett and Barry Loewer, Cambridge: Cambridge University Press.

—— (2006). "Is Role-Functionalism Committed to Epiphenomenalism?" *Journal of Consciousness Studies* 13: 39–66.

Nagel, Ernest (1961). *The Structure of Science*, Harcourt, Brace and World, New York.

—— (1970). "Issues in the Logic of Reductive Explanations", in Nagel, *Teleology Revisited*, New York: Columbia University Press, 1979.

Putnam, Hilary (1967). "Psychological Predicates", repr. under the title "The Nature of Mental States" in Putnam, *Mind, Language, and Reality: Philosophical Papers*, vol. ii (Cambridge: Cambridge University Press, 1979). Also reprinted in numerous anthologies, e.g., *Philosophy of Mind: Classical and Contemporary Readings*, ed. David J. Chalmers, Oxford: Oxford University Press, 2002.

Ross, Don, and David Spurrett (forthcoming). "What to Say to a Skeptical Metaphysician: A Defense Manual for Cognitive and Behavioral Scientists", *Behavioral and Brain Sciences*.

Sklar, Lawrence (1967). "Types of Intertheoretic Reduction", *British Journal for the Philosophy of Science* 18: 109–24.

Smart, J. J. C. (1959). "Sensations and Brain Processes", *Philosophical Review* 68: 141–56. Repr. in numerous anthologies, e.g., *Philosophy of Mind: A Guide and Anthology*, ed. John Heil, Oxford: Oxford University Press, 2004.

6

CP Laws, Reduction, and Explanatory Pluralism

Peter Lipton

Scientific descriptions are pitched at different levels. Some of these levels line up in an intuitive hierarchy, where one level is 'macro' relative to another that is 'micro'. The relationships between macro and micro include whole to parts, entity to constituents, and functional property to realisations. Many scientific explanations remain at a single level, but some cross levels. Reductive explanations, in particular, may be the explanations of macro effects in terms of micro causes.

There is a natural line of thought to the conclusion that reductive explanations are better than explanations that remain entirely at the macro level. There are reasons to think that even if the laws of nature at the micro level are strict, at the macro level all we have are hedged or cp (*ceteris paribus*) laws, and that cp laws do not support good explanations, or at least not as good as the explanations that are available at a level ruled by strict laws. In this essay I explore this line of thought and conclude in favour of explanatory pluralism. CP laws may underwrite good explanations, and the best explanation may be macro, reductive or micro, depending on the question and the context.

I begin by exploring two good reasons for the claim that macro laws are cp laws. One is Jerry Fodor's argument from multiple realisation; the other is Hempel's argument from provisos. These features also underwrite a kind of anti-reductionism, a rejection of the view that macro laws can be replaced by micro laws. I then consider the relationship between reduction and reductive explanation. In the last part of this essay, I attempt to defend cp laws from the claim that they suffer from various liabilities that preclude them from supporting good scientific explanations. In particular, I focus on the two objections that cp laws may fail to provide good explanations because they are contingent, and because they miss out causes.

I am grateful to the other participants in the 2005 NAMICONA Conference on Reductive Explanation in Aarhus, Denmark for their responses to the talk that was the precursor of this chapter and to the editors of this volume for comments on a draft.

MULTIPLE REALISATION AND PROVISOS

In a seminal discussion, Jerry Fodor (1974) showed how multiple realisation leads both to anti-reductionism and to the view that macro laws are cp laws. The multiple realisation idea is that although macro properties may be realised by micro properties, different instantiations of the same macro property may be realised by different micro properties. To use Fodor's example, while each macro monetary exchange has a physical (even if only electronic) micro manifestation, different monetary exchanges of the same monetary type will be very different physically. Sciences at different levels are dividing the same world up in different ways, and the relationship between macro properties and corresponding micro property will generally be one–many.

On a strong reading, reduction requires that macro properties can be identified with micro properties, and macro laws replaced by micro laws. On this reading, multiple realisation immediately entails anti-reductionism, since what reduction requires is precisely what multiple realisation denies, namely that each macro property correspond to the same micro property or cluster of micro properties. Here the model might be the identity of water with H2O: this is the kind of one-to-one matching that typically does not obtain between macro properties—properties like that of being a monetary exchange—and micro physical properties.

Multiple realisation also both explains why we might expect macro laws to be cp laws, even if the micro laws are all strict, and helps to clarify what cp lawhood comprises. Consider the property that figures in the antecedent of a macro law. Where multiple realisation applies, this will correspond to a disjunction of micro properties. The same holds for the macro consequent property. So the macro law corresponds to a large set of micro conditionals, each linking one of the realisations of the macro antecedent to one or more of the realisations of the macro consequent. Fodor plausibly suggests, however, that we would have to be lucky for every actual and possible antecedent realiser to yield a consequent realiser. What is more likely is that some antecedent realisers will be 'isolated', failing to cause a consequent realiser. This may happen generally for this realiser type, so that it never causes the consequence property, or just sometimes, because this realiser is particularly susceptible to interference, blocking the expression of the consequent property (Roberts 2004). And where there are isolated realisers, the macro law will have exceptions: it will only hold cp.

Thus multiple realisation supports both anti-reductions and the cp character of macro laws. And if macro laws are cp laws (and micro laws are taken to be strict), this provides an additional argument for anti-reductionism. For if macro and micro properties lined up as reduction requires, and the micro laws are strict, then macro laws would turn out to be strict as well: they would inherit the strictness of the micro laws that undergird them. So reduction must fail.

We can also get to anti-reductionism and to macro cp laws from a different though related starting point: provisos (cf. Earman and Roberts 1999). In Carl Hempel's (1988) account, provisos are a particular kind of presuppositions of theoretical inference, needed to make deductive contact between theory and prediction. To use his gravitational example, the Newtonian theory, along with relevant information about masses, motions, and positions at one time does not alone permit the deduction of positions and motion at any other time, for the simple reason that the theory says nothing about non-gravitational forces. To secure the inference requires a proviso to the effect that in the case in question no such forces are in play. As Hempel explains, provisos are a kind of assumption of completeness in a particular case, an assumption that the theory in use is not leaving anything out. Provisos are thus contingent claims about particular situations to the effect that there are no forces or factors in play other than those the theory describes, a claim that the theory itself does not make. They are thus in a way like initial conditions, but of a highly theoretical sort: they speak of forces, not of positions, masses and velocities.

Although it shares the focus on additional premises, as Hempel points out the provisos point is not the same as the familiar Quine–Duhem thesis (Duhem 1914, ch. 6; Quine 1951) that deductive falsification of a hypothesis is not in general possible because of the need for background hypotheses. For provisos are not general background hypotheses but specific and contingent claims of completeness or absence of additional factors in a particular case. Hempel's point is also different from Putnam's (1975) appeal to auxiliary premises. Putnam is here indeed discussing provisos, but his point is that they are often known to be false: we know that there really are other forces present but we decide that they can be ignored. Hempel is making a different point. He is happy to suppose that the requisite provisos are true; his emphases are rather on their particular and contingent character, and on the fact that they often can only be expressed in a theoretical vocabulary.

There is one more contrast that it is useful to draw here, and that is with cp laws. For although the need for provisos is closely related to the existence of cp laws, Hempel's case for provisos does not rest on a claim that laws are cp. The gravitational example shows this, since gravitational laws are strict, yet a proviso is still required in order to apply them. Moreover, whereas in the case of cp laws there is often a difficulty in specifying just when the generalisation holds—otherwise presumably the generalisation could be made strict by building the exception specification into its antecedent—Hempel's case does not rest on the inexpressibility of the proviso's content. As he observes, Newton's second law $f=ma$ is a law governing total and not just gravitational force, so the proviso can be expressed within the Newtonian vocabulary by means of the claim that the total force is the same as the gravitational force.

The need for Hempelian provisos provides another route to anti-reductionism. For if, as Hempel suggests, provisos can often only be expressed in the macro vocabulary, then it will not be possible to replace the macro theory with a micro theory: the need for macro talk will persist. This route to anti-reduction does not overtly appeal to multiple realisation, since even if it were possible to identify every macro property in a theory with a micro property, the ineliminability of macro predicates in provisos would still block a strong reduction. One way of thinking about it is this. Even if the macro laws were replaceable by means of property identification to micro laws, the application of the theory requires provisos, so if these must be framed in macro properties, the application of theory has not left the macro level behind. Admittedly, this is only so if the macro predicates needed in the provisos are different from those in the macro theory: otherwise the presumed identification of the macro properties in the theory would also obviate the need to appeal to macro properties in the provisos. But it does seem that the macro properties needed in provisos will indeed sometimes fall outside the properties to which the theory itself appeals, since the function of provisos is precisely to certify the absence of forces that the theory does not address. This is not the case in Hempel's Newtonian example, since the second law addresses all forces, not just the gravitational force, but it appears that it will be the case for many other theories.

As I have emphasised, one of the interesting aspects of provisos is that they are required for the application of theory, even when the laws in the theory are strict. But the need for provisos also provides a route to the conclusion that macro laws will tend to be cp laws (cf. Earman and Roberts 1999, 447). For even if the micro laws are strict, they will require provisos in order to recover the macro regularities. The intuitive idea is that the macro laws correspond to a package consisting of both micro laws and provisos: the macro laws have those provisos 'built in'. (Though the macro laws may be associated with additional, external provisos when they are applied as well.) But provisos are *contingent*, and this means that the macro laws that depend on them will themselves have actual or possible exceptions: they will be cp laws.

Neither multiple realisation nor the typical need for provisos strictly entails that a given macro law must be a cp law. For it might be that, in the case of a particular macro law, although properties it cites are multiply realised at the micro level, there are no isolated antecedent realisers. And it might be that, in a particular case, a macro regularity is fixed by strict micro laws without the need to build in any contingent provisos. But it does seem that these conditions will seldom if ever be satisfied, so these two routes—from multiple realisation and from provisos—do take us naturally to the view that macro laws are cp laws. Moreover, in addition to providing a reason to hold that macro laws will at least tend to be cp laws, these conditions help to explain why this is the case. For they locate two sources for the contingency that cp laws suffer and strict laws avoid. The first is the contingency of the way the macro antecedent property is realised in particular cases; the second is the contingency of the absence of disturbing forces, the absence vouchsafed by the contingent proviso.

The two routes also give us two different pictures of what a cp law comprises. One picture is that a cp law is a description of how things would behave if only one force were in play in a world with many forces (cf. Lipton 1999). In the case of a specific force law, such as Newton's gravitational law, it may be strict. But if the law describes behaviour, such as the movement of the planets, then it will be a cp law, since the inference from the force law to the behaviour depends on those contingent, specific provisos. Multiple realisation gives us a different picture. Here the law has exceptions not because of the possibility of additional forces, but because of an isolated realiser: there are some possible instances of the antecedent macro property that just don't have the power that the other realisations enjoy. So we could speak of two kinds of cp laws here, though two aspects would probably be a better way of putting it, since a single macro law will probably have both features. Although it may only be an analogy, perhaps it is helpful here to consider the generalisation that birds fly. One kind of exception are birds whose wings have been clipped; another are penguins. The first case corresponds to the failure of a proviso; the second to an isolated realiser.

REDUCTIVE EXPLANATION AND CP LAWS

Whether we start with multiple realisation or with provisos, we end up with the same package: macro cp laws and anti-reductionism. This could be bad news. The fact that the macro laws are only cp laws may suggest that macro explanations are not much good, so they need to be reductively replaced by micro explanations that invoke strict micro laws; but anti-reductionism rules this out. We will shortly consider whether cp laws really are an explanatory liability, but first we have to clarify what anti-reductionism does and does not rule out. For 'reductive explanation' can mean different things, and not all of them are ruled out by the anti-reductionism that multiple realisation and provisos support.

Presumably not every explanation couched in micro terms counts as a reductive explanation: there must be some relation to the macro realm. But there are many different relations possible. It could be a translation of a macro explanation into a corresponding micro explanation, by means of property by property identities. But a reductive explanation might rather involve giving the micro constitution of a macro phenomenon. Or it might involve giving the micro mechanism that underlies a macro process. Here the macro explanation is not replaced but complemented. The macro explanation gives the why, and the micro explanation gives the how. As Fodor puts it, 'the point of reduction is *not* primarily to find some natural kind predicate of physics coextensive with each kind predicate of a special science. It is, rather, to explicate the physical mechanisms whereby events conform to the laws of the special sciences' (1974, 435). We may also think about reductive explanations that straddle the micro–macro divide, by giving micro causes of macro phenomena: we explain macro phenomena in micro terms.

The anti-reductionism that multiple realisation and provisos support is thus compatible with several forms of reductive explanation. One way of putting it is that not all reductive explanations require reduction. Thus multiple realisation and the need for provisos are both compatible with giving explanatory micro causes of macro phenomena. Particular realisations of the antecedent property of a macro cp law may explain particular instantiations of the consequent macro property. And the need for provisos couched in the macro vocabulary is again compatible with the specification of micro causes and micro mechanisms. Various types of reductive explanation are thus available in the context of cp laws. My remaining question, then, is whether macro cp laws have an explanatory liability that such reductive explanations would resolve.

The putative liabilities of cp laws are diverse. Four concern content, deduction, contingency, and causation. The content worry is that cp sentences have no empirical content, because to say that all Fs are G, cp is only to say, disappointingly, that all Fs are G except those that aren't. The deduction worry is that, even if cp laws do have empirical content, they will not support deductive explanations, since the fact that all Fs are G, cp and that this is an F does not entail that this is a G. The contingency worry is that cp statements are not really laws and therefore do not really explain, because they lack the nomological necessity of true laws that scientific explanation requires. Finally, there are worries about causes. At the extreme, one might worry that cp statements do not give causes at all. This worry might be motivated by a Humean conception linking cause with constant conjunction, since the cp law is not a fully constant conjunction: it has exceptions. Less extremely, even if a cp law does give some causal information, it does not give the 'full cause'. And even if one does not hold that explanation requires a full cause, one may worry that cp laws suffer an explanatory liability on this front because they may not even give the 'dominant' cause (Earman and Roberts 1999, 451–2).

I will not consider here the vexed question of the semantics of cp sentences, except to suggest that the route from multiple realisation and provisos to cp laws seems to help both to assuage the worry that cp sentences have no content and to clarify in what that content consists. Nor will I dwell on the deduction worry, except to say that although a deduction from a cp law on its own will not go through, the addition of a proviso may permit a deductive explanation, and anyway explanation does not require deduction. Many good causal explanations, even in science, fail to meet that standard. But I do want to say a little more about the worries over contingency and missing causes.

CONTINGENCY AND MISSING CAUSES

Multiple realisation and provisos are signs of contingency in cp laws. In the case of multiple realisation, where there are isolated realisers, then even if this F is a G, it might not have been, because this F might have had a different realisation by an isolated realiser and so not been a G. As for provisos, they are themselves contingent, so insofar as there is a proviso built into a cp law, that law will also be contingent. There might have been other forces in play. And it is anyway independently plausible that cp laws have a kind of contingency that strict laws avoid. One familiar symptom of the necessity of strict laws is that they, unlike accidental generalisations, entail corresponding counterfactuals. Thus if it is a law that all Fs are G, then not only are all Fs in fact G, but if this non-F had been an F, it would have been a G too. Cp laws do not support counterfactuals in this way, for even if it is a law that all Fs are G, cp, it does not follow that if this non-F had been an F, it would have been a G. Perhaps it would have been an exception instead (Lipton 1999). Given how rarely if ever all else is equal for some cp laws, the nearest world where there is an additional F may well be one where it is not G.

The contingency of cp laws and hence of the putative explanations that rely on them raise two questions. The first is whether the contingency could be avoided by moving to the micro level. The answer appears to be that while the contingency of laws might be thus avoided, the contingency of explanation would remain. The contingency of laws that arises from isolated realisers could be eliminated by going down to a level where the laws are expressed in terms of particular realisers that are not isolated. And, as we have seen, the need for provisos does not in itself show that a law cannot be strict or necessary, so this does not preclude necessity in the micro laws either. But the need for provisos does appear to show that contingency applies to micro explanations, since those explanations will depend on the laws and the provisos together, not the laws alone.

So the answer to the first question seems to be that contingency in explanation cannot be eliminated by moving to the micro level, at least insofar as the micro laws, strict and necessary though they may be in themselves, require provisos to be applied in explanation. The second question is whether contingency in cp laws is an explanatory liability. It is not clear that it is. After all, there is contingency in all singular causal explanations, since even if the law is strict, presence of the cause will be contingent. And insofar as the phenomenon to be explained is itself contingent, one would expect the explanation to be contingent as well.

Indeed contingency can be seen as an explanatory virtue. Not all causes make a difference, because of the possibility of overdetermination. But a good causal explanation should cite a cause that does make a difference, something without which the effect would not have occurred. And this suggests that in a good causal explanation it must make sense to suppose that the cause did not occur, which is to suppose a kind of contingency.

In this respect micro explanations are sometimes worse than macro explanations. One way this may happen is because they may suggest a misleading contingency that is avoided by keeping explanation at the macro level. To use Alan Garfinkel's example, we can explain why a rabbit was eaten by a fox by citing the high fox population, along with the Lotka–Volterra cp law in ecology giving the dynamics of predator–prey populations, a macro explanation. Alternatively we could explain the death of this rabbit by specifying the location of the guilty fox just before he pounced, a micro explanation (Garfinkel 1981, ch. 2; cf. also Jackson and Pettit 1990). As Garfinkel observes, the micro explanation has a peculiar liability that the macro population explanation avoids, a problem that arises from overdetermination at the micro level. The problem is that, given that the fox population was high, if that fox had not eaten the rabbit, another fox probably would have. The micro explanation falsely suggests that the rabbit's death was contingent on the location of that particular fox, when it wasn't. The explanation in terms of the high fox population, by contrast exhibits a genuine and virtuous contingency, since if the fox population had been lower, the rabbit would probably have survived.

CP laws do encode a kind of contingency that is absent from strict laws, but that contingency does not in itself preclude good explanation, because explanatory causes typically exhibit just the same kind of contingency. And macro explanations may have explanatory virtues that a corresponding reductive explanation would lack. This may be so because there is overdetermination at the micro level that compromises explanation, as we have just seen with the fox and the rabbit. This overdetermination can itself be seen as a form of multiple realisation. There are many micro ways a rabbit can be eaten, by this fox, by that one, or by a third. This form of multiple realisation makes possible a kind of overdetermination that compromises the micro explanation, a liability the macro explanation avoids.

Multiple realisation is also the source of another potential explanatory advantage of macro explanation, an advantage of generality and unification. Realising causes that are unrelated at the micro level are tied together at the macro level, and displaying this unity often provides an explanatory benefit that the contingency of the macro laws does not compromise. Consider the question of why the same side of the moon always faces the earth. This phenomenon ought to be surprising, since it requires that the period of moon's orbit around the earth be exactly the same as the period of the moon's spin around itself, yet these two periods appear completely uncoupled. (As you can ascertain with any two handy objects on your desk, or indeed with your fists: if the moon were not spinning, the side facing the earth would be constantly changing.) A lovely macro explanation of this phenomenon is that the moon is not a perfect sphere but slightly oblong, and whenever its long axis does not point exactly towards the centre of the earth there will be a net restoring gravitational force, twisting it into line, since the pull on the far end of the moon will perforce be somewhat less than the pull on the near end. This explanation in terms of the overall shape of the moon could in principle be replaced by a micro explanation in terms of the details of the distribution of tiny mass segments that make up the moon, but this would entail an explanatory loss of generality, since the macro explanation accounts for the fact that synchronised orbits are in fact typical of satellites or planets that are close to their primary.

I do not wish to give the impression that macro explanations are always superior to their micro reductive explanatory counterparts. It all depends, and one of the things it depends upon is the fine structure of the why-question being asked. One aspect of this fine-structure is the contrastive form of many why-questions. We ask not simply 'Why this?' but 'Why this rather than that?', where the choice of foil helps to determine what would count as a good explanation (Garfinkel 1981, ch. 1; Lipton 2004, ch. 3). Thus while my musical tastes might explain why I went to see Bob Dylan rather than Yo Yo Ma last night, they do not explain why I went to see Bob Dylan rather than staying at home. And sometimes the choice of foil will favour a micro explanation. Thus, as Garfinkel observes, although the high fox population gives the better answer to the question of why that rabbit died at that time rather than surviving, it is the appeal to micro facts about the movements of the guilty fox that explains why the rabbit died at that time rather than at another time.

Macro phenomena are governed by cp laws: these laws are contingent and have exceptions. As we have seen, however, that does not prevent them from supporting good explanations where they do apply, and indeed sometimes those explanations are preferable to the micro explanations governed by strict laws that might in principle replace them. But what about the exceptional cases, where things are not cp? These arise because of isolated realisers and because of the violation of provisos. In these cases the explanatory limitations of cp laws seem clear: surely a law that says what happens when all things are equal does not explain what happens when things are not equal. But this seems to me a mistake.

Many cp laws can be seen as describing one force in a world of many forces. And many provisos can be seen as saying that, in a particular situation, one force is the only one in play. But causal explanations never describe all the causes of the phenomenon being explained, so the cp law may perform an explanatory function even when other forces are in play, that is even where the cp clause is not satisfied. Indeed the cause given by the cp law need not even be the main or 'dominant' cause, because it is not always the dominant cause that explains. In the case of contrastive explanation, for example, what counts is not how dominant the cause is, but whether it 'makes a difference' between the fact and foil. Consider the fact that there are cats' eyes marking the lanes on

British roads. Why is this? Presumably the dominant cause is something like the fact that they significantly reduce accidents. Another cause, though surely not the dominant cause, is that it snows very little in Britain, since the use of cats' eyes precludes the use of snowplows, because of the way they stick up out of the road surface. Yet if the contrastive question is why there are cats' eyes in Britain but not in Denmark, then a good answer is that there is little snow in Britain.

So it is not the case that cp laws only explain in situations where all else is equal: their scope is substantially wider than this. For even where all else is not equal, and we have what is strictly an exception to the cp law, the cp law may still provide an explanatory cause. And that may be so even when it is not the dominant cause. In other cases, to be sure, the exception is not explained by the rule, and what does the explanatory work is information about the interference that prevents the expected effect from coming off, the perturbation that modifies the result, and so on. Here micro causes are often what is required, since the macro theory does not have the conceptual resources to describe the nature of the interference. Thus while the normal operation of a computer may be explained at a macro computational level, its failure to run may need to be explained in terms of a broken wire. The same often applies when it comes to giving the detailed mechanism that underlies the macro activity: this 'how' of the mechanism can only be described at the micro level. Macro and micro explanation often complement each other.

In this essay I have tried to get a little clearer on how, in different ways, both the facts of multiple realisation and the need for provisos make a case for cp laws at the macro level and for the impossibility of reducing macro theories to strict micro laws. Multiple realisation, laws, reduction: this is metaphysics. I've gone on to consider what the metaphysical picture tells us about the forms that scientific explanation should take. And here the main moral is: not much. For on the one hand, the impossibility of micro reduction does not preclude explaining macro phenomena in micro terms; and on the other hand the cp status of macro cp laws does not preclude their use in explanation. A good scientific explanation sometimes requires macro causes, sometimes micro causes, and sometimes a combination of the two. When it comes to scientific explanation, we should be pluralists.

REFERENCES

Duhem, P. (1914). *The Aim and Structure of Physical Theory*, New York: Antheneum (1954).

Earman, J. and Roberts, J. (1999). '*Ceteris Paribus*, There is No Problem of Provisos', *Synthese* 118, 439–78.

Fodor, J. (1974). 'Special Sciences, or The Disunity of Science as a Working Hypothesis', *Synthese* 28, 77–115. Repr. in R. Boyd, P. Gasper and J. D. Trout (eds.), *The Philosophy of Science* (Cambridge, Mass.: MIT, 1991), 429–41. Pagination from reprint.

Garfinkel, A. (1981). *Forms of Explanation*, New Haven: Yale University Press.

Hempel, C. (1988). 'Provisos: A Problem Concerning the Inferential Function of Scientific Theories', *Erkenntnis* 28, 147–64.

Jackson, F. and Pettit, P. (1990). 'Program Explanation: A General Perspective', *Analysis* 50, 107–17.

Lipton, P. (1999). 'All Else Being Equal', *Philosophy* 74, 155–68.

—— (2004). *Inference to the Best Explanation*, London: Routledge.

Putnam, H. (1975). 'The "Corroboration" of Theories', in his *Mathematics, Matter, and Method*, Cambridge: Cambridge University Press, 250–69.

Quine, W. V. O. (1951). 'Two Dogmas of Empiricism', *Philosophical Review* 60, 20–43.

Roberts, J. T. (2004). 'There are no Laws of the Social Sciences', in C. Hitchcock (ed.), *Contemporary Debates in Philosophy of Science*, Oxford: Blackwell.

7

Must a Physicalist be a Microphysicalist?

David Papineau

1. INTRODUCTION

I take myself to be a physicalist. I hold that all facts, including such prima facie non-physical facts as mental and biological facts, metaphysically supervene on the physical facts.

However, I do not have any views about the relationship between macroscopic and microscopic facts. I am neutral on such questions as whether big things are always made of small things.

Recently I have become worried about this combination of views. This is because many other philosophers seem to think of physicalism as some kind of commitment to the primacy of the microscopic. In their view, physicalism doesn't just say that everything is physical. It also says that everything is *micro*scopically determined.

Here are some representative quotations:

[Physicalism is] the doctrine that actually (but not necessarily) everything non-microphysical is composed out of microphysical entities and is governed by microphysical laws (Pettit 1994, 253; see also Pettit 1993).

Any thing of any level except the lowest must possess a decomposition into things belonging to the next lower level. In this sense each level, will be as it were a 'common denominator' for the level immediately above it (Oppenheim and Putnam 1958).

The bottom level is usually thought to consist of elementary particles, or whatever our best physics is going to tell us are the basic bits of matter out of which

Versions of this chapter were read at the NAMICONA conference in Aarhus in May 2004, the Kline Colloquium in Columbia in November 2004, and in King's College London in January 2007. I would like to thank all those who made comments on those occasions, incuding Tim Crane, Helen Beebee, Frank Jackson, Peter Menzies, Philip Pettit, Barry Loewer, Keith Allen, Jennifer Hornsby, Richard Samuels, and Gabriel Segal.

all material things are composed. As we go up the ladder, we successively encounter atoms, molecules, cells, larger living organisms, and so on. The ordering relation that generates the hierarchical structure is the mereological (part–whole) relation: entities belonging to a given level, except those at the very bottom, have an exhaustive decomposition, without remainder, into entities belonging to the lower levels (Kim 1998).

[Physicalism requires] a *mereological structure*, ordered by the part–whole relation . . . (Schaffer 2003).

Perhaps I have been missing something. Despite my lack of interest in the issue, maybe physicalism does entail that everything is microphysically determined.

But there is another possibility. Perhaps there are two separable theses associated with physicalism, and the philosophers just quoted are unjustifiably running them together. This is what I shall argue in this paper. I shall distinguish physicalism per se from a further thesis about microphysical determination, and I shall argue that these two theses are independent. Physicalists don't have to be Microphysicalists.[1]

2. TWO THESES

Let me start with what I take to be the basic content of physicalism.

(P) All facts metaphysically supervene on the physical facts.

For clarity, I shall capitalize this thesis henceforth as 'Physicalism'.

Now consider this further claim about the nature of the physical facts themselves.

(M) All physical facts metaphysically supervene on the microphysical facts.

I shall call this thesis 'Physical Microscopism'.

On the surface, it certainly looks as if these two theses could be independent. Physicalism is a doctrine about the relationship between prima facie non-physical things and physical things. It says that the mental, biological, meteorological and other prima facie non-physical things—that is, those things that can be directly identified using mental, biological, meteorological and other non-physical vocabulary—are not in fact ontologically distinct from physical things. Physicalism thus tells us how prima facie non-physical realms relate to the physical realm.

Physical Microscopism, by contrast, doesn't say anything about the relationship between the physical and other realms. Rather it is a doctrine about how things

[1] The distinction between Physicalism and Microphysicalism was originally defended in Hüttemann and Papineau 2005. Here I want to revisit some of the issues raised in that earlier paper.

go *within* physics itself. It says that all physical facts are fixed by microphysical facts. It doesn't say anything about prima facie non-physical things.[2]

The theses expressed in the quotations above can be viewed as the *conjunction* of Physicalism and Physical Microscopism. Let us define 'Microphysicalism' as the thesis that

(A) All the facts metaphysically supervene on the microphysical facts.

Microphysicalism so defined is equivalent to the conjunction of (P) and (M).

To verify this equivalence, note first that, if (P) everything supervenes on physical facts and (M) all physical facts supervene on microphysical facts, then (A) everything supervenes on microphysical facts, by the transitivity of supervenience. Conversely, if (A) everything supervenes on microphysical facts, then immediately (M) everything *physical* supervenes on microphysical facts, and also (P) anything prima facie non-physical supervenes on microphysical facts and so a fortiori on physical facts.

The Microphysicalist doctrines quoted above are thus committed to the conjunction of Physicalism and Physical Microscopism.[3] By the same coin, there are philosophers who *deny* both Physicalism and Physical Microscopism. Not only do they defend the traditional dualist view that non-physical realms like the mental are ontologically separate from the physical realm, but they also maintain holist doctrines about the physical realm itself, insisting that certain kinds of physical wholes are metaphysically more than the sum of their microphysical parts. (Thus Crane and Mellor's influential 'There is No Question of Physicalism' (1990) defends a version of this extreme anti-Microphysicalism.)

However, I shall be arguing that it is not mandatory to tie Physicalism to Physical Microscopism in this way. By way of preliminary support for this claim, note that the other two combinations of assertion and denial of Physicalism and Physical Microscopism also make perfectly good initial sense.

Thus there is the possibility of defending Physical Microscopism while rejecting Physicalism. I would have thought that this was Descartes's view, for example. Even though Descartes is a paradigm dualist about the relation between the mental and physical realms, within physics itself he certainly looks like someone who thinks that the microphysical facts at least fix all the *physical* facts. We might also expect some contemporary dualists, such as David Chalmers, similarly to

[2] In Hüttemann and Papineau 2005 we talked about 'Levels Physicalism' and 'Part–Whole Physicalism' rather that 'Physicalism' and 'Physical Microscopism'. My rationale for the change of terminology is that it is unhelpful to present Physical Microscopism as a species of physicalism, given that its claims are internal to the physical realm.

[3] It is true that the above quotations speak of decomposition into microphysical entities, where I have defined Microphysicalism in terms of supervenience on microphysical facts. I have switched to the latter formulation because it seems to me both more general and more precise. It certainly includes cases where the existence of some macroscopic entity is determined by the existence and arrangement of its microphysical parts, but it also covers other kinds of determination of macroscopic facts by microphysical ones. The specific issue of decomposition into *spatial* parts will be the focus of sections 10 and 11 below.

uphold this combination. There is no obvious reason why their commitment to an ontologically separate mental realm should force them to any kind of holism within physics itself.

The other possibility is Physicalism without Physical Microscopism. This is the option that interests me. The Microphysicalist quotations above suggest that once you are a Physicalist, then this will carry Physical Microscopism in its train. But why should this follow? Suppose I am a Physicalist about the mind. I think that the mental level is determined by the physical level. There is nothing more to the mind than the brain. Why should this commit me to any view in particular about the way things go within physics? Why shouldn't I hold that physical wholes transcend what is determined by their microphysical parts? Such a within-physics holism would seem perfectly consistent with my rejection of Cartesian dualism. Can't I still identify mental facts with macrophysical facts, even if I think that those macrophysical facts transcend what is determined by microphysical parts?

This anyway is the possibility that will concern me in the rest of this paper. Can one be a Physicalist without embracing Physical Microscopism? Equivalently, must a Physicalist be a Microphysicalist?

3. MOTIVATIONS FOR MICROPHYSICALISM

Why might anybody think that Physicalism requires Physical Microscopism? Are the Microphysicalist views expressed in the earlier quotations just an oversight, betraying insufficient thought about the nature of Physicalism? Or is there some more principled reason for linking Physicalism to Physical Microscopism?

I can think of two possible reasons for forging this link. The first is to do with the *meaning of 'physical'*. The second relates to the availability of *arguments for Physicalism*. Let me consider these possible reasons now, as they will allow me to introduce some points that will be useful later. I shall take them in turn.

The difficulties involved in defining 'physical' are well known. As Carl Hempel (1969) pointed out many years ago, Physicalists cannot simply define this term in terms of the categories recognized in contemporary Physics Departments. This is because current physics is a work in progress, so to speak—future discoveries will no doubt add to and subtract from the categories recognized by current physical theory. So a 'Physicalism' that asserts that everything supervenes on currently recognized physical categories will almost certainly prove false. Nor is it much of a solution, Hempel added, to define 'physical' by reference to the categories that will be recognized by *future* Physics Departments—at the ideal end of enquiry, perhaps. To the extent that we currently lack any clear idea of what those categories will be, this would remove any substantial content from Physicalism.

In the face of this dilemma, one possible solution is to define 'physical' in terms of 'microphysical'. That is, we might read 'physical' as encompassing only what is microphysically determined. Philip Pettit understands 'physical' in this way. The passage quoted earlier is part of an argument designed to show that 'physical' can be defined as 'composed out of microphysical entities and governed by microphysical laws'. By this proposal, Pettit hopes to counter the view that there is no good way of understanding 'physical' and that 'Physicalism' is therefore an empty doctrine.

Now, if we do define 'physical' as Pettit does, then Physical Microscopism will become a definitional truism. All physical facts will inevitably supervene on microphysical ones, for if they didn't they wouldn't be 'physical'. And therewith the Physicalist claim that everything is physical will automatically collapse into the Microphysicalist thesis that everything is microphysically determined.

However, there are alternatives to Pettit's definition of 'physical' as microphysically determined. These will leave it open whether or not everything physical is microphysically determined, and therewith allow for versions of Physicalism that are not committed to Physical Microscopism.

For a start, there is the option of defining 'physical' negatively, as covering anything that can be directly identified *without* using some distinguished terminology. For example, we might count as 'physical' anything that can be directly identified using non-mental terminology. Or we might define it somewhat more restrictively, as anything that can be directly identified without using mental *or* biological terminology. This is the way of understanding 'physical' that I myself favour. In my book *Thinking about Consciousness* (2002) I argue for an understanding of 'physical' as *inorganically identifiable*. The idea here is that we start with a distinguished inventory of mental and biological terms, and then pick out the physical realm as anything that can be directly identified without using those terms. (Note that the physical realm is here anything that *can* be so identified, not things that can *only* be so identified. Physicalists will of course hold that some parts of that physical realm can *also* be identified using mental or biological terms.)

Some philosophers favour a yet further option, one that takes off from Hempel's dilemma. The idea here is to appeal to the categories represented by current Physics Departments, but to allow some wiggle room for future developments. So we might think of 'physical' as referring to all those categories that bear some *resemblance* to the categories recognized in contemporary Physics Departments. For example, 'physical' might be understood as equivalent to something like 'displaying mathematically simple and precise behaviour'. I shall call this the 'resemblance' conception of 'physical' in what follows.

I shall not choose between these different understandings of 'physical' in this paper. It will be enough for my purposes to show that they allow various senses in which Physicalism might hold without Microphysicalism. But it will be useful to make one further point about the meaning of 'physical'. Suppose we have fixed on one of the above definitions of 'physical'. It will be convenient for the purposes of this paper to understand 'physical' recursively, in the sense of including any categories that supervene on the so-defined physical realm, even if they do not themselves fit the base definition. For example, suppose we equate 'physical' with 'inorganically identifiable'. Then it may be that facts about insects supervene on the physical realm so-defined, but that there is no way of stating insect facts using inorganic terminology. (Suppose that insect facts are 'multiply realized' at the inorganic level, in a way that precludes any uniform inorganic specifications of such facts.) Even so, I will take the supervenience of the insect facts on the physical facts to qualify them as 'physical'.

This recursive way of understanding 'physical' would not necessarily be appropriate for all philosophical purposes. For instance, if our focus were on physical *explanation*, it would be confusing to hold that certain facts were physically explainable just because they could be explained in terms of entomological facts that supervene on physical facts, even though there was no question of specifying those entomological facts in physical terms. But our interest here is with ontology, not explanation, and in particular with which categories supervene on the physical facts and which do not. Given this, it will suit my expository needs to count anything in the former category as 'physical'.

I turn now to the other possible reason for equating Physicalism with Microphysicalism, namely, the demands of providing an *argument* for Physicalism. Even if there are ways of understanding 'physicalism' that do not automatically collapse Physicalism into Microphysicalism, it could nevertheless be that the only way of *arguing* for Physicalism argues for Physical Microscopism too.

Thus consider this inductive argument: all facts so far subject to scientific scrutiny have turned out to supervene on the microphysical facts; so all the facts supervene on the microphysical facts. Some philosophers take this to be the primary rationale for embracing Physicalism. (Cf. Rey 2002.) Now, if this kind of inductive argument were the only available argument for Physicalism, then clearly any justification of Physicalism would justify Microphysicalism too. Our rationale for thinking that all facts supervene on the physical facts would essentially depend on the lemma that they all supervene on the microphysical facts. So our rationale for Physicalism would endorse Physical Microscopism along the way.

However, the above inductive argument is not the only possible argument for Physicalism.[4] There are alternatives that are quite free of any assumptions about microphysical goings-on. Thus consider the 'causal argument' that goes: prima facie non-physical facts like mental and biological facts have physical effects; all physical effects have physical causes ('the causal completeness of the physical'); so

[4] Which is just as well for Physicalism, if you ask me—after all, only a very limited range of facts have been shown actually to supervene on microphysical facts (as opposed to being assumed to so supervene on the basis of a prior commitment to Microphysicalism).

those prima facie non-physical facts must supervene on physical facts (or we would have unacceptable overdetermination). This is the argument for Physicalism that I myself favour. As we shall see below, this argument need not commit us to any claim that all the physical facts supervene on the *micro*physical facts. The crucial premise—the causal completeness of the physical—need only claim that all physical effects have *physical* causes, not that they have microphysical causes. And then this argument will only commit us to the conclusion that prima facie non-physical facts must supervene on physical facts, not that they must supervene on microphysical facts. The causal argument will thus remain available even to those Physicalists, like myself, who wish to remain neutral on the issue of Physical Microscopism.[5]

4. SPECIES OF EMERGENCE

My aim is to show that we can deny Microphysicalism without denying Physicalism. That is, I want to show that Microphysicalism might fail, not because there are non-physical facts, but rather because some physical facts fail to supervene on the microphysical facts. In such a case, we would have a violation of Physical Microscopism, but not of Physicalism.

I won't be concerned here to make a positive case for any such violations of Physical Microscopism. As I said at the beginning, my first commitment is to Physicalism, not to any views about microphysical determination. So my aim is only to establish conditional claims of the form: even if certain facts are emergent vis-à-vis the microphysical realm, Physicalism can still be true. I shan't defend the antecedents of these conditionals. My interest is not in microphysical emergence as such, but rather in the fact that Physicalists don't always *need* to reject microphysical emergence.

Of course, not all kinds of microphysical emergence are compatible with Physicalism. Cartesian dualism, for example, posits microphysically transcendent facts that would clearly violate Physicalism. This is because Cartesian minds would not only transcend the microphysical realm, but the physical realm too. To support my thesis, I need microphysically emergent facts that would remain genuinely physical.

[5] In the context of the philosophy of mind, some philosophers defend Physicalism via an 'inference to the best explanation', rather than by appeal to the causal argument. Their thought is that there are many well-established synchronic correlations between mental states and brain states, and that Physicalism is a 'better explanation' of these correlations than dualist epiphenomenalism (Hill 1991, Hill and McLaughlin 1999). To my mind, this starts the argument in the middle rather than at the beginning, by simply assuming the relevant mind-brain correlations. The point to note here is that we wouldn't posit such correlations if we were interactive dualists (for then we wouldn't think dualist mental states needed any help from synchronic neural correlates to produce physical effects). So we need the causal argument, not the proposed inference to a best explanation of correlations, to eliminate interactive dualism.

Some of the microphysically emergent facts I consider below will fail to support my thesis. This is because it will prove difficult to avoid the conclusion that they would not count as physical. In the face of these particular species of microphysical emergence, Physicalists cannot of course stand neutral. They must reject any emergent facts that would transcend the physical realm, just as they must reject Cartesian minds. Fortunately, as we shall see, there are good arguments for denying those variants of microphysical emergence that would also transcend the physical realm.

5. HUMEAN SUPERVENIENCE

Microphysicalists claim that all the facts, including the macrophysical facts, supervene on the microphysical facts. The strength of this claim depends on what gets included in the 'the microphysical facts'. Austere understandings of the microphysical facts make for strong versions of Microphysicalism. Such strong versions will be comparatively easy to deny. By contrast, the more that gets included in 'the microphysical facts', the less easy it will be to show that there are facts that transcend the microphysical facts.

A particularly strong version of Microphysicalism would correspond to David Lewis's doctrine of 'Humean Supervenience' (Lewis 1986):

> (HS) All the facts are metaphysically determined by the intrinsic properties of spacetime points plus the spatiotemporal relationships between those points.

This asserts that any world which agrees with the actual world on the 'Humean mosiac' of spacetime points and their intrinsic properties will contain all the facts that are present in the actual world. This is an extremely strong doctrine. It countenances no 'external relations' between spacetime points except their spatiotemporal relationships. Every other relational fact is fixed by the intrinsic properties of the points and the way these points are arranged in space and time.

Suppose we agree that the intrinsic properties of spacetime points are all physical properties. Humean Supervenience will then amount to a very strong form of Microphysicalism. Because it is so strong, it is easy for it to be false. In particular, it will be false if a non-Humean view of laws is true. The Humean view is that laws depend on nothing more than the 'constant conjunctions' of particular facts displayed by the actual world. So any view on which laws transcend such facts of constant conjunction will contradict Humean Supervenience. Any such view implies that a world can agree with this world on the Humean mosaic yet differ on the laws.

I take this to illustrate a minimal sense in which one can be a Physicalist while rejecting Microphysicalism. If we equate Microphysicalism with Humean

Supervenience, then anybody who rejects a Humean view of laws will be rejecting Microphysicalism. But nobody, I take it, would want to argue that a non-Humean view of laws amounts to a violation of Physicalism. This would only follow if non-Humean laws must in some sense themselves be non-physical, and there seems no reason to hold this. Certainly many actual Physicalists embrace this kind of non-Humeanism about laws without feeling that it somehow undermines their Physicalism.

Still, I don't suppose that this point will worry any of the philosophers who think that Physicalism requires Microphysicalism. This is because they are unlikely to understand Microphysicalism as making the extreme claims of Humean Supervenience, and in particular as requiring a Humean view of laws. Just as Physicalists in general will say there is nothing non-physical about non-Humean laws, so those who equate Physicalism with Microphysicalism are likely to say that there is nothing non-*Micro*physical about non-Humean laws either. They will thus be happy to add non-Humean laws to Lewis's Microphysicalist supervenience base, and thereby weaken the relevant supervenience doctrine: to fix all the facts, it is not enough just to fix the intrinsic properties and spatiotemporal arrangements of spacetime points—we must also fix the laws that govern the causal interactions between those points. These laws themselves need not supervene on the properties and arrangements of spacetime points.

This doesn't mean that those who want to equate Physicalism with Microphysicalism will place no restrictions at all on the laws present in a given world. They will typically insist that the only basic laws are *microphysical* laws. There may be genuine macroscopic laws, but if so they will be derived from the microscopic laws. As Pettit puts it, '. . . once the microphysical conditions and the microphysical laws have been fixed, then all the crucial features of a world like ours will have been fixed; viz., all the other laws that obtain at the world . . .' (1993, p. 219). From this point of view, while we might have to add non-Humean laws to get an adequate Microphysicalist supervenience base for all facts, it will be enough to add *microphysical* non-Humean laws. There are no further laws that are not determined by microphysical laws plus arrangements of microphysical initial conditions. So now we have another Microphysicalist supervenience thesis, one that places restrictions specifically on laws.

(L) All the laws are metaphysically determined by microphysical laws and microphysical initial conditions.

6. BROAD-STYLE EMERGENT LAWS

I now want to consider whether a Physicalist can deny (L) and yet remain a Physicalist. That is, would the existence of macroscopic laws that are not dependent on microphysical laws and microphysical initial conditions somehow contradict Physicalism?

This will prove a less than straightforward matter. In this section I shall argue that there is no immediate reason why Physicalists should not countenance macroscopic laws that do not depend on microscopic ones. However, the situation is complicated by considerations to do with force fields. I shall consider these complications in the next section.

A first question to address is what exactly qualifies a law as microphysical. We can take a microphysical law to be one that applies inter alia to small physical systems. (We needn't worry about what precisely qualifies a physical system as 'small'—the issues will come out the same wherever we draw this line.)

Note that there is nothing in this definition of a microphysical law to require that it applies *only* to small physical systems. It may be that microphysical laws are formulated in such a way that they apply uniformly to both small and large physical systems.

Thus consider the law of gravitation. This says that, in any isolated physical system made up of bodies $B_1, \ldots, B_n$, each body B_k will be subject to the vector sum of the forces due to the other B_js ($j \neq k$) (namely, $Gm_km_j/r^2{}_{jk}$—where m_j is the mass of the other body B_j, r_{jk} is the distance between B_j and B_k, and G the constant of universal gravitation). Now, this law qualifies as a microphysical law because it tells us what would happen in a very small localized system comprising a few tiny particles. But at the same time it is formulated in an entirely general way. So it also tells us what would happen to a large falling body near the surface of the earth, say. We don't need any new principle to tell us what will happen to such a body. We simply apply the same gravitational law that applies to very small systems to the more complex set-up comprising the falling body and the earth.

Now, there seems no principled reason why all basic laws should be microphysical in this sense. Thus consider 'emergent laws' of the kind C. D. Broad (and other 'British Emergentists') envisaged. These are laws that (a) apply to specific large-scale physical initial conditions, (b) don't follow from microphysical laws, and (c) are essential to the appearance of certain physical effects. For example, imagine that, when the molecules constituting animal cells are in the physical context characteristic of a developing embryo, they start behaving in ways that aren't predictable given only the microphysical laws. Or, again, suppose that the molecules comprising neurotransmitters behave in a similarly unpredictable way when they are in the physical environment of a functioning brain.[6]

[6] Note how clause (c) is needed to ensure that emergent laws are genuinely independent of microphysical laws. To see why, consider Jerry Fodor's version of non-reductive physicalism, as outlined in his influential 'Special Sciences' (1974). Fodor there posits special laws that (a) apply to specific large-scale physical initial conditions; (b) don't follow from microphysical laws. But Fodor is not denying that his special laws supervene on the microphysical laws plus particular microphysical initial conditions. This is because Fodor does not think that his special macroscopic laws describe any *independent causal influence* governing particular outcomes. In each *particular* case, the generation of physical results can be fully accounted for by the way microphysical laws govern

Emergent Broad-laws would thus violate (L). They would give us a kind of macroscopic law that is not metaphysically determined by microphysical laws and initial conditions. There could be two possible worlds that agreed in their microphysical laws and microphysical initial conditions yet differed in their large-scale emergent laws—for example, one might have a law about special molecular movements to be found in developing embryos, while another might lack any such law.

The question now is whether this kind of emergence would threaten Physicalism. Would Broad-style emergence transcend the physical realm and call into being something non-physical? Or would it merely be a violation of Physical Microscopism that transcended the *micro*physical but leaves Physicalism intact?

At first pass, there is no obvious reason why Broad-laws should be viewed as requiring anything non-physical. Broad-laws would mean that certain large-scale complexes enter into laws that don't follow from basic microphysical laws and which make a real difference to the evolution of physical systems. But there would seem no immediate reason not to count both these large-scale complexes and the laws they enter into as *physical*. After all, nothing said so far requires these complexes to be anything more than large-scale arrangements of small physical parts. And nothing said so far requires the emergent laws to do anything except relate these physical initial complexes to physical results. (True, if 'physical' by definition required governance by microphysical laws, as in Pettit's definition of 'physical', then the physical complexes entering into emergent laws would come out as 'non-physical'. But they won't if we adopt either the 'resemblance' or 'inorganically identifiable' conceptions of 'physical', as seems more natural in this context.)

What about the *argumentative rationale* for Physicalism? Would this survive the existence of emergent Broad-laws? Again, there seems no immediate reason why Broad-laws should stop us arguing for Physicalism. Maybe they would if the only argument for Physicalism somehow proceeded via a demonstration that all physical laws supervene on microphysical ones. However the causal argument for Physicalism sketched above makes no such assumption. Rather it hinges on the causal completeness of the physical realm, which says nothing about

the microscopic parts of the system. True, Fodor supposes that the microprocesses responsible for such outcomes will be *different* in different instances of the special law—that is why his special laws don't follow via a classic Nagelian reduction from microphysical laws. But, even so, there will be *some* microprocess that is responsible for the outcome in each particular case, and so what happens in general will be fixed by microphysicial laws plus the overall distribution of particular microphysical facts. This is where Broad-style emergent laws differ from Fodor's special laws. With genuinely emergent laws, but not with Fodor's laws, we get particular outcomes that wouldn't occur were the evolution of particular systems governed by microphysical laws alone. (Fodor's picture might make one wonder why all his variable realizations should conform to the same macropattern, if they involve such different microprocesses. But that is another issue. See Papineau 1993, ch. 2, Block 1997.)

microphysics, but only that every physical effect has a fully sufficient *physical* cause. Broad-laws seem in perfectly good accord with this assumption. True, such laws would mean that some physical effects essentially result from macroscopic physical causes in ways unpredictable on the basis of microphysical laws alone. But for all that, they are still physical effects with sufficient (macro)physical causes. And so the causal argument will still tell us that any mental causes of those physical effects cannot be metaphysically distinct from those (macro)physical causes.

7. SPECIAL FIELDS

Despite the points made in the last section, there are further considerations that complicate the question of whether emergent Broad-laws are consistent with Physicalism.

Modern relativistic physics implies that causal influences exerted over spacetemporal distances must be mediated by the propagation of force fields. Relativity theory precludes any causal influences travelling faster than the speed of light. So there will be temporal gaps between any separated causes and effects. In typical cases this temporal interval will mean a violation of the conservation of energy. The standard solution is to suppose that the causes work locally, not at a distance, by propagating force fields which in turn produce the distant effects. These fields can then be viewed as embodying the relevant energy during the temporal delay between distal causes and effects (Lange 2002, ch. 5).

This argues that any Broad-laws would be associated with the emergence of special fields generated by the specific macroscopic initial conditions appearing in those laws. It is not to be taken for granted that these fields will count as 'physical', even if the macroscopic initial conditions that generate them do. To the extent that they would, Physicalism will remain intact, and the special fields would at worst violate the within-physics supervenience required by Physical Microscopism. But if the extra fields were non-physical, then they would automatically invalidate Physicalism.

To see more clearly what is at issue here, return to the suggestion that organic molecules behave in a distinctive manner in a developing embryo, or that neurotransmitters do the same when in a functioning brain. These behaviours would give us reason to posit 'vital' and 'mental' force fields respectively. And these fields would be genuinely extra to basic physical force fields like gravitation and electromagnetism, given that Broad-style laws give rise to physical effects that cannot be accounted for by more basic force fields.

The question is now whether fields like these would count as 'physical' or not. This turns out to be a rather messy question. I earlier considered three ways of defining 'physical': (a) metaphysically supervenient on the microphysical; (b) inorganically identifiable; and (c) resembling currently recognized physical categories. At a first approximation, the last of these make special force fields come out as physical, the second argues that at least some are non-physical, while the first delivers no clear verdict.

Let me briefly run through these options. (a) *'Physical' = 'supervenient on the microphysical'*. At first sight it might seem as if special force fields won't be 'physical' on this definition, because they aren't supervenient on the aggregates of microphysical facts that generate them: after all, there are worlds containing those facts that lack the relevant Broad-laws and so the fields. But that doesn't necessarily decide the issue, for special force fields will still standardly supervene on the local values of the fields themselves: fix the field values at all spacetime points and you fix all the field facts. So special force fields will be micro*scopically* determined. But does this mean they are micro*physically* determined? It depends on whether local values of special force fields count as physical or not. And this would seem to require a verdict from some other criterion of physicality, such as our second and third definitions. (b) *'Physical' = 'inorganically identifiable'*. On this definition, it matters what type of special fields are at issue. If they are mental or vital force fields, then they will presumably count as *non*-physical. Referring to them as 'mental' or 'vital' force fields clearly doesn't give us a way of referring to them directly in inorganic terms. Of course, we could always form new terms to name such fields. But these terms will arguably be 'organic' too, insofar as they refer specifically to entities that are found only in living bodies and never elsewhere. However, not all special fields associated with Broad-laws need be so exclusively attached to organic circumstances. There could be fields that arose specifically in certain complex inorganic chemical molecules, say. These fields would then come out as *physical* on the second definition. (c) *'Physical' = 'resembles current physical categories'*. As I suggested earlier, a natural way to fill this out is to require that putatively physical entities should display 'mathematically simple and precise behaviour'. Any special force fields associated with Broad-style laws would be likely to satisfy this requirement. The principle of the conservation of energy is relevant here. Given this principle, any increases in kinetic energy occasioned by some force field must be compensated by a loss of potential energy with respect to that field, and vice versa. It is hard to see how this requirement could be satisfied if the evolution of any special fields were not governed by some definite mathematical principle that allowed us to define potential energy. To this extent, then, the third definition would count any Broad-style special fields as *physical*.

Overall, then, it looks as if special force fields associated with complex *inorganic* circumstances will come out as 'physical' on any definition, but that vital or mental force fields will only be 'physical' given the resemblance definition of 'physical', and not if 'physical' means inorganically identifiable. No doubt there is more to say on whether special force fields should count as 'physical'. But I do not propose to pursue this issue any further. To the extent that special force fields do qualify as 'physical', the associated Broad-laws will illustrate my thesis that you can deny Microphysicalism without denying Physicalism: such laws will violate the Microscophysicalist thesis (L), yet will not take us beyond the physical realm. On the other hand, special force fields that count as 'non-physical' will be no good for my thesis, since their associated Broad-laws will not only violate Microphysicalism but Physicalism too.

Of course, this means that Physicalists must resist any force fields of the latter kind. But this presents no great difficulty. Whichever definition of 'physical' is in play, the only force fields that threaten physicalism are vital and mental fields. I take it that there is no good reason to believe in any such fields. Until the end of the nineteenth century, most scientists took vital and mental fields for granted, along with other special fields. But modern research has not supported their view. In particular, twentieth-century physiology has given no indication that there are any processes inside living bodies that cannot be fully accounted for in terms of more familiar physical forces. (Cf. Papineau 2002, appendix.)

8. PERSISTING OBJECTS

I turn now from laws to another kind of fact that might fail to supervene on the microphysical facts, namely facts about persisting objects, like molecules, stones, brains, beetles and bicycles. These are objects that retain their identity through time: a stone at one time can be identical to a stone at another time. It will turn out that there is plenty of room for Physicalists to deny that facts about persisting objects are microphysically determined without compromising their Physicalism.

As with laws, a strong form of Microphysicalism about persisting objects would assert Humean Supervenience:

(O) All facts about persisting objects are metaphysically determined by the intrinsic physical properties and spatiotemporal relations of spacetime points.

Some contemporary philosophers endorse this claim. More specifically, they hold that facts about persisting objects depend on nothing but appropriate relations of spatiotemporal continuity among 'time-slices' (and that facts about 'time-slices' depend on nothing but the intrinsic physical properties and spatial relations of spatial points at the time in question). We can think of a time-slice as conveying an instantaneous 'snapshot' of the putative object. The strong Microphysicalist view at issue is thus that a persisting stone, say, is determined by a sequence of stone-type 'snapshots' that over time trace a continuous stone-type 'worm' through space.

However, this strong Microphysicalist view is denied by at least as many contemporary philosophers as uphold it. In support, they standardly invoke Kripke's 'rotating disc' argument.[7] Consider a homogeneous disc made of

[7] Kripke's argument is given in unpublished lectures. See also Armstrong 1980.

completely smooth matter. A sequence of time-slices will reveal where the disc is centred at each moment, but will not reveal whether it is rotating or not. In both cases, the time slices will simply be 'frozen' snapshots of homogeneous matter. So both a rotating disc and a non-rotating disc would display the same sequence of homogeneous time-slices. Yet intuitively there is a difference between these two alternatives. It seems to follow that there are facts about the disc that are not fixed by relations of spatiotemporal continuity among its time-slices.

This then gives us one sense in which Physicalists might fail to be Microphysicalists about persisting objects without compromising their Physicalism.[8] They can deny that persisting objects are sums of time-slices. For it certainly doesn't look as if this denial will somehow automatically undermine their Physicalism. After all, there seems no reason why Physicalists should withhold the term 'physical' from molecules or stones—or discs, for that matter—just because they think that these persisting objects fail to supervene on time-slices. Persisting objects like these would seem to be the paradigm of physical objects, whether or not they supervene on time-slices.

Perhaps there are few Microphysicalist philosophers who wish to uphold a strong Humean Supervenience thesis about persisting objects (just as few wish to uphold a strong Humeanism about laws). Still, the point I have just made also applies to various weaker Microphysicalist supervenience theses about persisting objects. There are in fact a range of possible weaker such Microphysicalisms, differentiated by what they add to time-slices in search of an adequate supervenience base for persisting objects. Thus there are philosophers who hold that the way to stick the time-slices together, so to speak, is to add instantaneous velocities to the supervenience base (Tooley 1988). Others favour the addition of primitive relations of singular causation (Zimmerman 1997).[9] Yet others appeal to 'non-supervenient relations' between the time-slices (Hawley 2001).

[8] In Hüttemann and Papineau (2005) we appealed to a different idea to defend the possibility of Physicalism without Microphysicalism about particular facts. We argued that the macroscopic properties of objects are not *asymmetrically* determined by their microscopic properties, since the macroscopic properties determine the microscopic ones as much as vice versa. Thus consider a system composed of three bodies, of masses m_1, m_2 and m_3 respectively. These individual masses determine that the whole has a mass of $m_1 + m_2$, $+m_3$. But, by the same coin, the mass of the whole plus the mass of the first two bodies determines the mass of the third. (Cf Hüttemann 2004.) I stand by the idea that there is a symmetry of determination here. However, it no longer seems to me that this contradicts Microphysicalism. Why shouldn't Microphysicalists simply concede this kind of object-relative symmetry of determination? They can still explain why it is appropriate to think that macrophysics depends on microphysics, rather than vice versa, by pointing out that a world matching ours in microphysical detail will match it in macrophysical respects too, while the converse is not true—for the obvious reason that our world contains many 'free-floating' microphysical features that aren't properties of objects that also have macrophysical features.

[9] Interestingly, it looks as if these singular causal relations need to be prior to laws, not derivative from laws and particular non-causal facts. It won't help to add laws that don't generalize over singular causal relations to the supervenience base, not even non-Humean causal laws: if we don't yet

We need not dissect these strategies in any detail here. The important point for my purposes is simply that there seems plenty of room to dispute these weaker Microphyicalisms too, without thereby contradicting Physicalism. For a start, any supervenience thesis of the above form will be denied by 'three-dimensionalists', that is, those philosophers who deny that persisting objects have time-slices as temporal parts, and so a fortiori will reject any claim that persisting objects are time-slices 'glued together' by such things as instantaneous velocities, singular causation or non-supervenenient relations. And even among 'four-dimensionalists', who do recognize time-slices, none of these suggestions for gluing them together will have majority support. Yet, as before, there seems no reason why somebody denying any of these Microphysicalist theses should be deemed thereby to have compromised their Physicalism. As I said above, things like molecules and stones are paradigms of physical objects. We needn't stop viewing them as such just because we deny one or more theses about how they are constituted out of temporal parts.

9. BRAINS, BEETLES AND BICYCLES

Maybe molecules and stones are still paradigms of physical objects, even if they fail to supervene on time-slices and relations between them. But what about other kinds of persisting objects, including organic entities like brains and beetles, and artefacts like bicycles? Here it is not so clear that their status as 'physical' will survive their failure to supervene on time-slices plus 'glue'. And, if their physical status doesn't so survive, then this will argue that Physicalism about these entities does require some kind of four-dimensional Microphysicalism about persisting entities after all.

Let us suppose, for the sake of the argument, that three-dimensionalism is true, and that there is no way of 'gluing together' persisting objects out of time-slices. Given this, it is by no means obvious that objects like brains, beetles and bicycles will still qualify as physical.

Recall how we earlier considered three different notions of 'physical': (a) microphysically determined, (b) resembling current physical categories, and (c) inorganically identifiable. Under the hypothesis of three-dimensionalism, brains, beetles and bicycles clearly won't qualify as physical because they are microphysically determined by time-slices and their relations. Nor do they seem likely to qualify because they resemble current physical categories. As to the requirement of inorganic identifiablity, brains and beetles certainly won't satisfy this; moreover, it's not even clear that inanimate artefacts like bicycles will qualify, given that it is arguably essential to such artefacts that they are made by an intelligent designer.

have any particular qualitative differences between the stationary and rotating discs, such laws won't distinguish them. Cf. Zimmerman 1998.

This suggests that Physicalism isn't compatible with three-dimensionalism after all, and that we need some doctrine of supervenience on time-slices and relations to ensure that organic and artefactual persisting objects do not transcend the physical realm.

However, there is a further line of thought that promises to preserve the physical status of such objects even in the face of three-dimensionalism. For such objects might well supervene on their *spatial* parts even if they don't supervene on their temporal parts. And if those spatial parts are physical, then this will restore the physical status of brains, beetles and bicycles after all, even without any four-dimensional supervenience on time-slices.

The thought here is that organic and artefactual objects will surely supervene on facts about atoms, molecules or other small material constituents, whatever view we take about temporal parts. Could you have two identical arrangements of molecules, and one constitute a beetle, or a bicycle, and the other not? It seems unlikely. And we have already argued, in the last section, that the physical status of paradigm physical objects like molecules will not be undermined by their failure to supervene on time-slices. So this argues that beetles, brains and bicycles will retain their status as physical even if four-dimensionalist supervenience fails. All persisting physical objects, big and small, may fail to supervene on temporal parts, but as long as organic and artefactual objects supervene on small spatial parts, and those small spatial parts are physical, then organic and artefactual objects will count as physical too. (Note how the recursive understanding of 'physical', flagged in section 3 above, matters here. Brains, beetles and bicycles may not qualify as physical in their own right, so to speak, but they will qualify derivatively, in virtue of their supervenience on their small spatial parts, plus the physicality of these parts.)

So the thought is that Physicalists can reject Microphysicalist four-dimensionalism and yet maintain their Physicalism by insisting that organic and artefactual persisting objects will still count as physical in virtue of the physicality of the spatial parts that they supervene on. A natural question to ask at this point is *why* there should be such supervenience on spatial parts, if there is a failure of supervenience on temporal parts. Does not my putative three-dimensionalist Physicalist owe us some *argument* for the claim that organic and artefactual persisting objects supervene on their spatial parts? However, such an argument is not hard to find. A version of the standard causal argument for Physicalism makes it very hard to see how organic and artefactual objects could fail to supervene on their spatial parts without generating an unacceptable species of systematic overdetermination.

To see how this would go, note that causes involving organic and artefactual objects characteristically have physical effects. (They dislodge stones, leave tracks, and so on.) At the same time those physical effects can surely be fully accounted for by causal processes involving only the small spatial parts of those objects. (The impacts of the molecules in those objects will fully account for the dislodging of the stones and the leaving of tracks.) So, if the organic and artefactual objects were metaphysically distinct from their molecular parts, in the sense of not supervening on them, we would have two ontologically independent causes for the relevant effects, which would be absurd.[10]

So my putative three-dimensionalist Physicalists can offer a good argument in support of their crucial claim that organic and artefactual objects supervene on their small physical parts. At this point, however, we might well wonder why a similar argument won't undermine their three-dimensionalism. If persisting objects can't transcend their spatial parts without generating unacceptable overdetermination, then how come they can transcend their *temporal* parts? Why won't this imply unacceptable overdetermination too, on the grounds that effects of causes involving the persisting object will already have full causes involving the temporal parts of that object?

However, I take it that somebody who is persuaded by the arguments for three-dimensionalism will deny the completeness premise assumed here. After all, they deny that persisting objects have temporal parts, and so a fortiori will not allow that there are already a full set of causes involving such temporal parts. Rather, they will insist that the only particular entities that feature in causes are persisting objects, like molecules and stones, or beetles and bicycles, not any supposed 'time-slices' of those objects. So for them there will be no question of the effects of molecules and stones also being determined by facts involving temporal parts.

These last comments illustrate a general point. I have taken the canonical argument for physicalism to be the causal argument: putatively non-physical causes have physical effects; all physical effects have physical causes; so avoiding (strong) overdetermination requires the putatively non-physical causes to supervene on the physical ones. Now, if we could replace the second premise with a stronger claim that all physical effects in some sense have *microphysical* causes, then obviously the argument would deliver the conclusion that all putatively non-physical causes must supervene on causes which are microphysical in that sense. Correlatively, Physicalists who wish to deny that putatively non-physical causes are microphysical in some given sense must deny that all physical effects have

[10] Some readers might be wondering, Kim-style, whether even the supervenience of persisting objects on their spatial parts is enough to avoid unacceptable overdetermination, if such supervenience falls short of identity. In the context of the relation between mental and physical properties, Kim (1993) uses this thought to argue in favour of type identity and against non-reductive supervenience. In the present context, however, there seems no question of *identifying* persisting objects with their spatial parts (given that the objects are one and the parts are many). Trenton Merricks concludes from this that the only way to avoid unacceptable overdetermination in this context is to *eliminate* persisting objects in favour of their spatial parts (2001). Myself, I think that these considerations cut the other way, and cast doubt on Kim's initial assumption that supervenience without identity generates unacceptable overdetermination. (Cf. Bynoe forthcoming.) Note that we can still insist that 'strong overdetermination' by two non-supervenient causes is unacceptable (as required for the causal argument for Physicalism) even if we allow 'weak overdetermination' by two supervenient causes. (Cf. Bennett 2003.)

microphysical causes in the relevant sense. The possibility of three-dimensionalist Physicalists illustrates the general point. It is specifically because they deny the relevant microphysical completeness thesis—that all physical effects have sufficient causes composed of time-slices—that they are able to deny the metaphysical thesis that all physical causes must supervene on time slice facts.

10. A MICROPHYSICALIST FORK

It might seem to some readers as if the main point has now been conceded to those who hold that Physicalism implies Microphysicalism. After all, haven't I just agreed that Physicalism requires all facts about persisting objects to supervene on facts about small spatial parts like atoms and molecules? And wasn't this always the most natural reading of the view that Physicalism implies Microphysicalism (at least as it relates to particular facts rather than laws)? Thus recall the wording of the quotes with which I started, which spoke mostly of 'composition' by microphysical entities. Such talk of 'composition' can be read in various ways, but the most obvious way is as implying that the existence and properties of large persisting objects supervene on the existence and properties of their small spatial parts.

Let us briefly take stock of the dialectical situation. I brought in the idea of supervenience on small spatial parts to show how an anti-time-slice three-dimensionalist can uphold the physical status of organic and artefactual objects. The thought was that even three-dimensionalists will have good reason to uphold supervenience on small spatial parts, and that this will preserve the physicality of brains, beetles and bicycles. Without such supervenience, however, three-dimensionalists are in danger of violating Physicalism, for it is not clear, given their three-dimensionalism, what will ensure the physicality of organic and artefactual objects.

Given this, it looks as if Physicalists must at least embrace this final Microphysicalist thesis:

(C) Facts about persisting objects supervene on the intrinsic physical properties of (and causal and spatial relations between) their spatial parts.

Maybe this thesis itself isn't indisputable. In principle, there is room to argue that facts about bicycles and beetles do in fact transcend facts about their spatial parts. And maybe this won't automatically generate unacceptable overdetermination—perhaps the relevant microphysical causal completeness thesis can be questioned, on the grounds that whole objects like bicycles and beetles do sometimes have physical effects that aren't also caused by their small spatial parts. (Cf. Owens 1992.) But none of this looks any good to Physicalists, for if *they* deny the Microphysicalist (C), then it seems that they will lose their reason for saying that organic and artefactual objects are physical.

In short, it looks as if either Physicalists must accept Microphysicalist thesis (C)—or deny it and thereby undermine their Physicalism. Either way, there doesn't seem any room for a Physicalist to avoid this last version of Microphysicalism.

Even so, I am now going to argue that Physicalists can deny (C) consistently with their Physicalism. This is because quantum mechanics gives us strong reason to deny (C), but doesn't therewith undermine the physical status of brains, beetles and bicycles.

11. QUANTUM HOLISM

Prepare two electrons in the singlet state and send them off in opposite directions. The left hand electron will have a 50% chance of showing spin-up in the x direction, and 50% chance of showing spin-down. The same is true of the right hand one. They are—let us suppose—a light year apart, and in consequence have no current causal connection. Yet there will be a further fact about this joint system that does not supervene on the facts so far mentioned. The joint state of the two electrons is 'entangled'. If the left hand electron is spin-up, the right hand one will be spin-down, and vice versa. This is a 'non-local' fact about the joint system, in the sense that it cannot be viewed as the sum of local facts about the separated electrons.

This kind of non-locality needs to be distinguished from the non-local *action at a distance* that some interpretations of quantum mechanics posit to explain what happens when measurements are made on distant 'entangled' objects. Thus suppose you measure the left-hand electron in the above situation and observe spin-up. You will then know that any measurement on the other electron will display spin-down. Some interpretations of quantum mechanics cannot avoid concluding that the measurement on the left-hand electron instantaneously produces real effects at the location of the right-hand electron. Other interpretations, in particular Everettian interpretations, claim to avoid any such non-local action at a distance. However, the non-locality I am concerned with here is independent of what happens in measurements, and so of these different interpretations of quantum mechanics. Rather it involves the structure of the quantum wave function before any measurements are made. It arises directly from the fact that the wave function for multiple particles can contain information beyond what it implies for any localized properties of the particles. This species of non-locality is thus unavoidable in any interpretation of quantum mechanics that views the quantum wave function realistically.[11]

[11] Some philosophers take this quantum non-locality to show that 3N-dimensional 'configuration space' (where N is the number of particles in the universe) eclipses ordinary 3-dimensional space as the fundamental framework of reality. (Cf. Albert 1996.) And others argue that this restores

Non-local entanglement is ubiquitous in the real world. I illustrated it above by considering a system of two separated electrons. But it will also be present in systems comprising basic physical persisting objects, like atoms and molecules. The joint state of the local components of such composite systems will characteristically contain information additional to that implied by the local properties of the components (see e.g. D. Lewis 2004, section I).

This point thus undermines our final Microphysicalist thesis (C). There are facts about persisting objects like atoms and molecules that transcend the intrinsic physical properties of their spatial parts plus the spatial and causal relations between them.

Note, however, that this denial of thesis (C) certainly doesn't look as if it undermines Physicalism. (Cf. Esfeld 1999.) The properties of atoms and molecules may be irredeemably holist because of quantum non-locality, but these properties are surely still physical. We don't want to say that the total spin of a number of electrons doesn't count as 'physical' just because it isn't determined by the local properties of the individual electrons. (I suppose that this would follow if we made satisfaction of Microphysicalist thesis (C) a defining requirement for 'physical'—but this implication surely simply counts against that reading of 'physical'. Certainly the relevant holist properties will come out as 'physical' on the inorganic and resemblance understandings of 'physical'.)

Can a Physicalist really deny the Microphysicalist thesis (C)? The worry in the last section was that brains, beetles and bicycles—not atoms and molecules—might end up as non-physical if they don't supervene on their small physical parts, as ensured by thesis (C). Still, there seems no reason why organic and artefactual objects should end up as non-physical just because their composite atoms and molecules have quantum holist properties. After all, those properties will still be physical (for the reasons I have just given) and facts about brains, beetles and bicycles will still supervene on them (here I revert to the assumption—contrary to the in-principle alternative aired towards the end of the last section—that all the physical effects of organic and artefactual objects will already have complete causes among the physical properties of their atomic and molecular parts).

What if the failure of Microphysicalist thesis (C) is more radical, and the quantum holism extends beyond atoms and molecules to larger entities, perhaps even to brains, beetles and bicycles themselves? That is, what if such larger entities also have properties that cannot be inferred from the local properties of their component atoms and molecules? At this point differing views on the interpretation of quantum mechanics come into play. Some will deny that there are any such macro-holist properties, because of what happens when the wave

a version of Humean Supervenience, on the grounds that all facts supervene on the intrinsic 'local' properties of points in configuration space plus 'spatial' relations between these points (Loewer 1996). However, it is debatable whether quantum mechanics really implies that ordinary 3-dimensional space is superseded by configuration space (P. Lewis 2004).

function 'collapses'. Others will hold that there are such properties, and will offer some explanation for why they are so difficult to detect. But we can by-pass these issues here. Let us simply suppose, for the sake of the argument, that quantum non-locality does extend beyond atoms and molecules, and that certain larger entities have properties that do not supervene on the local properties of their spatial parts. This still doesn't look as if it is going to undermine Physicalism. Any such large-scale quantum-based non-local properties will still count as physical (given that they will (a) occur in inorganic contexts as well as organic ones, and (b) display mathematically simple and precise behaviour). And facts about organic and artefactual objects will still supervene on physical properties including those non-local quantum properties (given that the physical effects of organic and artefactual objects will have a full set of causes among such physical properties).

So it seems that Physicalists can deny Microphysicalist thesis (C) after all. Quantum non-locality gives us cases which violate thesis (C) but do not take us beyond the realm of the physical. Even if this non-locality sometimes involves objects larger than atoms and molecules, it still won't transcend the physical realm. It thus turns out that Physicalists can deny even this last minimal version of Microphysicalism without compromising their Physicalism.

REFERENCES

Albert, D. 1996. 'Elementary Quantum Metaphysics' in Cushing, J., Fine, A. and Goldstein, S. (eds.). *Bohmian Mechanics and Quantum Theory: An Appraisal* Dordrecht: Kluwer.

Armstrong, D. 1980. 'Identity Through Time' in van Inwagen, P. (ed.). *Time and Cause*, Dordrecht: Reidel.

Bennett, K. 2003. 'Why the Exclusion Problem Seems Intractable, and How, Just Maybe, to Tract It', *Noûs* 37: 471–97.

Block, N. 1997. 'Anti-Reductionism Slaps Back', *Noûs*, suppl. vol. (Tomberlin, J. (ed.), *Philosophical Perspectives* 11. *Mind, Causation and World*), 107–32.

Broad, C. D. 1925. *Mind and its Place in Nature*. London: Routledge.

Bynoe, W. forthcoming. 'Composition without Overdetermination: A Reply to Merricks'.

Crane, T. and Mellor, D. H. 1990. 'There is No Question of Physicalism', *Mind* 99: 185–206.

Esfeld, M. 1999. 'Physicalism and Ontological Holism', *Metaphilosophy* 30: 319–37.

Fodor, J. 1974. 'Special Sciences or: The Disunity of Science as a Working Hypothesis', *Synthese* 28: 77–115.

Hawley, K. 2001. *How Things Persist*. Oxford: Oxford University Press.

Hempel, C. 1969. 'Reduction: Ontological and Linguistic Facets', in Morgenbesser, S. et al. (eds.), *Essays in Honor of Ernest Nagel*. New York: St Martin's Press.

Hill, C. 1991. *Sensations*. Cambridge: Cambridge University Press.

—— and McLaughlin, B. 1999. 'There are Fewer Things in Reality than are Dreamt of in Chalmers' Philosophy', *Philosophy and Phenomenological Research* 59: 444–54.

Hüttemann, A. 2004. *What's Wrong with Microphysicalism?* London: Routledge.
—— and Papineau, D. 2005. 'Physicalism Decomposed', *Analysis* 65: 33–9.
Kim, J. 1993. *Supervenience and Mind: Selected Philosophical Essays.* Cambridge: Cambridge University Press.
—— 1998. *Mind in a Physical World.* Cambridge Mass.: MIT Press.
Lange, M. 2002. *The Philosophy of Physics.* Oxford: Blackwell.
Lewis, D. 1986. Preface to his *Philosophical Papers*, vol. ii. Oxford: Oxford University Press.
—— 2004. 'How Many Lives Has Schrödinger's Cat?' *Australasian Journal of Philosophy* 82: 3–22.
Lewis, P. 2004. 'Life in Configuration Space', *British Journal for the Philosophy of Science* 55: 713–29.
Loewer, B. 1996. 'Humean Supervenience', *Philosophical Topics* 24: 101–27.
Merricks, T. 2001. *Objects and Persons.* Oxford: Oxford University Press.
Owens, D. 1992. *Causes and Coincidences.* Cambridge: Cambridge University Press.
Oppenheim, P. and Putnam, H. 1958. 'Unity of Science as a Working Hypothesis', in Feigl, H., Scriven, M. and Maxwell, G. (eds.), *Concepts, Theories, and the Mind-Body Problem, Minnesota Studies in the Philosophy of Science*, Minneapolis: University of Minnesota Press, vol ii, 3–36.
Papineau, D. 1993. *Philosophical Naturalism.* Oxford: Blackwell.
—— 2002. *Thinking about Consciousness* Oxford: Oxford University Press.
Pettit, P. 1993. 'A Definition of Physicalism', *Analysis* 53: 213–23.
—— 1994. 'Microphysicalism without Contingent Macro-Micro Laws', *Analysis* 54: 253–57.
Rey, G. 2002. 'Physicalism and Psychology: A Plea for Substantive Philosophy of Mind', in Gillet, C. and Loewer, B. (eds.), *Physicalism and Its Discontents.* Cambridge: Cambridge University Press.
Schaffer, J. 2003. 'Is There a Fundamental Level?' *Noûs* 37: 498–517.
Tooley, M. 1988. 'In Defence of the Existence of States of Motion', *Philosophical Topics* 15: 225–54.
Zimmerman, D. 1997. 'Immanent Causation', *Noûs*, suppl. vol. (J. Tomberlin, (ed.), *Philosophical Perspectives* 11. *Mind, Causation, and World*), 433–71.
—— 1998. 'Temporal Parts and Supervenient Causation: The Incompatibility of Two Humean Doctrines', *Australasian Journal of Philosophy* 76: 265–88.

8

Why There *Is* Anything Except Physics

Barry Loewer

In the course of defending his view of the relation between the special sciences and physics from Jaegwon Kim's objections Jerry Fodor asks

> So then, why is there anything except physics? That, I think, is what is really bugging Kim. Well, I admit that I don't know why. I don't even know how to think about why. I expect to figure out why there is anything except physics the day before I figure out why there is anything at all, another (and presumably related) metaphysical conundrum that I find perplexing. (Fodor 1998, p. 161)

Why is Fodor perplexed and Kim (allegedly) bugged by the existence of anything, i.e. any sciences, other than physics? I think the explanation is this. Fodor and Kim both believe

(1) All items belonging to the ontologies of the special sciences (all special science individuals, events, properties etc.) are constituted or realized by or in some way made up out of the microphysical entities, properties, and quantities that are the subject matter of fundamental physics.

and

(2) The dynamical laws of microphysics are complete in the domain of microphysics.[1]

Fodor but not Kim also maintains that

(3) There are autonomous special sciences with their own natural kinds, laws, explanations, causal relations, confirmation relations that are *not reducible* to those of physics.

This chapter is a companion piece to my "Why Is There Anything Except Physics?" (Loewer 2008) and tries to partly answer that question. Earlier versions of this paper were given at the University of Missouri, Brown University, Columbia University, and at the Conference *Being Reduced* in Aarhus. I am grateful to members of those audiences and to Katalin Balog, Tim Crane, and the editors Jesper Kallestrup and Jakob Hohwy of *Being Reduced* for comments on an earlier version. My ideas on the matters discussed in this paper arise from hours and hours of discussion with David Albert to whom I am enormously grateful.

[1] It is not completely clear what either Fodor or Kim thinks the fundamental laws of physics are like but they seem to think of them as involving causal relations between types of local physical properties. As I later discuss this is not the way physicists think of fundamental laws.

Exactly what anti-reductionists mean by "reducible" is often not clear. But this much can be said about Fodor's view of the relationship between special sciences and physics. He thinks that each special science taxonomizes nature into natural kinds in terms of its own proprietary vocabulary. What makes a special science a *science* is that it contains lawful regularities stated in its proprietary vocabulary that ground explanations and counterfactuals. He is clear that what makes a special science regularity *lawful* is a fact that is irreducible to the laws and facts of fundamental physics (and other special sciences).[2] That is, the lawfulness of special science regularities is a fact about the world as basic as and independent of the lawfulness of the laws of fundamental physics. Fodor's view can be illustrated with the help of a souped up version of Laplace's demon. The demon knows all the physical facts obtaining at all times and all the fundamental dynamical laws of physics, has perfect computational powers and also a "translation" manual connecting special science and physical vocabularies. The demon is thus able to tell which microphysical situations correspond to, for example, a philosophy conference and is able to determine which generalizations about philosophy conferences are true and which are false. It can do the same for all the special sciences. It will also be able to tell which special science regularities hold under counterfactual initial conditions and so which hold in all physically possible worlds (i.e. all the worlds at which the fundamental laws of physics obtain). But on Fodor's view the demon *will not* be able to discern which regularities are laws.[3] Because of this "blindness" the demon will be missing those counterfactuals and explanations that are underwritten by special science laws and so will not have an understanding of special science phenomena. Although the demon will be able to predict and explain the motions of elementary particles (or whatever entities are physically fundamental) from the state of the universe at any time and so could have predicted the stock market crash of 1929 it will not understand why it crashed. To do that it would need to know economics.[4]

Even without further clarifying (3) one can see that there is a tension among the three claims.[5] According to (1) the subject matters of all the special sciences are ultimately constituted/realized by microphysical entities (fields, elementary particles, strings, etc.) and events (changes in the positions

[2] Fodor identifies lawful regularities by the usual criteria of supporting counterfactuals and being confirmable by their instances. His view is that the laws of a higher level science are reducible to those of a more basic science only if the kinds of the higher level science can be identified with those of the more basic science. However, he sheds little light on what a *kind* is other than that they are properties that occur in laws. I discuss how to understand Fodor's anti-reductionism in Loewer (2008).

[3] See Loewer (2008) for a defense of this way of understanding Fodor's account of the relationship between special sciences and physics.

[4] Kitcher (2001) makes this point with the example of "Arbuthnot's regularity" that more males than females are born each year in London. I discuss Kitcher's argument later in this paper.

[5] Kim certainly sees the tension although he develops it in terms of causation rather than laws. Since I think causation is not a fundamental physical notion I think this is a mistake. See Kim (2005 and 2007) and Loewer (2007*a* and *b*; and 2008).

and momenta of particles, changes in field values, etc.).[6] Completeness of the dynamical microphysical laws means that the fundamental laws completely specify the dynamical evolution of the microphysical state of the universe (or of an isolated sub-system); i.e. for every time t, if the fundamental dynamical laws are deterministic and if S(t) is the state of isolated system Σ at t then S(t) and the laws determine a unique state S(t′) for Σ at t′; if the laws are probabilistic then, for every t, S(t) and the laws determine the chances at t of the evolution of future states.[7] It follows from (1) and (2) that special science regularities (including probabilistic regularities) are made true by physical facts and laws. It is hard to resist the conclusion that those special science regularities that are lawful derive their status as laws from the fundamental laws of microphysics. Where else could it come from?

A reduction of a special science law to fundamental physics would show how it is that the laws and facts of fundamental physics make certain special science regularities obtain and why some of them are laws. But, as Fodor observes, successful reductions of special science laws to physics are, at best, very scarce.[8] Although most biologists think that living organisms are constituted by microphysical entities obeying only microphysical laws no one has any idea of how, for example, the Hardy-Weinberg law (or any other biological law or psychological law) is made a law or even made true by physical facts and laws.

Fodor thinks that nothing is more obvious than that there are special science laws. One of his often cited examples, Gresham's law, says that if two kinds of money in circulation have the same denominational value but different intrinsic values, the money with higher intrinsic value will be hoarded and eventually driven out of circulation by the money with lesser intrinsic value. It apparently explains the hoarding of gold (i.e., "good money") in Germany in the 1920s in terms of the introduction of quantities of paper money (i.e., "bad money") into the German economy. Fodor has an argument that apparently shows that Gresham's law doesn't derive its lawfulness from microphysical laws. He observes that special science kinds, for example, *money*, are multiply and heterogeneously realized by physical kinds. Money can be made of no end of physically distinct materials (and also be electronically and psychologically realized). And he observes that special science laws are implemented by many

[6] The natures of constitution and realization are complicated matters. Necessary conditions on constitution and realization are: A macro-entity X is *constituted* by configuration C of micro-entities (particles or fields related in such and such ways) at time t only if, given the fundamental laws, C's existence at t metaphysically necessitates X's existence at t. If X has property F at t then this instance of F is *realized* microphysically only if there is a history of microphysical states that, given the laws, metaphysically necessitates that X has property F at t.

[7] This characterization needs to be modified for relativistic space-times (in which there is no "state at a time") and to take into account various other complications that are not relevant to the issues in this paper.

[8] The best cases of reductions are laws of chemical combination to quantum mechanics and thermodynamics to classical or quantum mechanics.

distinct kinds of physical processes. Monetary transactions can involve no end of physically distinct processes (writing checks, making verbal promises, over the internet, etc.). Other than providing the matter out of which the various kinds of money are made and the implementing causal processes it looks (to Fodor) like physics has little to do with explanations in economics, psychology, biology or any of the special sciences. He (and many others following him) takes the fact that special science laws typically involve kinds that are multiply realized and that special science laws are typically multiply implemented to show that they cannot be reduced to physics.[9] Fodor observes that

> The very existence of the special sciences testifies to reliable macro-level regularities that are realized by mechanisms whose physical substance is quite typically heterogeneous. . . . Damn near everything we know about the world suggests that unimaginably complicated to-ings and fro-ings of bits and pieces at the extreme micro-level manage somehow to converge on stable macro-level properties. (1998, p. 160)

He finds it "*molto mysterioso*" that the motions of the particles to-ing and fro-ing in accordance with $F = ma$ (or whatever the fundamental dynamical laws prove to be) lawfully end up converging on special science laws. It is not difficult to get into this mood. How do the particles that constitute an economy "know" that their trajectories are required (*ceteris paribus*) to enforce Gresham's law?

One response to the tension generated by 1–3 is to deny that the dynamical laws of physics are complete. This is the response of emergentists who think that there are special science dynamical laws or causal relations that shape the evolution of certain systems in ways that are not accounted for by laws of physics.[10] According to emergentism some special science laws are as metaphysically fundamental as laws of microphysics. On one variety of emergentism special science laws override the fundamental laws of microphysics in certain circumstances.[11] Another variety claims that there are gaps left by the fundamental laws of microphysics that may be filled by special science laws. On either of these views there are irreducible special science laws that in certain situations "direct" the motions of particles and the undulations of fields and so account for how those motions converge on special science regularities. In my view emergentism is not at all plausible. Despite occasional claims to the contrary physics has accumulated much evidence that there are fundamental dynamical laws of microphysics that are complete (even if they are not now known) and no

[9] Fodor's argument seems to be that if two distinct laws implement a higher level law then the lawfulness of the higher level law involves a kind of unity that isn't accounted for by the lower level laws. There is a lot wrong with this argument. One problem is, as we will see, when it comes to fundamental microphysical dynamical laws there are not many laws but, on most proposals, a single law of the evolution of state.

[10] By emergentism I mean the view that there are fundamental laws involving macro-properties. The macro-properties involved in such laws may themselves be physical and may be realized microphysically.

[11] On this view the laws of physics hold only as long as these circumstances don't obtain.

evidence that the fundamental laws can be overridden or are gappy in the way these versions of emergentism require.[12]

Fodor's own response to the tension among 1–3 is also a kind of emergentism but of a very peculiar kind. He grants that every special science system is microphysically constituted and that the dynamical laws of physics are complete but he claims that the laws of physics are *explanatorily* and *modally* incomplete. He adds that there are explanations and counterfactuals expressible in the language of a special science that are not necessitated by the laws and facts of fundamental physics. On his view special science counterfactuals and explanations require for their truth irreducible special science laws. So while a regularity expressed by a special science law is not independent of physics (i.e. it is implied by microphysical laws and facts) its status as a law is metaphysically independent of physics. It follows that the motions of the micro-constituents of a special science system are over-determined by both fundamental physical and special science laws even though special science counterfactuals and explanations are not determined by the physical laws and facts. So an economic interaction conforms both to Gresham's law and to the physical laws that govern the micro-entities that constitute the economic system but only Gresham's law supports the counterfactuals that underlie economic and intentional explanations of why it holds.

At first Fodor's view looks like it resolves the tension in a way that allows all of 1–3 to be true. However, I argue in a companion to this paper that Fodor's view is metaphysically and epistemologically implausible. The gist of my criticism is that if (1) and (2) are true then, contra Fodor, special science counterfactuals *are* necessitated by fundamental physical laws and facts.[13] So if there are metaphysically independent special science laws then they can only overdetermine counterfactuals. Such overdetermination is very puzzling. Why would there be a redundant system for some parts of nature? Was the lawmaker worried that the microphysical laws might wear out? A corollary of microphysical determination of macro counterfactuals is that we can never know whether or not

[12] The most serious worries about whether our universe contains a complete set of fundamental laws comes from the problem of reconciling general relativity with quantum mechanics and whether quantum theory itself can be understood as specifying objective laws. While many physicists are content to understand quantum mechanics instrumentalistically there are a number of interpretations that construe it as specifying objective laws (see Albert 1992). While the reconciliation problem remains it concerns regimes (black holes, the big bang) far from the concerns of the special sciences. Some philosophers, e.g. Nancy Cartwright (Cartwright 1999), claim that evidence for fundamental physical laws is obtained only in very special circumstances for very simple systems and doesn't provide support for the nomological completeness of physics. I can't get into this issue in this paper except to remark that a Nobel Prize is waiting for the scientist who demonstrates that the laws of physics that hold for microscopic systems fail for macroscopic systems. For a good discussion of Cartwright see Hoefer (2003).

[13] The fundamental microphysical laws that ground special science laws and counterfactuals include more than the dynamical laws. Why this is so is one of the main points of this paper. I get to it in a few pages.

there are metaphysically independent special science laws. All our experiments and observations would come out exactly the same way whether or not there are metaphysically independent special science laws. On Fodor's view it really is utterly mysterious why there should be anything except physics.

So we are confronted by a trilemma. On the one hand, there are reasons to think that special science laws are irreducible. On the other hand, there are reasons to think that both (1) and (2) are true. But (1) and (2) apparently leave no room for *irreducible* special science laws either as overriding or filling in gaps left by the fundamental laws or overdetermining microphysical events.

The questions of whether special science laws are reducible to or even can co-exist with dynamical laws of physics is even more difficult than Fodor thinks.[14] The problem is that all the candidates for the fundamental dynamical laws that physicists have taken seriously are so different from the typical special science dynamical laws that it is hard to see how it can be that if the world is governed by the former there can even be special science laws, let alone that they can be reduced to fundamental laws and facts.

The main relevant differences between fundamental dynamical laws and special science laws are these: The candidates for fundamental dynamical laws are (i) *global,* (ii) *temporally symmetric,* (iii) *exceptionless,* (iv) *fundamental (not further implemented),* and (v) *make no reference to causation.* In contrast, typical special science laws are (i*) *local,* (ii*) *temporally asymmetric,* (iii*) *multiply realized and implemented,* (iv*) *ceteris paribus,* and (v*) *often specify causal relations and mechanisms.*[15]

It is easiest to explain the features (i)–(v) of fundamental dynamical laws with the example of classical mechanics (similar points apply to relativistic mechanics and various versions of quantum mechanics). The basic ontology of classical mechanics (considered as a fundamental theory) consists of a space–time and point particles. The state of the universe (or an isolated subsystem) at a time t is given by a specification of the positions and momenta of the particles at t and a specification of the forces on the particles (which is given by a law connecting the positions of particles at t to the forces on the particles at t, e.g. Newton's gravitational law). The dynamical laws are specified by differential equations that characterize how the state evolves (the motion of particle k is given by $F = m_k a_k$). If we think of classical mechanics as the complete fundamental theory of the world then we will think that all material macroscopic (planets, storms, cats, humans) are constituted by point particles and that their movements are governed by these fundamental laws.

[14] Most of the discussion of whether the special science laws can be reduced to laws of physics is oblivious to these features of fundamental dynamical laws.

[15] The issues of stating determinism and whether the fundamental physical laws are deterministic are complicated (Earman 1986 and Loewer 2007*b*). Suffice it here to mention that there are proposals for the fundamental laws, in particular versions of quantum mechanics, that are deterministic and also versions that are probabilistic.

The dynamical laws of classical mechanics are complete and deterministic. Given the state at any time t they determine the state at any other time. The determination is *global* since the position and momentum of any particle at a time t + r is determined only by the global (i.e. the entire) state of that system at time t. That is, to know how any one particle moves at t + x one has to know something at each particle at t. The dynamical laws and a partial description of state at t (except in special cases) do not entail much about the state of the system at other times and, in particular, don't say much about what any particular particle will (was) doing at t + r. The classical mechanical dynamical laws are temporally symmetric since for every sequence of states s1, s2. . . sn that is compatible with the laws there is a temporally reversed sequence of states s*n, . . . s*2, s*1 where the sk and s*k are identical with respect to particle positions and particle momenta are reversed in direction. This means, for example, that since (we may suppose) a sequence of particle positions corresponding to a diver jumping off a diving board and landing in a pool is compatible with the dynamical laws then so is a sequence of states in which the diver is ejected feet first from the water and lands foot first on the board.[16] The Newtonian laws are exceptionless and obviously not multiply implemented since they are fundamental. Finally, "cause" is not a primitive relation of Newtonian mechanics. In a Newtonian world whatever causal relations among events exist are derivative and must supervene on the fundamental states and laws.[17]

Typical special science laws are very different from F = ma. One kind of special science law describes an aspect of the causal development, *ceteris paribus*, of macroscopic systems. For example, Gresham's law specifies that, *ceteris paribus*, introducing "bad" money into an economy *causes* the hoarding of "good" money. Some special science laws specify correlations among macro variables without specifying a causal relation. For example, *ceteris paribus* dropping atmospheric pressure is followed by stormy weather. Both of these examples (and many others) are temporally asymmetric and local.

The temporal asymmetry, locality of special science laws is difficult to reconcile with the temporal symmetry and globality of the fundamental laws. Note that the question isn't whether a special science regularity can be true given the fundamental laws. It is plausible that for a regularity like Gresham's there are certain initial conditions that the fundamental dynamical laws evolve so as to make it true. This had better be so if the fundamental laws are complete and Gresham's regularity is true. But there are also true but non-lawful regularities (e.g. that all the quarters in Smith's pockets (at all times) are quarters) that

16 There are fundamental processes involving the decay of certain elementary particles that are temporally asymmetric but this asymmetry has nothing to do with the temporal asymmetry of special science laws.

17 The same holds for other proposals for fundamental theories. The most well-known account of how causal relations supervene on more fundamental physical facts and laws is David Lewis's counterfactual account of causation (Lewis 1986).

the initial conditions are evolved to validate. Rather, the question is how a special science regularity can be *lawful* given the difference between it and the fundamental laws. How can there be temporally asymmetric and local special science laws when the fundamental dynamical laws are complete and temporally symmetric and global.

An obvious proposal is that those special science regularities that hold for *all* initial conditions are laws. But this isn't right. As I will shortly discuss typical special science laws are not true for all physically possible initial conditions. So where does the lawfulness of special science regularities come from? That is our question. And our problem is that it looks like there are special science laws, they are not metaphysically basic (as emergentists claim) and their lawfulness can't come from the fundamental dynamical laws. This should be enough to bug anyone.

A closely related question came up more than a century ago when physicists tried to account for how the special science of thermodynamics is related to fundamental physics. Examining this problem will lead us to a suggestion for how all special science laws are related to physics.

Thermodynamics concerns how certain macroscopic features of matter (gases, liquids, plastics, solids) including volume, temperature, pressure, energy, heat, work, entropy and so on are related to one another and how they evolve in certain systems. The dynamical laws of thermodynamics possess most of the features I listed for special science laws. The second law of thermodynamics says, in one of its forms, that the entropy of a macroscopic system increases over time. It is a *ceteris paribus* law since it holds only as long as the system is approximately energetically isolated. It is temporally asymmetric, local, and as multiply and heterogeneously realizable as it gets since it applies to gases, liquids, solids, electromagnetic fields and so on.

When physicists began to take seriously the idea that macroscopic systems are composed of molecules that (they thought) satisfy classical mechanics the question arose of how the temporally asymmetric thermodynamic laws can emerge from or even be compatible with the temporally symmetric fundamental laws. It was observed that there are physically possible initial conditions that realize an ice cube in warm water and are evolved by the fundamental laws to a state that realizes the ice cube melted and the water cooler. This process is entropy increasing. But there are also initial conditions that realize an ice cube in warm water where the laws evolve into a state that realizes a bigger ice cube in warmer water![18] However, the second evolution violates thermodynamic laws since it is entropy decreasing.[19] The puzzle that confronted physics when the hypothesis that material systems (gases, liquids and so on) are constituted by

[18] If S(t) is a state at t of a system consisting of an ice cube in warm water that evolves to a state S(t*) of a melted ice cube then the state S^(*t*) which consists of particles in the same relative positions as those in S(t*) but with reversed momenta will evolve into the state S^(*t*).

[19] There are a number of different formulations of the second law. See Sklar (1994) for a good discussion.

particles obeying classical mechanics was how it can be that, on the one hand, the fundamental dynamical laws are complete and temporally symmetric while there are laws of thermodynamics which take the form of dynamical laws governing macroscopic states and are temporally asymmetric? How does all the to-ing and fro-ing of molecules and fluctuations of fields manage to converge on the second law and other thermodynamic regularities?

The problem of reconciling the existence of temporally asymmetric laws of thermodynamics with temporally symmetric fundamental dynamical laws was first partly solved by Boltzmann. He observed that "most" of the micro-states (where the state is characterized by the positions and momenta of molecules of liquid water and ice) corresponding to an ice cube in warm water (and other non-equilibrium states) evolve towards the future into states in which the ice is melted and the water slightly colder (i.e. are entropy increasing). The sense of "most" that Boltzmann had in mind is this: Relative to the natural measure on micro-states the measure of the set of states exhibiting the melting of the ice is very nearly 1. He thought of this measure as corresponding to a probability distribution over the possible micro-states that realize a system satisfying thermodynamic conditions. It follows that for any system not in equilibrium (i.e. whose entropy is not maximum) the probability that its entropy is increasing is very nearly 1. But Boltzmann soon realized that the dynamical laws and probability distribution also entail that the probability that the ice cube was *previously* in a higher entropy state is also nearly 1, i.e. the ice cube spontaneously formed from water at a uniform temperature and grew bigger. This follows from the temporal symmetry of the dynamical laws. Of course this is an intolerable consequence so Boltzmann's "solution" can't be correct. There are various ways of responding to this paradox. The most promising proposal was suggested by Boltzmann himself, and has recently been given an elegant formulation by David Albert. Albert proposes that the laws include a claim that specifies that in the distant past (at the time of the big bang) the macro condition of the universe was one of very low entropy.[20] Although there are issues about exactly how to characterize entropy for the very early universe it is widely believed that current cosmological views agree that the entropy was very small. Albert calls the proposition that characterizes the macro-state of the universe at the time of the big bang "the Past Hypothesis" (PH). His proposal then is that the fundamental laws of the universe are the dynamical laws (and whatever plays the role of the force laws) and a law that specifies a probability distribution (or density) over possible initial conditions that assigns a value 1 to PH and is uniform over those micro-states that realize PH. I will call this probabilistic constraint on the initial conditions of the universe "PROB".

[20] Current cosmological theories also claim that the entropy of the macro-state of the very early universe was very very small. For a non-technical discussion see Greene (2005).

Following standard statistical mechanical reasoning Albert argues that the dynamical laws together with PROB entail probabilistic versions of the laws of thermodynamics (e.g. a probabilistic version of the second law). It is obvious that it follows from PROB and the dynamical laws that the entropy of the universe as a whole is very likely to increase as long as the macro-state's entropy is not maximum. Applied to parts of the universe the second law says that a system that becomes approximately energetically isolated and is not at equilibrium will be entropy increasing. The argument that Albert's proposal has this consequence can be illustrated as follows. Suppose that an ice cube is haphazardly dropped into a glass of warm water and the system S (the ice cube + glass of water) is approximately energetically isolated. Think of system S as "branching off" from a larger system $ (say a refrigerator that produced the ice cube and then ejected it into the bucket of water). Assume that $ satisfies the second law (i.e. the probability before the branching off that the entropy of $ increases is nearly 1). It is enormously likely (on the distribution determined by PROB) that there is no correlation between the micro-states of S and $; i.e. the state of S is "selected" at random from the states that realize the macro-state of $. It follows that it is enormously likely that the state of S is entropy increasing.[21] This line of reasoning can be pursued back to the time of the early universe where PROB posits a uniform distribution over the universe and so the second law holds.[22]

It is absolutely essential that PROB be understood as a law if it is to ground the increase of entropy as lawful. PROB is not a dynamical law but a law about initial conditions. This is why there is room to add it to the dynamical laws even when these are dynamically complete. It must be admitted that it is unusual to think of a constraint on initial conditions as a law, particularly a constraint on the initial conditions of the universe. Also, on most interpretations of objective probability it is impossible to make sense of a probability distribution over initial conditions of the universe.[23] But the probabilities posited by PROB must be objective if it is to ground lawful regularities. While I cannot get into a detailed discussion of this issue here I will mention two reasons. One is that an adequate account of counterfactuals (at least along the lines of David Lewis's account) needs to take PROB into an account and construe it as a law in order to ground the temporal

[21] The expression "branch system" is due to Reichenbach. He had the idea that the uniform statistical mechanical probability distribution should be applied to branch system at the moment it comes into existence and cannot be used to draw conclusions about the system prior to that time. There are problems with this idea (e.g. when does the system come into existence?). On Albert's account when a system branches off the probability distribution isn't the uniform one since it is constrained by the PH but like the uniform distribution it entails the high likelihood of entropy increasing.

[22] See Albert's discussion in (2000) for a bit more detail.

[23] Neither frequency nor propensity interpretations of probability are suitable. Frequency is inapplicable since there is only one initial condition. Propensity is inapplicable since propensities are dynamic.

asymmetry of counterfactuals. Second, the Best System account of laws deems it to be a law since adding it to the dynamical laws greatly increases informativeness with only a slight decrease in simplicity. Further, there is a natural extension of the best system account to include objective probabilities that does make sense of a probability distribution over initial conditions of the universe.[24]

The addition of PROB to the dynamical laws has consequences far beyond thermodynamics. One consequence that isn't much noticed but is quite important is that it justifies ordinary applications of classical mechanics to macro-systems.[25] When classical mechanics is used to predict (or explain) the motions of, for example, a cannon ball on the surface of the earth it is implicitly assumed that the micro-state of that cannon ball is a "normal" one in which it more or less maintains its shape until it strikes the something. But there are "abnormal" micro-states compatible with macro-descriptions of the cannon ball and its environment in which a few seconds after being shot it flies into three pieces each landing at different places. In fact there are all sorts of much more bizarre possibilities. Physicists neglect these possibilities since they implicitly and correctly assume that they are enormously unlikely. Their very low probability is a consequence of PROB.[26]

When PROB is added to the dynamical laws the result is completeness of the laws of physics in a sense that is stronger than dynamical completeness. Not only do the dynamical laws specify the evolution of state but every physical event and every regularity concerning physical events and every conditional probability involving physical events are assigned probabilities by PROB and the dynamical laws. It follows from PROB and the dynamical laws that there is an objective probability that a coin toss of a particular kind will result in heads conditional on the current macro-state, and an objective probability of a heat wave hitting the east coast on August 1, 2007 conditional on the current macro-state, and an objective probability that the introduction of bad money into the economy at t will subsequently lead to the hoarding of good money and so on. Of course, there is the *empirical* issue of whether the probabilities predicted by PROB and the dynamical laws are correct. That they are correct is supported by the fact that they underwrite thermodynamics. I provide some more reasons below.

My proposal is that lawful special science regularities are grounded in PROB and the dynamical laws. The case of thermodynamics shows how the probability distribution induced by PROB and the dynamical laws can ground temporally asymmetric, local, and multiply heterogeneously realizable probabilistic regularities. We can see all the to-ing and fro-ing of the molecules in an ice cube and the warm water into which it is dropped leads as a matter of law to the

[24] For a defense of these controversial claims see Loewer (2004 and 2006).

[25] This point is discussed in Albert (2008).

[26] Bizarre possibilities compatible with the macro-state involve very fine correlations among the positions and momenta of the particles that compose the projectile.

melting of the ice cube. So part of our puzzlement of how special science laws and complete dynamical laws can co-exist is relieved. Could it be that Gresham's law, the laws of natural selection, laws of intentional psychology and all other genuine special science laws are also grounded in PROB and the dynamical laws? It would be a very tall order to show that the dynamical laws and PROB imply a probabilistic version of Gresham's law (or any other special science law). No one will ever produce a deduction of a special science law since the special sciences are about entities and systems that are incredibly complicated from the perspective of physics and unlike the super Laplacian demon we don't have a translation manual that tells us which micro-states realize which special science properties. Nevertheless there is good reason to think that if SS is a special science law then its lawfulness is derived from PROB and the dynamical laws.

Here is a first stab at how this might work. Given PROB and the macro-state of the early universe certain regularities in addition to those entailed by the dynamical laws will have a high probability of holding. An example is the thermodynamic second law. As the universe evolves (as the micro-state evolves in accordance with the dynamical laws) the probability distribution conditional on the macro-state will also evolve. Let's say that the special science laws that hold at t are the macro-regularities that are associated with high conditional probabilities given the macro-state at t. That is Fs are followed by Gs *cp* is a law at t if P(Fs are followed by Gs/C&M(t*)) is near one. M(t*) is the macro-state at t, C is a stand-in for whatever *ceteris paribus conditions* are relevant. On this account the special science laws may change over time (new ones coming into existence and old ones going out of existence).

This account needs a lot of tinkering with if it is to capture those regularities that are deemed to be laws in the special sciences. My point in suggesting it is to show how PROB could ground special science regularities that have the problematic features of special science laws even though the dynamical laws are complete.

Of course the viability of this account depends on PROB's being true. So here are the reasons for thinking that it may well be true. First, it accounts for thermodynamic laws and the success of macro-classical mechanics. Second, it also seems to account for probabilistic processes that are not immediately connected to thermodynamics; for example Brownian motion and the behavior of gambling devices. Third, it looks like it provides a solution to our problem of the grounds of the lawfulness of special science laws.

By adding PROB to the fundamental dynamical laws the reductionist can answer an influential anti-reductionist line of argument that is alleged to show that physics misses nomological/explanatory structure that the special sciences supply. Philip Kitcher states the argument this way, citing:

the regularity discovered by John Arbuthnot in the early eighteenth century. Scrutinizing the record of births in London during the previous 82 years, Arbuthnot found that in each year a preponderance of the children born had been boys: in his terms, each year was a "male year". Why does this regularity hold? Proponents of the Unity-of-Science view can offer a recipe for the explanation, although they can't give the details. Start with the first year (1623); elaborate the physicochemical details of the first copulation-followed-by-pregnancy showing how it resulted in a child of a particular sex; continue in the same fashion for each pertinent pregnancy; add up the totals for male births and female births and compute the difference. It has now been shown why the first year was "male"; continue for all subsequent years. Even if we had this "explanation" to hand, and could assimilate all the details, it would still not advance our understanding. For it would not show that Arbuthnot's regularity was anything more than a gigantic coincidence. By contrast, we can already give a satisfying explanation by appealing to an insight of R. A. Fisher. Fischer recognized that, in a population in which sex ratios depart from 1:1 at sexual maturity, there will be a selective advantage to a tendency to produce the underrepresented sex. It will be easy to show from this that there should be a stable evolutionary equilibrium at which the sex ratio at sexual maturity is 1:1. In any species in which one sex is more vulnerable to early mortality than the other, this equilibrium will correspond to a state in which the sex ratio at birth is skewed in favor of the more vulnerable sex. Applying this analysis to our own species, in which boys are more likely than girls to die before reaching puberty, we find that the birth sex ratio ought to be 1.104:1 in favor of males—which is what Arbuthnot and his successors have observed. We now understand *why* [my italics], for a large population, all years are overwhelmingly likely to be male. (2001, p. 71)

Kitcher's point is that although Laplace's super demon could predict that each year more males than females are born from the complete micro-state and the dynamical laws (and the "translation" manual that specifies which physical states realize male births etc.) it would not really understand why Arbuthnot's regularity obtains. From the demon's perspective it would appear to be a gigantic coincidence since the initial micro-conditions that result in a majority of male births have nothing physically salient in common. On the other hand, "Fisher's law" that connects the survival rate of the sexes to their ratios at birth does explain the regularity and render it non-coincidental. Kitcher takes this to show that there is a lacuna in the physical laws that is filled by Fisher's law and more generally there are explanatory lacunae involving macro-regularities that are filled by special science laws. But if PROB is correct then it must also fill these lacunae. The reason is that if a regularity is lawful then it must also be likely and PROB is the arbiter of what is likely. If the super Laplace's demon knows PROB then it will be able to compute the probability of Arbuthonot's regularity given the macro-state of the world (or London) in 1683. That probability must be close to 1. If it weren't then it would be a coincidence that it turned out to be true. Further, it must be that if Fisher's law *is a law* then, starting at some time in the past (perhaps already at the big bang), the probability of Fisher's regularity given the macro-state at that and subsequent times must be close to 1. If this were not so then it could not be a law. And the same holds for all special science regularities that are genuinely lawful. So PROB (assuming it is correct) fills the explanatory lacunae that Kitcher noticed.

If the dynamical laws and PROB ground the lawfulness of all special science laws, does that show that special sciences are unnecessary or that special science laws are reducible to the laws of physics? It certainly doesn't show that they are unnecessary. There is no question of using PROB and the fundamental dynamical laws to make predictions since we are far from being super Laplacian demons. We need the special sciences to formulate lawful regularities in macro-vocabularies and to explain macro-phenomena. PROB is part of the explanation of why there are such regularities.

It is true that the account of special sciences I have described is reductionist in that it explains the lawfulness of special science laws in terms of the lawfulness of laws of physics including PROB. It thus reconciles the tension among 1–3 by denying the construal of 3 on which there are metaphysically independent special science laws. But the account isn't reductionist in some other ways. It doesn't entail that special science properties are identical to properties of fundamental physics and it allows for the multiply realizability, temporal asymmetry and so on of special science laws.

Question: "Why is there anything except physics?"
Answer: "Because there is physics!"

REFERENCES

Albert, David (1992). *Quantum Mechanics and Experience*, Cambridge, Mass.: Harvard Press.

—— (2000). *Time and Chance*, Cambridge, Mass.: Harvard Press.

—— (2008). *After Physics*. MS.

Cartwright, Nancy (1999). *The Dappled World: A Study of the Boundaries of Science*, Cambridge: Cambridge University Press.

Dyson, Freeman (2006). *The Scientist as Rebel*, New York: New York Review Books.

Earman, John (1986). *A Primer on Determinism*, Dordrecht: Reidel.

Elga, Adam (2006). "Isolation and Folk Physics", in *Russell's Republic: The Place of Causation in the Constitution of Reality*. Huw Price and Richard Corry, eds. Oxford: Oxford University Press.

Feynman, Richard (1965). *The Character of Physical Law*, Cambridge, Mass.: MIT Press.

Fodor, Jerry (1974). "Special Sciences and the Disunity of Science as a Working Hypothesis", *Synthese*, 28, 77–115.

—— (1998). "Special Sciences; Still Autonomous after All These Years", in *Philosophical Perspectives*, 11, *Mind, Causation, and World*, 149–63.

Greene, Brian (2005). *The Fabric of the Cosmos*, New York: Vintage Books, Random House.

Hoefer, Carl (2003). "For Fundamentalism", *Philosophy of Science*, 70, 1401–12.

Kim, Jaegwon (2005). *Physicalism, Or Something Near Enough*, Princeton: Princeton University Press.

—— (2007). "Causation and Mental Causation" in *Contemporary Debates in Philosophy of Mind*. Brian Mclaughlin and Jonathan Cohen, eds. Oxford: Blackwell, ch. 13.

Kitcher, Philip (2001). *Science, Truth, and Democracy*, Oxford: Oxford University Press, paperback edn. 2003.

Lewis, David (1986). *Philosophical Papers*, vol. ii, Oxford: Oxford University Press.

Loewer, Barry (2004). "David Lewis' Account of Objective Chance", *Philosophy of Science*, 71, 1115–25.

—— (2006). "Counterfactuals and the Second Law", in *Russell's Republic: The Place of Causation in the Constitution of Reality*. Huw Price and Richard Corry, eds. Oxford: Oxford University Press.

—— (2007*a*). "Mental Causation; or Something Near Enough", in *Debates in Philosophy of Mind*. Brian Mclaughlin and Jonathan Cohen, eds. New York: Blackwell publishing.

—— (2007*b*). "Determinism" in *The Routledge Companion to the Philosophy of Science*. Stathis Psillos and Martin Curd, eds. London: Routledge.

—— (2008). "Why Is There Anything Except Physics?" Forthcoming in *Synthese*.

Pietroski, P. and Rey, G. (1995). "When Other Things Aren't Equal: Saving Ceteris Paribus Laws from Vacuity", *British Journal for the Philosophy of Science*, 46: 81–110.

Sklar, Lawrence (1993). *Physics and Chance: Philosophical Issues in the Foundations of Statistical Mechanics*. Cambridge and New York: Cambridge University Press.

—— (1994). "Idealization and Explanation: A Case Study from Statistical Mechanics", in *Midwest Studies in Philosophy*, 18 (Philosophy of Science). P. French, T. Uehling and H. Wettstein, eds. South Bend, Ind.: University of Notre Dame Press, 258–70.

Weinberg, Steven (1992). *Dreams of a Final Theory*. New York: Pantheon.

9

Multiple Realization: Keeping It Real

Louise M. Antony

Jaegwon Kim's notorious "causal exclusion" argument is generally discussed in the context of the mental causation debate—the debate, that is, as to whether mental events can cause other events, or can cause them in virtue of their mentalistic properties (Kim 1993, 1999, 2000/1998). As I see it, however, it is an ontological challenge—to the view that mental properties are multiply realizable. The theory of multiple realizability (MR) was meant to show how one could resist reductionism without embracing dualism. The view combines two theses:

1) Mental properties are realized by physical properties.
2) Mental properties are multiply realizable.

Thesis (1) explains how mental properties can be causally efficacious, and thesis (2) certifies the autonomy of the mental from the physical, by blocking the reduction of a mental property to any particular physical property.

Philosophers have argued for MR on the basis of the intuition that it's not necessary to have a *brain* in order to have a *mind*. This intuition appears to be widely shared, both within and outside the academy. Popular culture abounds with extraterrestrials and artificial persons. The popular science fiction television series, *Star Trek: The Next Generation*, featured a gentle, thoughtful android named "Data"; in one episode, "The Measure of a Man", Data's status as a "sentient being" was challenged and successfully defended in a courtroom scene full of allusions to Shylock's speech in Shakespeare's *The Merchant of Venice*.

But will the intuition survive scrutiny? The thesis of MR is the natural concomitant to functionalism, the view that mental states are functional states. But about as soon as the doctrine of functionalism was articulated, skeptical voices began to sound. David Lewis, for example, pointed out that our ordinary concept of pain pushed simultaneously in two opposite directions: while we favored a functional characterization when we contemplated differently embodied, but similarly organized Martians, we treated sameness of physical state as criterial in the case of terrestrial creatures (Lewis 1978). Ned Block mischievously considered a robot controlled collectively by the citizens of China, choreographed so as to replicate the functional organization of a single human brain: would we really think such a golem had a mind?

More recently, Ruth Millikan has challenged the possibility of a substantive science built around functional kinds. When objects are typed according to abstract functional properties, she argues, the only "laws" that cover them will be the analytical truths that fall out of the functional definitions of the properties themselves. The "similarities" posited by functionalist typologies are not objective, but merely reflect shifting human interests (Millikan, 1986, 1999). In a rare point of convergence between the two thinkers, Noam Chomsky concurs with Millikan: "there is no interest in taking 'mental types' to be non-biological, any more than there would be in defining 'chemical' or 'optical types' that share some properties of chemical and optical aspects of the world". The question whether androids or aliens "really have minds", Chomsky avers, is precisely as interesting as the question whether airplanes "actually fly"—both are matters for decision, not discovery (Chomsky 2003, 261). (This from the person who is, arguably, the inventor of computationalist, and hence, functionalist psychology!)

Kim is really mounting the same sort of challenge, only more urgently. The causal exclusion argument, when applied to allegedly multiply realizable properties, shows not just that MR is trivial or uninteresting, but actually incoherent.

To see this, let's start with an instance of the exclusion problem, where a mental event appears to be the cause of a physical event: I want to tune up my E♭, and so I lift the first finger on my left hand. In this case, the mental event M(x) of my wanting to tune up my E♭ results in the physical event P(y) consisting in the rising of my finger. We may presume, with Kim, that the realm of the physical is *causally closed*, that is, that every physical event that has a cause at all has a completely sufficient physical cause (the principle CC). Since P(y) is a physical event, by CC, it must have a physical cause. That, presumably, is a neurophysiological event, N(z). The question now arises: what is the relation between property M and property N? We get a dilemma: if M is distinct from N, then M is causally otiose (because the instantiation of N is causally sufficient for the instantiation of P). In order, then, for M to be causally efficacious, it must be identical with N.

Kim is happy to stop here, to endorse "strong" or "type–type" reductionism.[1] But defenders of MR will protest that they have direct arguments against this conclusion. If minds are multiply realizable, then it is possible for there to be an M-instance that is not an N-instance. In that case, M cannot be the same property as N, and the reduction fails.

To this argument Kim makes a diabolical rejoinder. He points out, first of all, that for two physical properties to count as distinct realizers, they must be associated with different sets of causal powers. Hence, to say that a property, e.g. M, is multiply realized is to say that its instances are causally heterogeneous. But in that case, M is not a natural kind property. It is not the sort of property that can provide a basis for generalization from one of its instances to another; it does not "carve nature at its joints". MR properties are not, in short, "projectible".

[1] As opposed to "weak" or "token" reductionism.

To Kim, this means that multiply realizable properties are not the sort of properties that can figure in substantive scientific inquiry, and for very much the same reason cited by Millikan and Chomsky—the "resemblances" among instances of putatively multiply realizable properties are only superficial:

> [M]any philosophers want to argue that [a mental property M] is an irreducible property that nonetheless can be a property playing an important role in a special, "higher-level" science. I believe, however, that this position cannot be sustained. For if the "multiplicity" . . . of realizers means anything, it must mean that these realizers are causally and nomologically diverse. . . . All this points to the inescapable conclusion that [M], because of its causal/nomic heterogeneity, is unfit to figure in laws, and is thereby disqualified as a useful scientific property. On this approach, then, one could protect [M] but not as a property with a role in scientific laws and explanations. You could insist on the genuine propertyhood of [M] as much as you like, but the victory would be empty. (Kim, 1999, pp. 17–18)

So here is the irony. It is the asystematicity of the set of realizer properties that was supposed to provide the best reason for countenancing higher-order, functional properties in the first place. Here's Fodor making the point:

> I am willing to believe that physics is general *in the sense that it implies that any event which consists of a monetary exchange* (hence any event which falls under Gresham's Law) *has a true description in the vocabulary of physics and in virtue of which it falls under the laws of physics.* But banal considerations suggest that a description which covers all such events must be wildly disjunctive. . . . What are the chances that a disjunction of physical predicates which covers all these events . . . expresses a physical natural kind? In particular, what are the chances that such a predicate forms the antecedent or consequent of some proper law of physics? [Emphases original] (Fodor 1974: 102)

But Kim's rejoinder would go like this: if the set of physical realizer properties of the economic property MONETARY EXCHANGE is "wildly disjunctive" and hence anomic when described in physicalistic terms, that same set cannot be made nomic simply by introducing a new *predicate*. If instances of two physical properties P and P* are diverse with respect to the causal powers they possess, then they cannot be made to form a kind by just redescribing them both as "M's".

Defenders of MR will protest, insisting that instances of disparate physical realizers of a multiply realizable property like M really *do* have something in common, namely, their "M-ness". The predicate "M" is needed precisely because the real regularities that hold among M-instances cannot be "captured" in the vocabulary appropriate at the level of the realizers. M-regularities are "invisible" at lower levels.

Talk of this sort, of regularities that are "invisible" from the perspective of the physical or biological sciences, and that need to be "captured" by higher-order vocabulary, is ubiquitous in the MR literature. But when we look closely, we see that not much attention has been paid to the question of when there really is an objective regularity, one that is "missed" by the lower-order sciences, and needs to be "captured" by new terms. The answer to this question is certainly not evident in the ontological architecture of a multiply realized property. Here is the canonical schematic:

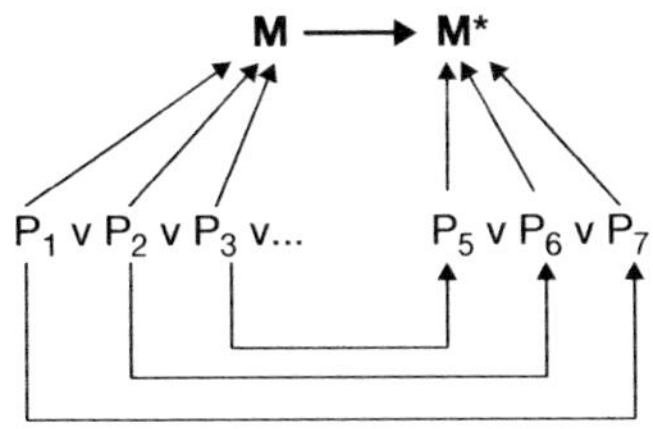

The problem is that we can easily cook up "regularities" and "properties" that are, intuitively, completely bogus, but yet fit the ontological profile characteristic of multiply realized properties.

Choose three pairs of causally related events, and make them as dissimilar as possible (so, for instance: (1) a soprano's singing a high C resulting in the shattering of a glass (does that really happen?), (2) my wanting to whistle a tune resulting in the pursing of my lips, and (3) my daughter's pounding the pad with the mallet at the carnival causing the bell to ring). Label each of the causally relevant properties, C_1, C_2, and C_3; and label each of the properties instantiated as effects, E_1, E_2, and E_3. Now let's define two higher-order properties, **C** and **E**, as follows: an object has property **C** just in case it has either C_1, C_2, or C_3; and an object has property **E** just in case it has either E_1, E_2, or E_3. We now have a new "regularity" that cannot be expressed in the vocabulary of C_i's and E_I's, but that can be expressed in our new terms: **C**'s cause **E**'s.

I trust no one will be tempted to take seriously the suggestion that we need to add "**C**" and "**E**" to our vocabularies, lest we "miss" the "regularity" thus described. Yet the ontological structure of the situation is exactly isomorphic to cases of "genuine" multiple realizability:

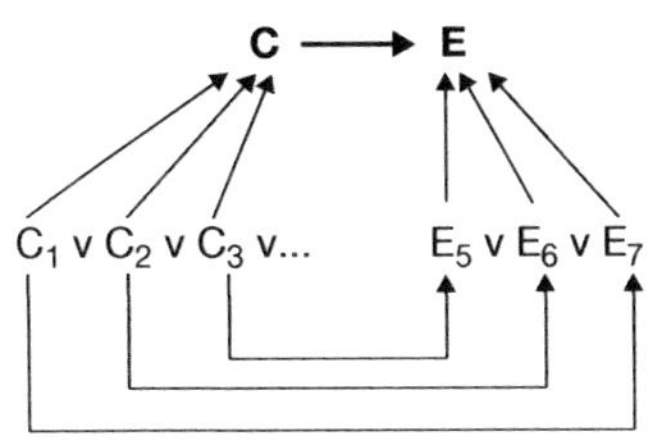

The defender of MR needs to say much more about what makes for a real regularity in order to meet Kim's challenge.

What the preceding has shown, I think, is that there are actually two distinct critical strands in Kim's challenge to MR. The first could be called the *Incoherence Challenge*: this is the charge that it is incoherent to hold that one and the same set of objects or events is anomic at one level of description, but nomic at a different level of description. The second I'll call the *Conventionality Challenge*: here the charge is that nomicity should depend on objective similarity, and not merely on how things are described. I think both these challenges can be met, so that we can find a third way between the horns of Kim's dilemma, and vindicate MR. Along the way, I'll have some things to say about predicates, properties, nomicity, and reduction.

Let me start with the Incoherence Challenge. The problem here is the claimed mismatch in nomic status between two necessarily co-extensive properties: a higher-order property, which is supposed to be nomic, and a lower-order, disjunctive property, which is supposed to be anomic. This problem has an obvious solution: drop the claim that the lower-order disjunctive property is anomic.

But my suggestion may seem, from the point of view of a partisan of MR, deeply counterproductive. In the first place, isn't it a given that disjunctive properties are *not* nomic? And in the second place, if lower-order disjunctive properties actually are nomic, what argument is there anymore against strong reduction? Doesn't my proposed concession give away the game altogether? Finally, won't this maneuver simply strengthen the Conventionality Challenge—doesn't it just admit that higher-order properties are no more principled than the wild disjunctive properties they were to replace?

First things first: is there reason to think that disjunctive properties can never be nomic? Many philosophers have presumed that arguments developed by David Armstrong against disjunctive universals show exactly that (Armstrong 1978). So let's look at those.

The first argument is that there need be no "real resemblance" among objects that satisfy a disjunctive condition. (I'll assume that "real resemblances" are patterns of similarity tracked by nomic properties.) So, for example, Armstrong points out that there is nothing that ravens and writing desks have in common simply in virtue of their each possessing the property of being a raven or writing desk. This observation is certainly correct. But showing that many disjunctive properties are not nomic hardly shows that none are. And there can be no such demonstration, because it is easy enough to find examples of disjunctive properties that are nomic. Consider, for example, the property of being a cow or a bull. The animals that possess this property are exactly the individual members of the species BOS TAURUS (family Bovidae, subfamily Bovinae), and the species is a biological natural kind *par excellence*. It just happens that English has not lexicalized the species name, and has only names for male and female individuals. In the case of other animal species this is not true; we have "mare" and "stallion", but also "horse". This lexical accident, however, does not bear directly on the question whether cows and bulls really have something in common—they obviously do.

At best, what Armstrong has shown is (to speak loosely) that universals are not closed under disjunction—there's no guarantee that a disjunction of predicates each of which expresses a universal, itself expresses a universal. This leaves it completely open, however, that there be some disjunctive predicates that do express universals—or, in my parlance, express nomic properties.

So the mere fact that a predicate is disjunctive in form does not entail that the property it expresses fails to track real resemblances. The converse is also the case: it doesn't follow from the fact that a predicate is lexically simple that it expresses a property that tracks a real resemblance. This should be obvious from the example above, where I introduced the predicates "**C**" and "**E**"—it's altogether too easy to invent lexically simple expressions for the existence of such an expression to carry any metaphysical weight.

This brings me to the question of what a property is, anyway—or at least to the question when we've got a single property rather than two. Properties are clearly intensional entities of some sort—two properties may be completely co-extensive in the actual world, but have divergent extensions in other possible worlds. But are properties *hyper-intensional*? The extension of the disjunctive predicate "cow-or-bull" is necessarily co-extensive with the predicate "member of species *bos taurus*". But do these two predicates express the same property? This is obviously a huge topic, and not one that I can address adequately here. Let me just say this: if we are realists about properties at all, then it makes sense to allow that different linguistic expressions can express the same property, in just the way that different names can refer to the same object. This consideration, together with the ones marshaled above, suggests that we do not want a criterion of property identity so fine that we must acknowledge a new property for every distinct predicate.

It seems a natural step, then, to think of properties as individuated by their extensions in all possible worlds, or even to go the further step, following Lewis, of identifying properties with sets of possibilia. If we do that, then talk of "disjunctive *properties*" becomes inapt. Sets have no logical structure; it can only be the *predicates* that express them that have logical structure. So a linguistic reform is needed. I'll now express my proposal the following way: Every higher-order mentalistic predicate is necessarily co-extensive with, and thus expresses the *same property as*, the lower-order disjunctive predicate formed by alternation of physical realizers across possible worlds.

But if, as I've been arguing, we cannot look to the lexical/syntactic form of the predicate that expresses a property in order to see if it's nomic, what can we look to? In particular, what makes it the case that some disjunctive predicates express nomic properties, while others do not?

It will be helpful at this point to remember the history of the notion of "projectibility". As the notion was introduced by Goodman, it applies in the first instance to *predicates*. A predicate is projectible, Goodman said, if and only if it is *entrenched* within a linguistic community. Entrenchment is a sociolinguistic phenomenon: a predicate is entrenched just in case it is used successfully by members of a community to project properties from some sample of objects to other things in the target domain. Now Goodman was a nominalist, and he was, by modern lights, a deflationist about laws, so he rejected the suggestion that there was any nomic structure underlying the phenomenon of entrenchment—say, the existence of laws involving the properties expressed by the entrenched predicates. But we needn't honor Goodman's scruples in order to make use of his concepts of entrenchment and projectibility. We can ask what explains the entrenchment of a given predicate, and can countenance the following answer: the best explanation of a predicate's entrenchment in a given community is often that the property expressed by that predicate is genuinely nomic.

To make this a little more precise, let's adopt the following conventions: (1) "Entrenchment" is an observable socio-linguistic property, one that a predicate can have to a greater or lesser degree, and that the same predicate can possess to a high degree at one time or in one community, and to a low degree at another time or in another community. (2) A *predicate* will be said to be "projectible" just in case it (a) is entrenched in some community and (b) can in fact be used to state correct predictions and robust (although possibly *ceteris paribus)* generalizations. (3) A *property* will be said to be projectible if and only if it is expressed by some projectible predicate, in some language, for some intentional beings. (4) A property is *nomic* if it participates in objective lawful regularities.

Given these stipulations, we can now say the following: typically, but not necessarily, entrenched predicates will be projectible. That is, predicates that are entrenched permit and will continue to permit the formulation of correct predictions and robust generalizations. ("Witch" may have been entrenched for a while, but it is not, as it turns out, projectible.) The explanation for the projectibility of a predicate, and hence, in many cases, for its entrenchment, is that the property expressed by that predicate is nomic. Finally, all projectible properties are nomic, but not all nomic properties need be projectible. There may well be nomic properties that neither we, nor the members of any other linguistic community, are ever able to express by means of a projectible predicate.

Here's the situation, then, with respect to higher-order properties and lower-order disjunctive properties. Every higher-order predicate is necessarily co-extensive with some lower-order, possibly infinitely long, disjunctive predicate. Because they are necessarily co-extensive, they express the same property. Hence, it is impossible for one of these to express a nomic property and the other *not* to express a nomic property. (So much for the Incoherence Charge.)

But notice that the following is certainly possible, and indeed almost certainly true: the higher-order predicate and the lower-order disjunctive predicates can differ with respect to *entrenchment*, and hence with respect to their *projectibility*.

Lower-order disjunctive predicates have many features that make it overwhelmingly unlikely that they could ever become entrenched within human communities. For one thing, they may well be infinite, and then they will take too long to *say*. But there are many other features such predicates will have that will make them unsuitable for use by human beings:

> the list of disjuncts will be unprincipled: typically, no human being will know which items to put on the list;
>
> each disjunct in the disjunctive predicate will itself embody a welter of detail, typically more than any human being will have access to;
>
> the detail may concern matters about which human beings are generally ignorant (e.g., the neurophysiological detail that would presumably figure in disjuncts expressing the properties realizing a mental state).

In short, the lower-order disjunctive predicates we've been considering simply will not be suited to human beings' purposes in formulating observations and projecting hypotheses.[2]

So lower-order disjunctive predicates can safely be presumed to be unprojectible. This does not mean, of course, that they do not express projectible properties. If, as in the case we are imagining, a non-projectible lower-order disjunctive predicate is necessarily co-extensive with a well-entrenched mentalistic predicate, then the two predicates express the same property. And if the best explanation of the entrenchment of the higher-order mentalistic predicate is that the property it expresses is nomic, then the unentrenched, unprojectible disjunctive predicate, no less than the entrenched higher-order predicate, expresses a nomic property.

We are now, finally, in a position to return to the second of Kim's challenges, the Conventionality Challenge. The worry was that the expedient I adopted to meet the Incoherence Challenge—allowing that disjunctive properties could be nomic (or, as I'd now say, disjunctive *predicates* could *express nomic properties*)—would make it all the more difficult to answer the objection that the regularities "needing" capture by higher-order vocabulary are only artefacts of conventional linguistic practice. But in fact, the floodgates did not open when I allowed that disjunctive predicates *could* express nomic properties. We can make an invidious distinction among disjunctive predicates: some do and some do not express nomic properties. Of the ones that do express nomic properties, a good many will be those that are necessarily co-extensive with the higher-order predicates that are well entrenched in our community.

This all makes good sense of the arguments of Fodor and Putnam I alluded to before. Both philosophers appealed to the *disutility* of purely physicalistic descriptions of things covered by higher-order predicates. Fodor emphasized the disutility of lengthy (possibly infinite) unsystematic disjunctive predicates, and

[2] I argue in much more detail for the presumptive non-projectibility of these predicates in Antony 1999, and Antony 2003.

Putnam emphasized the disutility of extremely detailed predicates. Neither sort of predicate could ever serve human purposes of prediction and explanation, and thus could never become entrenched in a human society. Fodor took this unsuitability as indicative of the ontological status of the properties expressed by the disjunctive predicate, but we do not any longer need to endorse this conclusion. Entrenchment of a predicate is presumptive evidence of the nomicity of the property expressed, but non-entrenchment—indeed, non-projectibility—of a predicate should *not* be taken as presumptive evidence against the lawfulness of the property it expresses. (Consider: every non-basic nomic predicate will be co-extensive with *some* disorderly predicate.) Because the unwieldy disjunctive predicates are necessarily co-extensive with their associated higher-order predicates, the properties expressed by each must match with respect to lawfulness. Indeed, I've suggested, the properties expressed by the two predicates are identical.

The practical ineliminability of mentalistic vocabulary—of the canonical vocabulary of both folk and scientific psychologies—can now be seen to have ontological consequences. It's not *just* a fact about us that such vocabulary is useful. The vocabulary wouldn't be useful (in the precise ways that it is, grounding serious empirical prediction, for example) if it didn't track real patterns in the world, if it didn't mark out real resemblances among things. *That* such vocabulary is useful, is an empirical fact that demands explanation. The best explanation, I'm suggesting, is that there really are laws involving the properties expressed by mentalistic terms.

There remain two loose ends. First of all, I have not yet responded to the second of Armstrong's objections to the idea of disjunctive universals, or, rather, as I'd now put it, to the idea that disjunctive predicates can express nomic properties. This is the "causal powers" objection. The second dangler concerns reductionism: if I acquiesce in the identification of properties expressed by higher-order predicates with those expressed by lower-order disjunctive predicates, haven't I sacrificed the autonomy of the mental? Haven't I thereby identified mental properties with physical properties—what the strong reductionist was after all along?

I'll start with Armstrong's objection. "There is some very close link between universals and causality," he writes. How close a link? Armstrong tells us that different universals must bestow different causal powers on the objects that instantiate them; otherwise, we could have no knowledge of universals. But an object that has universal C would gain no new powers in virtue of having (the putative universal) C v M. Hence, C v M cannot be a distinct universal from C.[3] (This argument of Armstrong's taps the same intuition as Kim's appeal to "Alexander's Dictum" in the causal exclusion argument. There, recall, Kim argued that because a multiply realized property "inherits" its causal powers, on any given instantiation, from its lower-order realizer property, it has no causal

[3] Armstrong (1978).

powers of its own, and therefore cannot be countenanced as a real property.) To this objection I would like to make a "lawyerly" response: my client didn't do it, I say, and anyway, he was insane at the time.

My client didn't do it. Notice that the epistemological rationale Armstrong cites for the principle that distinct universals must bestow distinct causal powers is satisfied as long as two putatively distinct universals *differ* in the causal powers they bestow. There's no justification for the requirement, implicit in Armstrong's argument, that a "new" universal *adds to* whatever causal powers the object already possesses. There is, therefore, no reason why a property corresponding to a higher-order predicate couldn't be a universal associated with the intersection of the causal powers of all of its lower-order realizers.

He was insane at the time. I think the above response is sufficient. But if one insists on wholly new causal powers in order to countenance the properties I'm lobbying for, they can be provided. Remember that the projectibility of a mentalist predicate entails epistemic access, on the part of creatures like ourselves, to things grouped as mental. But epistemic access is a *causal* phenomenon. Mental things have the power to produce recognition in us, and this power is *not* one that's "inherited" from lower-order properties. The generalizations of folk psychology are, epistemically speaking, realization-independent. I recognize someone as being in pain, or as believing something, or as wanting something, in virtue of their instantiating mental universals, not neurophysiological ones. These latter properties are epistemically inaccessible to me, except *via* my access to the mental universals, together with knowledge of the correct realization theory. We thus have a case for there being a new causal power distinctive of mental universals: the ability to affect certain kinds of epistemic agents in certain ways.

That leaves just the worry about reductionism. Notice, to start, that in light of the criterion of property identity I've adopted, we need a new way of understanding reductionism. The old way involved putative relations between "mental properties" and "physical properties". But how are we to classify the properties I've been discussing? One and the same property, I contend, is expressed by a higher-order mentalistic predicate and by a lower-order disjunctive physicalistic predicate. But the same relation will hold between so-called "biological properties", "chemical properties", "geological properties", and so on. If we want to frame an issue about reductionism, it must be done in terms of a relation between various bodies of vocabulary.[4] So reconstrued, the thesis of strong reductionism about the mental says this: every mentalistic predicate is necessarily co-extensive with some *proprietary* predicate of a lower-order or lower-level science.

[4] This way of thinking of reductionism, by the way, is not such a departure from the original notion, à la Oppenheim–Putnam, of reduction, which was held to be a relation among *theories* and the laws stated within those theories. See Oppenheim and Putnam 1958.

This is not an *ad hoc* formulation. It's necessary to limit the reducing predicates to the proprietary predicates of the reducing theories to avoid trivializing the thesis of reductionism. If physicalism is true, then we know that every state of affairs has some true description couched entirely in the vocabulary of (the completed) physics. But most such states of affairs—the ones of interest to us at least—will appear from the perspective of fundamental physics to be unsystematic assemblages of stuff. It is highly significant that physics has no way of representing in a concise and intelligible way what—for example—all diamonds have in common. Physics must simply itemize the various distributions of energy over space-time (or strings, or whatever it is this week) that happen to constitute the various things that we have no trouble representing compactly in the proprietary language of mineralogy.

If we wish to express some truth that we would ordinarily express in a higher-order vocabulary—take Putnam's example: "rigid round pegs of 1″ diameter will not fit through square holes of a rigid material with sides of 1″"—we would have to rig up ungodly complicated combinations of fundamental physical facts, undoubtedly involving Boolean constructions of predicates of unbelievable complexity. As Putnam points out, there will be micro-differences between any two round pegs that will not matter at all for purposes of predicting fit with a particular hole. And these micro-differences will be no less significant, from the physical point of view, than any other set of differences between any other two pegs. It therefore would do us no good, if our interests are in generalizing from the behavior of one peg to the behavior of others, to try to work with the complete and fundamental physical picture. Proprietary predicates, in other words, are predicates that are or can become entrenched with a community. They represent the contours of resemblance discernible at a given level of abstraction. Such contours prescind from differences of detail apparent at a higher level of resolution, and therein lies their utility.

Multiple realizability, I conclude, has done everything it was supposed to do, Kim's argument notwithstanding. Mental properties (speaking loosely) are objective and autonomous from physical properties. We can be confident that they are objective because they are expressed by projectible predicates. We know them to be autonomous because the entrenched mentalistic predicates that express them are demonstrably not co-extensive with any proprietary predicates of any lower-order science.

REFERENCES

Antony, Louise (1999). "Multiple Realizability, Projectibility and the Reality of Mental Properties." *Philosophical Topics* 26/1: 1–24.

—— (2003). "Who's Afraid of Disjunctive Properties?" *Philosophical Studies* 13: 1–21.

Armstrong, David (1978). *A Theory of Universals: Universals and Scientific Realism*, vol. ii (Cambridge: Cambridge University Press).

Chomsky, Noam (2003). "Reply to Lycan." In L. Antony and N. Hornstein (eds.), *Chomsky and His Critics* (Oxford: Blackwell Publishers).

Fodor, Jerry (1974). "Special Sciences." *Synthese* 28: 97–115.

Kim, Jaegwon (1993). "Multiple Realization and the Metaphysics of Reduction." In *Supervenience and Mind* (Cambridge: Cambridge University Press).

—— (1999). "Making Sense of Emergence." *Philosophical Studies*, 95/1–2 (August): 1–36.

—— (2000/1998). *Mind in a Physical World* (Cambridge, Mass.: MIT Press). Paperback Edition.

Lewis, David (1978). "Mad Pain and Martian Pain." In *Readings in the Philosophy of Psychology*, vol. i (Cambridge, Mass.: MIT Press).

Millikan, Ruth (1986). "Thoughts Without Laws: Cognitive Science with Content." *Philosophical Review* 95: 47–80.

—— (1999). "Historical Kinds and the 'Special Sciences'." *Philosophical Studies* 95: 45–65.

Oppenheim, Paul, and Hilary Putnam (1958). "The Unity of Science as a Working Hypothesis." *Minnesota Studies in the Philosophy of Science*, 2: 3–36.

10

Causation and Determinable Properties: On the Efficacy of Colour, Shape, and Size

Tim Crane

1. INTRODUCTION

This paper presents a puzzle or antinomy about the role of properties in causation. In theories of properties, a distinction is often made between *determinable* properties, like red, and their *determinates*, like scarlet (see Armstrong 1978, volume ii). Sometimes determinable properties are cited in causal explanations, as when we say that someone stopped at the traffic light because it was red. If we accept that properties can be among the relata of causation, then it can be argued that there are good reasons for allowing that some of these are determinable properties. On the other hand, there are strong arguments in the metaphysics of properties to treat properties as *sparse* in David Lewis's (1983) sense. But then it seems that we only need to believe in the most *determinate* properties: particular shades of colour, specific masses, lengths and so on. And if we also agree with Lewis that sparse properties are 'the ones relevant to causal powers' (1983: 13) it seems we must conclude that if properties are relevant to causation at all, then all of these are determinate properties.

I call this 'the antinomy of determinable causation'. On the one hand, we have a good argument for the claim that determinable properties can be causes, if any properties are. I call this the *Thesis*. But on the other hand, we have a good argument for the claim that only the most determinate properties can be causes, if any properties are. I call this the *Antithesis*. Clearly, we need to reject either the

Work on this chapter was made possible by a fellowship at the Collegium Budapest, Hungary, and by support from the AHRB's Research Leave Scheme. Thanks to participants at the 2004 NAMICONA special science causation workshop in Aarhus, to participants at a workshop on mental causation at Macquarie University in 2004, and to audiences at the Universities of Edinburgh, the LSE and Warwick. Special thanks to Jordi Fernandez, Jakob Hohwy, and (especially) Jesper Kallestrup for their helpful written comments.

Thesis or the Antithesis—or we need to find a *Synthesis*. At the end of this paper I will indicate my preferred solution.

Although the antinomy can be framed purely in terms of physical properties (e.g. mass), it also connects with the debate about special science causation in a number of interesting ways. First of all, and most obviously, the special sciences seem to deal in determinable properties too, so they should be concerned with any threat to their causal efficacy. Second, and more specifically, it has been argued by Stephen Yablo (1992) that we should think of the relationship between 'higher-level' properties and basic physical properties in terms of the determinable–determinate relationship. The basic idea is that just as being red is a way of being coloured, so (for example) having one's brain in a certain specific condition is a way of being in pain. Yablo argues that this way of thinking of the relationship between higher-level (or special) properties and physical properties offers a solution to the problem of mental causation, the so-called 'exclusion problem'.[1] This problem is often framed at an intuitive level in terms of the idea of causal competition: how can a mental (or any higher level) property have any effects in the physical world, if physical causes (properties) are always enough to bring about all physical effects? Don't the mental properties 'compete' for causal efficacy with the physical properties, entering a competition that they cannot possibly win?

Yablo answers this question by applying the determinate–determinable distinction. For just as the redness of the traffic light and its simply being coloured do not 'compete' with one another for causal efficacy, so the brain state and the pain do not compete. This is not because these properties are identical, any more than redness and being coloured are identical. It is rather that in any given case, being in a particular brain state *just is* a way of being in pain. With this account of the relationship between properties, plus an account of causation, Yablo attempts to solve the causal exclusion problem (*cf.* Macdonald and Macdonald 1986 for an earlier, related solution).

Ingenious though it is, Yablo's solution is threatened by the antinomy of determinable causation. For unless determinable properties can be causes, Yablo's solution will not work. It turns out that the ramifications of the antinomy touch any theory which treats any higher-level or special science properties as determinables.

The remainder of this paper divides into four parts. In the next part I lay out some background assumptions about properties, determinates and determinables, and causes and effects. In the third I present an argument for the Thesis: determinables can be causes. Then I present an argument for the Antithesis: only the most determinate properties can be causes. In the final section I suggest how the antinomy might be resolved.

[1] There is a vast literature on this problem by now. For some important recent discussions, see Kim 1989, Kim 1998, Bennett 2003, Kallestrup 2006.

2. DETERMINATES, DETERMINABLES AND PROPERTIES AS CAUSES

By 'property' I understand any general feature or quality or characteristic of things. I will talk about 'properties' in a general way, without prejudice as to whether they are universals, sets, tropes or some other kind of entity altogether. There will be other reasons to distinguish between different conceptions of properties, and we may find reasons for being committed to one or another controversial thesis about them. But for the time being I will simply try and state the obvious.

I assume here that if they exist at all, properties are distinct from the words we use to talk about them. The words we use to talk about properties are sometimes grouped together as 'predicates'. In fact, we also use words which are not, strictly speaking, predicates to talk about properties. 'Red', for example, seems to be the name of a property, whereas 'is red' or '*x* is red' is a predicate. The natural thing to say is that 'red' is the name of the property which we predicate of something when we say that it is red. (Those with Fregean scruples may ignore this talk of names of properties; nothing turns on it here.)

Some properties are related as determinate to determinable.[2] Colours are the standard textbook example. Shapes are another, sizes and weights are yet others. The basic idea is that the properties of being coloured, say, and being red are related in the same kind of way that the properties of being shaped and being triangular (or having a weight and weighing 5 kilos) are. Being red, being triangular and weighing 5 kilos are all *determinates* of the *determinables* colour, shape and weight. If an object has a colour, or a shape or a size, then it must have some specific, particular colour, shape or size: it cannot just be coloured, shaped or sized *per se* (or *simpliciter* as it is sometimes said). Similarly, if an object is red or square, it cannot just be red or square *per se* or *simpliciter*; it must be some specific shade of red or some specifically sized square. So just as red is a determinate of the determinable colour, so scarlet is a determinate of the determinable red. The determinate–determinable relation is therefore a relative one: many properties are neither determinables or determinates in themselves, but rather they are determinates of one determinable, and determinables of other determinates. Thus *red* is a determinate of the determinable *colour*, and a determinable of the determinate *scarlet*.

However, it makes sense to suppose that there are properties which have no further determinates. To use a useful term of Eric Funkhouser's, these are

[2] Classic texts on this subject are: Johnston 1921, Prior 1949, Searle 1959. Also important are Sanford 2006, Yablo 1992, and Armstrong 1997: 48–63. An excellent recent discussion is Funkhouser 2006.

'super-determinates' (Funkhouser 2006). Likewise, it makes sense to suppose that there are properties which are not determinates of any determinable. These are, similarly, 'super-determinables'. They could also be called 'absolute determinates' or 'absolute determinables'.

Three further features of the determinable–determinate relation are worth noting here. First, the relation is not exactly the same as many other 'determination' relations, like entailment, supervenience, or the genus–species relation. Take genus–species for example. To say that *human being* is a species of the genus *animal*, for example, is to say that being a human being is being an animal *plus* something else (say, being rational). But being red is not being coloured *plus* something else. Being red is simply a way of being coloured. In addition, the determinate–determinable relation is not simply an entailment relation (although of course 'This book is red' does entail 'This book is coloured'). The way we are understanding the relation, the proposition 'P or Q' is not a determinable of 'P'; and 'P and Q' is not a determinate of 'P'. Yet these are examples of entailment.[3]

Second, it is traditionally held that determinates of the same determinable at the same level are incompatible with one another. If an object is completely red, then it cannot be completely yellow. If an object is triangular, then it cannot be square. However, if an object is completely red it can be completely scarlet: determinables can be compatible with those properties which are their own determinates. But they obviously cannot be compatible with other determinates of those determinables with which they are already incompatible (e.g. yellow with scarlet).

Third, determinates of the same determinable can be different in varying ways. Shades of colour, for example, can fail to coincide in at least one of three ways, standardly called (these days) *hue*, *saturation*, and *brightness*.[4] Following Funkhouser (2006) I will call these 'ways things fail to coincide' the *determination dimensions* of a determinable. The determination dimensions of colour are as just described; the dimension of mass is measured in units of mass; the dimension of squareness is the lengths of the four sides; and so on. Essentially, the idea is that different determinates of a determinable are distinguished by the values of their various determination dimensions.

There are many more things in general one can say about the determinable–determinate relation, both as a way of distinguishing it from other 'determination' relations, and in terms of its application to other areas of metaphysics. But here I want to put these complexities to one side, and briefly introduce what Funkhouser calls 'super-determinates', since this will be important when we come to formulate the antinomy.

[3] So I prefer the treatment of this issue in Funkhouser 2006, as against Yablo 1992.

[4] The last two are sometimes called *chroma/purity* and *value* respectively. For an introduction to the structure of colour, see Byrne and Hilbert 1994.

W. E. Johnson, who first introduced the terminology of determinates and determinables, clearly thought that there are superdeterminates, no matter how difficult it might be in practice to specify them:

> The practical impossibility of literally determinate characterization must be contrasted with the universally adopted postulate that the characters of things which we can only characterize more or less indeterminately, are, in actual fact, absolutely determinate. (Johnson 1921: 185)

For Johnson, this is a 'postulate'. And although not all philosophers would agree with him (see Sanford 1970), many have found it plausible. D. M. Armstrong, for example, writes that

> A physical object is determinate in all respects, it has a perfectly precise colour, temperature, size, etc. It makes no sense to say that a physical object is light-blue in colour, but is no definite shade of light blue. (Armstrong 1961: 59)

Many difficulties arise out of the assumption of super-determinacy, however. One is the problem of vagueness. However, a belief in super-determinacy will be consistent with the vagueness of our concepts if one were prepared to insist (as Johnson does) that the world *itself* is perfectly precise and non-vague. The boundaries between things in the world could be entirely sharp, even if our colour concepts are irredeemably vague. I will assume here that the vagueness of colour concepts does not imply that colours themselves cannot be super-determinate.

In what follows, I will use the example of colour, and later I will discuss the possibility that there are super-determinate colours. But this is really just an illustration of the general problem; if it turns out that there are no super-determinate colours—i.e. that colours are not among the super-determinate properties of things in the world—then the antinomy can be formulated in terms of another example of determinable properties.

So much, for the time being, for the distinction between determinates and determinables. My final preliminary remarks concern the role of properties in causation. I have talked above about properties as causes, or as causally efficacious. I realize that some philosophers will object to this idea. Some might say that *events* are causes, not properties (Davidson 1967). Others will say that *facts* (Mellor 1995) or *states of affairs* (Armstrong 1997) or *tropes* (Ehring 1997) are causes. There seems to be a bewildering variety of entities appealed to as the relata of causation. Why am I focusing on properties? And what does it even mean to say that properties are causes?

Let me first remove one possible source of confusion. It is sometimes said that properties are abstract entities (see van Inwagen 2004). Understanding 'abstract' in a standard way—according to which abstract entities have no spatio-temporal location—then properties so understood cannot be causes, since causes must have spatial or (at least) temporal location.[5] Therefore, when I say properties are causes, I cannot also mean that properties are abstract objects. I mean properties as concrete entities, the shapes and colours of objects, which we can see and touch. Properties in this sense are as spatio-temporal as objects themselves.

Is this the same as saying that only *instantiated* properties are causes, or that only 'property instances' are causes? Yes; but we need to distinguish two ideas. The first idea is this. Property instances are instantiated universals. I accept Armstrong's (1989) *Principle of Instantiation*: there are no non-instantiated universals. Given this, the thesis that properties are causes is the thesis that instantiated properties are causes.

The second idea is that property instances are tropes, a different kind of entity altogether from properties considered as universals (Williams 1958; Campbell 1990). If this is the right view of property instances, then the question arises as to the relationship between these tropes and the 'general' properties of which they are instances. What is the relationship, for example, between the particular whiteness of my shirt and whiteness as such? Is the relationship set-membership, as is maintained by a reductive account of universals in terms of tropes? Or should we admit universals as well as tropes, so we need some other kind of account of instantiation (Lowe 2006)? These are difficult questions, but fortunately we do not need to answer them yet. For whatever view we have about the relationship between tropes, properties and universals, it will still be true that properties only have effects insofar as they are instantiated. The simple truth is that uninstantiated properties have no effects. And this is either because what has effects must exist in space and time, or because uninstantiated properties do not exist.

Properties in this sense are causes because whenever things have effects, they have those effects because of the properties they have. As Hume says in the *Treatise*: 'where several different objects produce the same effect, it must be by means of some quality, which we discover to be common among them' (Hume 1739–40: book I, part III, section XV). The ice broke, *inter alia*, because it was fragile and because the skater weighed 100 kilos. These are properties of the ice and the skater. You might prefer to say that they are facts—the fact that the ice was fragile etc.—or states of affairs—the state of affairs of the skater weighing 100 kilos. I don't mind you saying this, so long as you allow me to say too that it was the skater's weight—a weight he shares with other people—that was a cause of the ice breaking.

For the purposes of this paper, I do not need to establish that other entities cannot be causes, only that properties can. Followers of Davidson will say that *only* events can be causes, and so will reject one of the starting assumptions of this paper. But such philosophers cannot say either that the skater's weight or

[5] Those like Keith Campbell (1990) who call tropes 'abstract particulars' will understand 'abstract' in a different way.

the ice's fragility is literally a cause of the ice's breaking; and to my mind this makes their position very unappealing. The other theories mentioned can accept, by contrast, that properties are causes; even if they would rather describe this in terms of facts, states of affairs or tropes. The important point is that they would also accept what I mean by saying that properties are causes.

3. THESIS: THE EFFICACY OF DETERMINABLE PROPERTIES

Suppose a matador's cape is a certain shade of red (say, scarlet). And suppose that it is the colour of the cape which causes a bull, on a specific occasion, to be enraged. (This example is empirically false, of course, since bulls have monochromatic vision; but I keep it because it is simple, traditional and vivid.) Then we can say, along with the everyday platitude ('red rag to a bull'), that the bull became enraged because the cape was red.

Or was it because the cape was scarlet? On the face of it, we seem to encounter here an exclusion problem of the sort mentioned in section 1. If the scarlet is sufficient to enrage the bull, then how can the redness play any causal role? Certainly, being red is *entailed* by being scarlet, but this does not imply its efficacy. Being coloured is also entailed by being scarlet, but this does not imply that it is the mere fact that the cape is coloured which causes the bull to be enraged. The cape's redness looks like it is epiphenomenal, because it is excluded by the sufficient cause, the scarlet. To say that both the redness and the scarlet are causes seems to be unnecessary double-counting, possibly leading to an unwelcome overdetermination.

Stephen Yablo (1992) proposed a way out of this problem, and then applied it to the mental/physical exclusion problem. Yablo's discussion is rich and complex, but at its heart are the following ideas. Determinates do not generally compete for causal influence with their determinables. For even if a determinate (or super-determinate) is causally or nomologically *sufficient* for a certain effect, a determinable is often a better candidate for being the (or a) *cause* of that effect. This is because a cause must be (in Yablo's terminology) 'commensurate' or 'proportional' to its effects: it should 'incorporate a good deal of causally important material but not too much that is causally unimportant' (1992: 188). Mental properties stand to physical properties as determinables to determinates. Hence, mental properties are efficacious because the 'effect is relatively insensitive to the finer details of [the cause's] physical implementation' (1992: 189). Yablo's claims about mental properties and mental causation will not be touched on here. I think he is right that mental properties are causes; but this is not because they are determinables of which their physical realizers are determinates. I do not think that the mental and the physical stand in this kind of relation, but this is not the concern of this paper. This paper is concerned with causation as such, not with the mental/physical relation.

Yablo's conception of causation is expressed in terms of counterfactuals: he takes himself to be expanding on the apparent platitude that the cause is the 'thing that made the difference'. Effects are what he calls *contingent* upon their causes:

> If x caused y then: If x had not occurred, then y would not have occurred either.[6]

These 'would'-counterfactuals are interpreted in Stalnaker's way: ' "if it had been that P, then it would have been that Q" is true iff Q is true in the P-world best resembling actuality' (Yablo 1992: 274 n. 56).

Yablo describes the essence of his solution as follows:

> Suppose we stipulate that it contributed nothing to Socrates' demise that he guzzled the hemlock rather than simply drinking it. Then Xanthippe is mistaken when, disgusted at Socrates' sloppy habits, she complains that his *guzzling* the hemlock caused his death. Assuming that the drinking still would have occurred if the guzzling hadn't, [the counterfactual condition above] explains the error nicely. Even without the guzzling, the death would still have followed on the drinking. So while Socrates' death may have been contingent on his drinking the hemlock, it was *not* contingent on his guzzling it. (Yablo 1992: 188)

Abstracting away from a lot of detail, we can see that if you have such a counterfactual conception of causation, then it is easy to derive the causal status of determinables. For on Yablo's preferred semantics for counterfactuals, and assuming the truth of the (false) empirical claim about bulls, the following counterfactual, call it 'RED', is true:

> (RED) If the cape had not been red, then the bull would not have been enraged.

While the following, 'SCARLET', is false:

> (SCARLET) If the cape had not been scarlet, then the bull would not have been enraged.

The idea is that the closest world in which the cape had not been scarlet is one in which it would have been a slightly different shade of red, and hence the bull would still have been enraged. Red is more proportional to the bull's anger than scarlet, even though scarlet is (in the circumstances, let us suppose) sufficient.[7] The fact that the cape is scarlet contains 'too much that is causally unimportant'. Therefore redness is a better candidate to count as the cause.

[6] See Yablo 1992: 274. Yablo holds that the 'contingency' of effects on their causes is one necessary condition for causation; hence he differs from Lewis (1973) and many others in thinking that counterfactual dependence is a necessary condition of causation. For his way of dealing with problems of pre-emption (etc.) see Yablo 2004: 121 ff.

[7] We can assume determinism here for the sake of argument, although this is not essential.

In broad outline, then, we can see how a determinable property like redness can be a cause and not compete with its determinates. The exclusion problem for determinables is solved. Or so it seems. For I now want to argue that given some other plausible metaphysical hypotheses about properties, predicates and causation, determinable properties cannot be causes after all.

4. ANTITHESIS: ONLY SUPERDETERMINATE PROPERTIES ARE EFFICACIOUS

I begin by introducing what Lewis (1983) calls properties in the 'sparse' sense, or 'sparse properties'. The doctrine of sparse properties essentially involves a denial of the thesis that to every distinct (type of) property-word, there corresponds a distinct property. Not every distinct, non-synonymous word for a property introduces a new property. For the purposes of this discussion, predications can be distinguished by the meanings of the predicates expressed therein, or by the concepts expressed when predicating something of an object. So when I talk of 'predications' I refer to types of application of predicates to objects, unified by the meanings of the words involved.

It is uncontroversial that we should distinguish between property-words (general terms or predicates) and the properties they refer to—just as we should distinguish between names and what they refer to. But this does not itself imply that there is no one-one correspondence between property-words and properties. The following is a possible view: each object has one and only one name, each property has one and only one distinct property-word associated with it (a general term or a predicate), yet objects and properties are distinct from names and property-words. Of course, we know that what this view says about names is false. Objects have many names; some objects have no names; some names refer to no objects at all. But how do we know that this view is false of properties and property words?

One obvious answer is that there are property words (general terms or predicates) to which no property corresponds. If there is no such thing as phlogiston, then there is no such thing as the property of being phlogiston. Yet the word 'phlogiston' has a meaning, and predications of the property of being phlogiston have a meaning (most of them are just false, that's all). So in this case, at least, we know that there is a general term which corresponds to no property whatsoever.

To this it might be responded that properties are necessary existents; so even though it is not actually instantiated, the property of being phlogiston still exists, since the property itself exists in all worlds. This is sometimes said to be a difference between properties and objects: properties exist necessarily and (some) objects do not. I myself find this an implausible view of properties; but fortunately we need not refute it in order to criticize the idea that properties and predicates correspond one–one. For even if properties are necessary existents, they need not correspond one–one with predicates.

To see this, consider the debate over whether there are 'disjunctive' properties. It is perfectly meaningful to say, for example, that a wine is red or white, and hence that the predicate '*x* is red or white' can be applied to it. But we are not obliged to say that a particular bottle of red wine has, in addition to the property of being red, the property of being red or white. This seems like over-counting properties. Surely it is better to say that the wine has one property, redness, and it is because of this that it is true to say that it is red or white. Anything which is red or white is either red or it is white. The disjunctive predication does not correspond to any disjunctive property. And this could be true even if properties were necessary existents.

This does not show that there are no disjunctive properties; only that we do not need to postulate them in order to explain why a disjunctive predication is true. But nonetheless it gives us enough of an understanding of the idea that properties may fail to correspond one–one with predicates, and once equipped with this idea we can move on to consider what role properties might have in our theorizing about causation, without them having to correspond one–one to predicates.

So one reason to reject disjunctive properties is that we do not need them in giving an account of what is true and why. There is an important and simple connection between the ideas of predication, property-hood, and truth. The properties of a thing are the ways it is, its general characteristics or qualities. When a predication of a property is true, it is true because of the way that thing is (and perhaps its relations to other things too). It is because the wine is a certain way—*red*—that it is true to predicate 'is red' of it. But it follows that it is also because the wine is that way that it is true to predicate 'is red or white' of it. The redness of the wine itself is enough to explain why it is true that it is red or white. We do not need the wine to have a further property, the property of being red or white.[8]

The central idea here is just the simple one that although there are many colour predications of things, there is a sense in which a uniformly coloured object only has one colour. After all, this is part of what it means to call it uniformly coloured. Although a uniformly coloured object may be said to have many colours in one sense—many distinct colour-descriptions are true of it—there is also a sense in which it only has one colour. In this sense, the colours of objects (if they exist at all) are sparse.

When a predication is true, it is the instantiation of a property which makes it true. This 'truth-maker' idea is, I think, one main motivation for believing

[8] I would also say the same thing about conjunctive properties: the wine does not have the property being red and dry, only the property being red and the property being dry. But opinions differ on this: see Oliver 1992 and Mellor 1992. Perhaps I should make it explicit that by 'white' in this context I mean some transparent non-red colour which so-called 'white' wines have.

in sparse properties. The same property (or instantiation of a property: see section 2 above) can make true many distinct types of predication. Now this truth-maker principle is difficult to spell out in detail. Armstrong has argued for an unrestricted version of the principle, while others (such as Lewis and D. H. Mellor) have denied that all truths have truth-makers, even though they do accept something like the idea. Here I do not endorse the thesis that all truths have truth-makers. Rather, I endorse a weaker thesis: that *if a predication has a truth-maker, its truth-maker is the instantiation of a sparse property*.

The first role for sparse properties, then, is as truth-makers. The second is their role in causation. In introducing the terminology of sparse properties, Lewis distinguishes Armstrong-style universals from properties in his own special sense: 'almost all properties are causally irrelevant, and there is nothing to make the relevant ones stand out from the crowd' (Lewis 1983: 13). By 'property' here, Lewis simply means the extension of a predicate. He accordingly distinguishes between properties as such, which are abundant, and *natural* properties, which are sparse. Natural properties are 'the ones whose sharing makes for resemblance, and the ones relevant to causal powers. Most simply, we could call a property *perfectly* natural if its members are all and only those things that share some one universal' (Lewis 1983: 13). Perfectly natural properties are sparse, and they are the ones responsible for the causal powers of things which have them. Ignoring the distinction Lewis makes between perfectly natural properties and universals, I will express the connection between sparseness and causation as follows: only sparse properties are the causally efficacious properties. If a property has effects, then it is a sparse property.

Why think only sparse properties have effects? Lewis says that they are the ones 'relevant to causal powers' but is this just a stipulation, or can some argument be given for it? I think an argument can be given. Consider first the case of disjunctive properties. The colour of a wine might have causal powers; it might cause Vladimir to buy it when faced with a choice in the wine shop, for example. Suppose Vladimir wants a red wine, and chooses this particular bottle because it was red. The redness of the wine is therefore a cause of his action. Given that the wine is red, it is also true that it is red or white. But how can its *being red or white* have any effects on Vladimir's action? He did not choose it because it was red or white, he chose it because it was red. In general, we can say that if the wine's colour has any effects at all, then it is the *actual* colour which matters, not the disjunction of that colour with a colour which it does not have. For how can a colour *not* possessed by something play any role in what that thing causes?

Perhaps it will be obvious in this case that *being red or white* cannot have any effects, because whiteness is nowhere instantiated in this situation. But this point cannot be applied to all non-sparse properties, unless we have some independent reason for thinking that only sparse properties exist.[9] Some philosophers (Armstrong 1997, Mellor 1993) do hold that view, and it does have some plausibility. However, I will not commit myself to it here; instead I will argue that only sparse properties are causes, even if there are also (epiphenomenal) abundant properties.

To get to this conclusion, we need to make explicit some assumptions about causation: that it is relational, and that its relata are properties (or property instances). When we make a true causal claim, we are describing a real relation between cause and effect.[10] So if a causal truth has a truth-maker, this truth-maker must be itself relational: it must relate cause and effect. The relata of the causal relation will then be the truth-makers for the relata of the causal truth. Causation, then, is a relation between truth-makers. And by our truth-maker principle proposed above, these truth-makers are sparse. Therefore the relata of the causal relation are sparse.

The view that causation takes place at the level of truth-makers should be welcome to any realist about causation who believes in truth-makers. Causation is a mind-independent relation between instances of properties in the world. How causes and effects are then described is another matter. Causes can be picked out in a number of different ways, and only some of those ways will make explicit their identity as sparse properties. Nonetheless, what are picked out are the sparse properties. The thesis that causes are causes no matter how they are described will be familiar from Davidson's (1967) classic discussion of causation, but it applies equally to those views which deny that causation relates events.

Do *all* sparse properties have effects? Lewis seems to think so, since he describes them as those 'relevant to causal powers', suggesting that they all are. Others would agree: those who agree with Shoemaker's (1979) view that properties are individuated by their causal powers, will hold that it is in the nature of any property that its possession by something which instantiated it was enough to dispose that thing to have certain effects. Of course, the claim would have to be restricted to empirical properties, rather than properties of numbers and other abstract objects. But if this Shoemakerian principle, applied to empirical properties, were correct, then we could say that all and only sparse properties are causes, or have causal powers. However, it is the 'only' direction which is important to the present argument.

The next stage is to apply these ideas about sparseness and causation to determinables and determinates. Consider a particular determinable property I have, say, my height. If I have a height, I must have a specific height. I am

[9] Sartorio (forthcoming) has an interesting argument for disjunctive causes, based on a situation where there are two actual causes of an effect, neither of which is sufficient for the effect, but which are not joint (i.e. conjunctive) causes. Her argument is construed in terms of events, however, and so does not touch the point made here about properties.

[10] *Pace* Mellor (1995) who denies that causation is a relation. Mellor has been effectively answered by Menzies (2003).

tall, but that too is a (species- or culture-relative) determinable: to be tall is to have a specific height within a certain range of specific heights. (Of course, it is vague what this range is. But that is not relevant here.) I am also over 150 cm; over 160 cm; and so on. Let's suppose that my height is exactly 185 cm. Then arguably *this* is what makes it true that I have a height; this is what makes it true that I am tall, and this is what makes it true that I am over 150 cm and so on. It is very plausible, then, that determinate properties are the truth-makers for the predications of determinables. Indeed, if there are any super-determinate properties, then these will be the ultimate truth-makers for any predications of less than super-determinate properties. For nothing more is *needed* in order to make all the determinable predications true. If it is true that I am exactly 185 cm tall, then this will be enough to guarantee the truth of the predications of all the other determinables.

Super-determinates, then, are sparse; and since predications of determinables have truth-makers, then these sparse properties will be the truth-makers for these predications (see Gillett and Rives 2005 for further defence of this claim). If it is true, as argued above, that only sparse properties are causally efficacious, then the conclusion follows that where properties with a determinable/determinate structure are concerned, only super-determinates are causally efficacious. So being red, being tall, having a height above 150 cm, being triangular, being heavy. . . none of these are really among the causally efficacious properties of things. The causally efficacious properties of things are always the super-determinates, not the determinables.

This is a conclusion which will be accepted by many philosophers (Armstrong 1997; Mellor 1993; Gillett and Rives 2005) many of whom think that there are in reality no determinable *properties* only determinable *concepts*. But the problem is that, as we saw in section 3, there are good reasons for believing that determinables can be causally efficacious. So something has to go.

5. RESPONSES TO THE ANTIMONY

The antinomy is the conflict between the Thesis and the Antithesis:

THESIS: *Determinable properties can be causally efficacious*

ANTITHESIS: *Where properties allow of a determinate–determinable classification, it is only the superdeterminate properties, and not their determinables, which are causally efficacious*

The argument for the Thesis is Yablo's. The essence of this argument is that our intuitive judgements about causes and effects often favour the counterfactuals which make the determinables causes. The argument for the Antithesis relies on two ideas: truth-makers for predications of determinables are sparse; and if a property is causally efficacious, then it is sparse.

I will now consider a number of responses to this antinomy. Assuming our starting point that properties are causes, there are three kinds of option available. One could reject the Thesis, the Antithesis or find some way of reconciling them (a synthesis). I will examine these options in reverse order.

Certainly it would be nice to find a reconciliation or synthesis. One strategy for reconciliation would be to identify an ambiguity in the use of the word 'cause' in the Thesis and in the Antithesis, and remove the appearance of conflict by insisting that they are using the word in different ways. In the mental causation debate, for example, a distinction is sometimes made between causal efficacy and causal relevance of properties.[11] Some physicalists attempt to preserve a belief in mental causation by saying that even though physical properties are the causally *efficacious* properties, mental properties can nonetheless be causally *relevant*. Perhaps this distinction can be applied independently of physicalism. In relation to our example from section 3, we might say that redness is causally *relevant* to the bull's anger, since this is what the counterfactual RED tells us: the counterfactuals are guides to what is causally relevant. RED tells us that redness is a causally relevant property. But the argument for the Antithesis tells us that it is the super-determinate shade of scarlet which is actually causally efficacious in producing the effect. Hence there is no real conflict between the Thesis and the Antithesis, since different causal notions are involved in each of them. Yablo's argument reveals causal relevance, while the argument of the Antithesis reveals causal efficacy.[12]

The success of this response depends on the plausibility of the distinction between causal relevance and causal efficacy. Without a fully developed account of causal relevance and its distinction from efficacy, the response can simply look like an insistence that in one sense, redness is the cause, and in another sense, scarlet is the cause. But this is a way of describing our problem, not a solution to it! Kripke (1977) has commented on philosophers' tendency to postulate an ambiguity whenever their theory runs into counter-example. Without a detailed account of causal relevance, plus an *independent* account of efficacy, there is a danger that this reconciliation strategy is a case of this tendency.

In an influential paper, Ned Hall (2004) has given an account of two concepts of causation, which he calls 'dependence' and 'production'. Dependence is just the familiar relation of counterfactual dependence between distinct events (2004: 257). Production is a relation between events which results in

[11] This kind of response (although writers differ in their terminology) is common in the mental causation debate: see Macdonald and Macdonald 1986, Jackson and Pettit 1988, Segal and Sober 1991. In the present context, it seems as if Funkhouser (2006) accepts something like this too.

[12] This proposal would not please Yablo (1992), since he identifies *causation* as a relation distinct from what he calls *causal sufficiency* and *causal relevance*. But this is hardly surprising since Yablo is not attracted to the ideas that lie behind the Antithesis.

a causal process which is intrinsic, transitive and local (2004: 252–3; 265). Dependence and production can come apart. The familiar examples of double prevention and causation by omission show how you can have dependence without production (my failure to water my plants causes their death because their death counterfactually depended on my failing to do this). And the familiar examples of late pre-emption show how you can have production without dependence (Suzy's rock causes the bottle to break, even though Billy's would have done so if she had missed, because there is a 'productive' process linking her throw with the breaking).

Hall gives us a detailed analysis of two notions which are plausibly contained within our everyday and more scientific thinking about causation. Could this account provide us with the notions needed to say in what sense the red and the scarlet are both causes? No. It seems to me that, whatever the merits of Hall's account, it cannot provide a resolution of our Antinomy. To be sure, the argument for the Thesis relies on the appeal of the notion of causation as dependence. But the argument for the Antithesis does not rely on anything like the notion of causation as production, as Hall construes it. The sense in which the super-determinate property is a cause does not entail that the relevant causal relation is transitive, for example. All that was appealed to in the argument was the idea of truth-making, and the idea of truth-makers as causes. These ideas, it seems to me, do not entail the conception of causation as production in Hall's sense. Hall's disambiguation does not provide us with a Synthesis.

I am not saying that there cannot be a Synthesis; but in the absence of any more concrete proposal, I would rather look elsewhere for a solution to our antinomy. For it turns out that one can give an account of the role of the determinable property in the explanation of effects without asserting any ambiguity in the ordinary word 'cause'.

Before dealing with this, I must dismiss the second possible response to the antinomy: to reject the claim that truth-makers must be super-determinate. On the face of it, this might seem intuitively plausible. Surely it is true that something is red simply because it is red; so what is wrong with stopping at the idea that the *redness* of things as such is one of the truth-makers of predications? This approach has some appeal, especially from the perspective of those (unlike Gillett and Rives 2005) who want to accept the existence of determinables as well as the existence of super-determinates. But for this response to be a general solution to the antinomy, it has to work in every case. Take the case of height. There is a potential infinity of true height predications which are true of me (of the form 'I am at least *n* cm tall'). If the absolutely super-determinate height property is not the truth-maker for all these predications, then I see no non-arbitrary way of distinguishing among this infinity which ones are the truth-makers and which ones aren't. And to say that I have an actual infinity of height properties and none of them is privileged is, in effect, to give up on the idea of sparse properties altogether.

To defend the idea that there is one truth-maker for the predication of an object's colour is in effect to defend the principle, mentioned above, that there is a sense in which a uniformly coloured object only has one colour. There may be another sense in which it has many colours—it is truly described as having many colours—but surely there is also a sense in which it only has one. As I said above, this is part of what it means to call it *uniformly* coloured. Once one has accepted this, then it is easy to see that the uniform colour is a sparse property in Lewis's sense. Given the additional claim about the efficacy of properties, the Antithesis follows.

I do not think, then, that we have been given any good reasons to reject the reasoning which led to the Antithesis. What we should do instead is to reject the Thesis. More specifically, what we should reject is the idea that there is any *straightforward* link between the truth of a counterfactual like RED and the causal efficacy of the determinable properties directly mentioned in them. We should not deny that these counterfactuals are true, nor that they are explanatorily useful. Rather, we should reject the claim that because a predicate 'F' or name 'Fness' occurs in a true counterfactual (of the RED type), this implies that Fness is a causally efficacious property.

If this view is to be adequately defended, we need to explain how counterfactuals like RED can be true, since they are not true because they directly report what the causally efficacious properties of things are. A full account of this matter would fall outside the scope of this paper. Here I can only give a general outline of an account.

To predicate a determinable property (like redness) of an object is, in effect, to specify that the object in question has a sparse property within some *range*. It is true that the bull charged because the cape was red; but that means that there is some property within a range (the range specified by the concept *red*) which the cape has. Suppose that the cause of the bull's charge was the fact that it was a superdeterminate shade of scarlet; that doesn't mean that SCARLET is true. For SCARLET, too, specifies a range of properties: all the determinates of scarlet. The point is that it isn't necessary for the bull to charge that the provocative property only comes from within this *latter* range. For, *ex hypothesi*, bulls charge at red things. (Notice here that the range is along only one of the dimensions of the determinable—hue or chroma—and not along all of them.)

In committing ourselves to a claim like RED, then, we are committing ourselves to the idea that *there is* a property within the relevant range on whose instantiation the relevant effect is counterfactually dependent. So although I would resist Jackson and Pettit's (1988) 'programme explanation' view, some of the examples they use in defence of their view can also be used to defend the present view. Consider a conductor who stops his performance in a concert because someone coughed. That someone coughed is sufficient explanation for why he stopped; but of course, it merely specifies that *there is* somebody who coughed, it does not say who it is. The role of the determinable property in the relevant counterfactual is analogous to the 'someone'. The determinable concept specifies the range of determinate properties which would produce the relevant effect.

Now the relevant counterfactual is implied by a generalization linking that kind of effect to properties within that range. In our example, there is the generalization, 'bulls charge at red things'; and this implies the counterfactual RED. Counterfactuals about determinables thus contain an implicit generality, and it is for this reason that determinable properties are suited for figuring in statements of laws of nature. Newton's second law, F = ma, is expressed in terms of the determinables' mass, force and acceleration, not in terms of determinate masses. But the law implies counterfactuals of the form, 'if x had mass *M* and force *F* were exerted upon it, it would accelerate at rate *A*' for specific values of *M*, *F* and *A*.[13] The law generalizes: it talks about all determinates of a given determinable. But individual causal interactions take place between the superdeterminate properties. If this picture is right, it turns out that much causation presupposes the existence of superdeterminate properties. If this is right, then sceptics about superdeterminates should therefore be sceptics about causation itself.[14]

6. CONCLUSION

Although my concern in this paper has not been with the mental/special sciences causation debate, the proposed resolution of the antinomy does have some consequences for that debate. One consequence is that the truth of counterfactuals of the general form 'if I hadn't had mental property M then I wouldn't have done X' cannot, without other assumptions, get you to any substantial conclusions about the causal efficacy of mental property M. Another consequence is that mental properties had better not be determinables with physical properties as their determinates, since this would make mental properties epiphenomenal on the conception of causation and sparse properties defended here. These consequences seem to me perfectly acceptable to someone who has this conception.

However, I do not pretend to have provided a knock-down argument for the Antithesis, or against the Thesis. It is still open for someone to reject

[13] *Ceteris paribus*, of course. Also, I should add that I am talking here about statements or formulations of laws; not the metaphysical structures (relations between universals) which Armstrong 1997 and others (e.g. Dretske 1977) call 'laws of nature'. How the present suggestion applies to these views is an interesting question, but not one I will address here.

[14] Of course, I have not given any specific account of causation in this paper, only of its relata. Those, like me, who wish to defend this kind of conception of the causal relata must give a consonant view of causation itself. For scepticism about such views, see Loewer (forthcoming).

sparse properties, and defend the counterfactual conception of causation embodied in the Thesis. But for someone who does believe in sparse properties and their efficacy, I claim the lesson is clear: they should give up the idea that counterfactuals like RED directly track the causal efficacy of properties.

There is, perhaps, a link to a more general issue in the philosophy of causation here. For some years now, many philosophers of causation have wrestled with the problems which pre-emption and redundant causation pose for counterfactual analysis.[15] Some of them have concluded that the analysis must be given up. Within the context of the metaphysics of sparse properties, and of a view on which properties are causes, it seems that the argument of this paper gives us another reason for doubting the counterfactual analysis: these counterfactuals, although they may be true, do not directly inform us about the causally efficacious properties of things.

REFERENCES

Armstrong, D. M. (1961). *Perception and the Physical World.* Cambridge: Cambridge University Press.

—— (1978). *Universals and Scientific Realism.* 2 volumes. Cambridge: Cambridge University Press.

—— (1989). *Universals: An opinionated Introduction.* Boulder, CO: Westview Press.

—— (1997). *A World of States of Affairs.* Cambridge: Cambridge University Press.

Bennett, Karen (2003). 'Why the Exclusion Argument Seems Intractable, and How, Just Maybe, to Tract it', *Noûs* 37: 471–97.

Byrne, Alex and Hilbert, David (eds.) (1994). *Readings on Color Volume I: The Philosophy of Color.* Cambridge, Mass.: MIT Press 1997.

Campbell, Keith (1990). *Abstract Particulars.* Oxford: Blackwell.

Collins, J., Hall, Ned and Paul, Laurie (eds.) (2004). *Causation and Counterfactuals.* Cambridge, MA: MIT Press.

Davidson, Donald (1967). 'Causal Relations', repr. in Donald Davidson, *Essays on Actions and Events.* Oxford: Oxford University Press 1980.

Dretske, Fred I. (1977). 'Laws of Nature', *Philosophy of Science* 39: 69–71.

Ehring, Douglas (1997). *Causation and Persistence.* Oxford: Oxford University Press.

Funkhouser, Eric (2006). 'The Determinable/Determinate Relation', *Noûs* 40: 548–69.

Gillett, Carl and Rives, Bradley (2005). 'The Non-Existence of Determinables: Or, a World of Absolute Determinates as Default Hypothesis', *Noûs* 39: 483–504.

Hall, Ned (2004). 'Two Concepts of Causation', in Collins, Hall and Paul (eds.) (2004), 225–76.

Hume, David (1739–40). *A Treatise of Human Nature.*

Jackson, Frank and Pettit, Philip (1988). 'Functionalism and Broad Content', *Mind* 97: 381–400.

[15] See, *inter alia*, Menzies 1989 and 1996; Schaffer 2000.

Johnson, W. E. (1921). *Logic.* Volume 1. Cambridge: Cambridge University Press.

Kallestrup, Jesper (2006). 'The Causal Exclusion Argument', *Philosophical Studies* 131: 459.

Kim, Jaegwon (1989). 'Mechanism, Purpose and Explanatory Exclusion.' In James E. Tomberlin (ed.) *Philosophical Perspectives 3: Philosophy of Mind and Action Theory.* 77–108. Atascadero, CA: Ridgeview. Repr. in Jaegwon Kim, *Supervenience and Mind.* Cambridge: Cambridge University Press 1993.

—— (1998). *Mind in a Physical World.* Cambridge, MA: MIT Press.

Kripke, Saul (1977). 'Speaker's Reference and Semantic Reference', *Midwest Studies in Philosophy* 2: 255–76.

Lewis, David (1973). 'Causation', *Journal of Philosophy,* 70: 556–67.

—— (1983). 'New Work for a Theory of Universals', *Australasian Journal of Philosophy* 61: 343–77, repr. in Lewis, *Papers in Metaphysics and Epistemology.* Cambridge: Cambridge University Press 1999.

—— (2000). 'Causation as Influence', *Journal of Philosophy* 97: 182–97.

Loewer, Barry (forthcoming). 'Mental Causation, Or Something Near Enough', in *Debates of Philosophers: Mental Causation.*

Lowe, E. J. (2006). *A Four Category Ontology.* Oxford: Oxford University Press.

Macdonald, Cynthia and Macdonald, Graham (1986). 'Mental Causes and Explanation of Action', *Philosophical Quarterly* 36: 145–58.

Mellor, D.H. (1992). 'There are no Conjunctive Universals', *Analysis* 52: 97–105.

—— (1993). 'Properties and Predicates', in Mellor and Oliver (eds.) (1997).

—— (1995). *The Facts of Causation.* London: Routledge.

—— (2000). 'The Semantics and Ontology of Dispositions', *Mind*: 109: 757–80.

—— and Oliver, Alex (eds.) (1997). *Properties.* Oxford: Oxford University Press.

Menzies, Peter (1989). 'Probabilistic Causation and Causal Processes: a Critique of Lewis', *Philosophy of Science* 56: 642–63.

—— (1996). 'Probabilistic Causation and the Pre-emption Problem', *Mind* 105: 85–117.

—— (2003). 'Is Causation a Genuine Relation?' In H. Lillehammer and G. Rodriguez-Pereyra (eds.) *Real Metaphysics.* London: Routledge.

Oliver, Alex (1992). 'Might there be Conjunctive Universals?' *Analysis* 52: 88–97.

Prior, Arthur N. (1949). 'Determinables, Determinates, and Determinants', *Mind,* 53: part I, 1–20; part II: 178–94.

Sanford, David H. (1970). 'Disjunctive Predicates', *American Philosophical Quarterly* 7: 162–70.

—— (2006). 'Determinates vs. Determinables', *The Stanford Encyclopedia of Philosophy* (Winter 2006 Edition), Edward N. Zalta (ed.), URL =<http://plato.stanford.edu/archives/win2006/entries/determinate-determinables/>

Sartorio, Carolina (forthcoming). 'Disjunctive Causes', *Journal of Philosophy.*

Schaffer, Jonathan (2000). 'Trumping Pre-emption', *Journal of Philosophy* 97: 165–86.

Searle, John (1959). 'On Determinables and Resemblance, II', *Proceedings of the Aristotelian Society Supplementary Volume* 33: 141–58.

Segal, Gabriel and Sober, Elliott (1991). 'The Causal Efficacy of Content', *Philosophical Studies* 18: 1–30.

Shoemaker, Sydney (1979). 'Causality and Properties', in *Identity, Cause, and Mind.* Cambridge: Cambridge University Press: 206–33.

van Inwagen, Peter (2004). 'A Theory of Properties', in *Oxford Studies in Metaphysics*, Oxford: Oxford University Press.
Williams, D. C. (1958). 'On the Elements of Being', *Review of Metaphysics* 7: 3–18.
Yablo, Stephen (1992). 'Mental Causation', *Philosophical Review* 101: 245–80.
—— (2004). 'Advertisement for a Sketch of an Outline of a Prototheory of Causation' in Collins, Hall and Paul (eds.) (2004), 119–38.

11

The Exclusion Problem, the Determination Relation, and Contrastive Causation

Peter Menzies

1. INTRODUCTION

This paper is concerned with the well-known exclusion argument against non-reductive physicalism (Kim 1989, 1998, 2005). The argument is so-called because it appeals to the following exclusion principle about causal relevance:

> If a property F is *causally sufficient* for another property G, then no property F* distinct from F is causally relevant to G.

The exclusion argument is intended to be a *reductio* of non-reductive physicalism: on the basis of the exclusion principle and other premises non-reductive physicalists accept, it attempts to establish the implausible conclusion that mental properties are causally irrelevant to physical properties.

This paper falls into two parts. The first part of the paper examines Stephen Yablo's (1992) influential objection to the argument that focuses on the exclusion

Versions of this chapter have been presented at the conference "Minds, Mobs, and Memories", organized by the Centre for Time, University of Sydney, in November 2006; and at the "Emergence" conference, organized by Cynthia and Graham Macdonald, Queens University, Belfast, in April 2007. My thinking about this topic has been helped by questions asked by members of the audience on those occasions, especially by Tim Crane, Uriah Kriegel, Daniel Nolan, Paul Noordhof, Laurie Paul, David Papineau, Philip Pettit, and Panu Raatikainen. At the Belfast conference, I benefited from some prepared comments on my paper by Ausonio Marras. I am also indebted to Jesper Kallestrup and Jakob Hohwy for written comments on the paper and to my postgraduate students Suzy Bliss, Wilson Cooper, and David Wilson for discussions about mental causation over a long period of time. The strategy of response to the exclusion argument pursued in this paper is similar in some respects to one line of argument in James Woodward's paper (Chapter 12 in this volume). Panu Raatikainen has also arrived independently at a similar line of argument in his unpublished paper "Mental Causation, Intervention, and Contrasts". The line of argument in this paper is different from that of some other papers of mine, especially Menzies (2003; 2007), which emphasize the model-relativity of causal discourse. How the new line of argument fits in with the old line of argument is a topic I hope to explore elsewhere.

principle. Yablo's objection turns on two crucial observations: first, that the relationship of mental properties to their underlying physical, neural properties is the relationship of determinable properties to determinate properties (that is, the relationship that a property such as red bears to more specific properties such as crimson and scarlet); and second, that determinables can still be causally relevant to some effect even when their determinates are causally sufficient for the effect. I argue that Yablo's objection is ultimately unsuccessful because, among other things, his first claim about the relationship between mental and physical properties is in all likelihood false.

Nonetheless, it is instructive to examine Yablo's arguments because they highlight some intuitive judgements about the causal efficacy of higher-level properties such as mental properties and provide a model for how to account for these judgements. The account of the causal efficacy of mental properties that Yablo provides is, unfortunately, limited in its application because it presupposes that mental properties are related to their underlying neural properties as determinables to determinates. In its place, I shall offer an alternative account of causation that emphasizes the contrastive character of causal claims. On this account, a causal claim like "F causes G" is really elliptical for a claim such as "F rather than not-F causes G rather than not-G". This alternative account, I claim, explains better than Yablo's own account why it is that a determinable property can be the cause of some effect even when one of its determinates is causally sufficient for the effect. Moreover, this account is broadly applicable to the question of whether high-level properties such as mental properties can be causes, independently of whether they are related to their underlying neural properties as determinables to determinates.

The second part of the paper examines a question that is raised by the discussion in the first part: Supposing that the contrastive account of causation falsifies the exclusion principle, as it is customarily formulated in terms of causal sufficiency, does it falsify a version of the principle formulated in terms of a double application of the concept of causation as follows:

> If a property F *causes* property G, then no property F* distinct from F *causes* G?

It would be natural to think that the contrastive account of causation would falsify this version of the exclusion principle as readily as the original version. But it is unclear whether this is so. Rather than concentrating on this general principle, however, I shall focus on two instances of the principle that are relevant to the exclusion argument; and I shall establish that the contrastive account of causation actually validates these two instances of the reformulated principle. This somewhat surprising result is a simple consequence of the contrastive account of causation.

In view of the fact that the relevant instances of the exclusion principle can be formulated so as to render them true statements, it is reasonable to revisit the question whether the exclusion argument poses a genuine and significant threat to non-reductive physicalism. In response to this question, I shall argue that even when reformulated in terms of more plausible instances of the exclusion principle, the exclusion argument is less than compelling. For the non-reductive physicalist can reject the argument's conclusion by challenging a different premise of the argument—the premise of the causal closure of the physical. This principle must be strengthened considerably if the exclusion argument is to be based on the relevant instances of the reformulated exclusion principle; but when the principle of the causal closure of the physical is strengthened in the required way, it is much less plausible than it appeared in its original version.

Here in detail is my plan for developing my two-part argument. The first part takes up sections 2 to 5 of the paper. Section 2 sets out a customary version of the exclusion problem and explains Yablo's objection to the exclusion principle. Section 3 explains why Yablo's account of the relation between determinables and determinates and his account of causation are unsatisfactory. Section 4 provides a brief introduction to the alternative contrastive account of causation; and section 5 deploys this account to show that mental properties can cause physical properties even though they are realized by neural properties that are causally sufficient for those physical properties.

The second part of my argument takes up the last two sections of the paper. Section 6 advances reasons for thinking that the relevant instances of an alternative version of the exclusion principle, formulated in terms of a double application of the concept of causation, are true. The final section 7 explores the implications of this result for the cogency of the exclusion argument, concluding that the non-reductive physicalist might reasonably challenge a strengthened principle of the causal closure of the physical.

2. THE EXCLUSION PROBLEM AND YABLO ON MENTAL CAUSATION

The exclusion argument can be formulated in slightly different ways. Yablo (1992: 247) discusses a formulation in terms of events, but notes that it can also be formulated in terms of properties. I shall discuss a formulation in terms of properties, as it seems to me that the most troublesome issues raised by the argument for non-reductive physicalism concern the causal relevance or efficacy of *mental properties*.

So formulated, the exclusion argument relies on a number of principles:

(1) *Exclusion principle*: If a property F is causally sufficient for a property G, then no property F* distinct from F is causally relevant to G.

(2) *Causal closure of the physical*: For every physical property G that has a cause, there is a physical property F that is causally sufficient

for G. (This deterministic principle could be replaced by a more accurate, indeterministic principle. But since the issue of determinism vs indeterminism is generally agreed not to be relevant to the soundness of the exclusion argument, I shall employ this simpler deterministic principle.)

(3) *Property dualism*: Every mental property F* is distinct from every physical property F.

Deploying these principles as premises, the argument runs like this: Suppose for the purposes of *reductio* that some mental property is causally relevant to a physical property, say a behavioural property. By the causal closure of the physical, we know that there is a purely physical property that is causally sufficient for the behavioural property. We also know, by property dualism, that this property is distinct from the mental property. But then inferring on the basis of the exclusion principle, we must conclude that the mental property both is and is not causally relevant to behavioural property, so reducing the initial supposition to absurdity. But the conclusion that a mental property cannot be causally relevant to a physical property is so highly implausible that we should reason that one of the principles (1) to (3) must be false. Since principle (1), the exclusion principle, and principle (2), the causal closure of the physical, are acceptable on independent grounds, we have reason to abandon (3), property dualism, which is one of the defining theses of non-reductive physicalism.

Yablo's defence of non-reductive physicalism against this argument involves challenging principle (1), the exclusion principle. He argues that the principle is not in fact independently acceptable, relying on two crucial observations in his criticism of the principle.

His first observation is that the relationship that mental properties bear to their underlying neural properties is the same as the relationship that determinable properties such as being triangular and being red bear to determinate properties such as being an isosceles triangle and being crimson. Yablo offers an intuitive explanation of this relationship: having a determinate property is a specific way of having the determinable property, so that to be crimson is to be a specific shade of red and to be an isosceles triangle is to be a specific kind of triangle. More formally, he offers necessary, but not sufficient, conditions for one property to be a determinate of another:

Property F *determines* property G only if:

(i) It is metaphysically necessary that for all x, if x has F, then x has G; and
(ii) It is metaphysically possible that for some x, x has G but lacks F.

Yablo argues that the strong supervenience of mental properties on neural properties implies that the first condition for the existence of a determination relation holds; and that the multiple realizability of mental properties by neural properties implies that the second condition for the existence of a determination relation holds. More generally, he argues that neural properties asymmetrically necessitate mental properties; and that the best explanation of this fact is that mental and physical properties are related as determinables to determinates. (Yablo admits that the assumption that neural properties metaphysically necessitate mental properties may be too strong. However, it focuses the essential line of his thought, he says, to work with this strong assumption (1992: 225 n. 26). Presumably, in making this assumption, he is bracketing functionalist views about mental properties' individuation in terms of causal roles and externalist views about the wide content mental properties. I will follow Yablo in bracketing these considerations from the discussion for ease of exposition.)

Yablo's second observation is that determinable properties are not excluded from causal relevance by their determinates. He motivates this observation in terms of an example. A pigeon is trained to peck at red things to the exclusion of things of other colours. The pigeon is presented with a red triangle and she pecks it. Yablo claims that the redness of the triangle is causally relevant to the pecking, even though the triangle's being a specific shade of red, say crimson, was causally sufficient for her pecking. More generally, Yablo states, "determinates do not contend with their determinables for causal influence" (1992: 259). He draws a useful analogy with an object's completely occupying a space: the fact that it occupies this space does not mean its parts are crowded out, since wholes and parts do not compete with each other for space. Likewise, Yablo suggests that determinables and determinates are not in competition for causal relevance and are "tolerant of each other's causal aspirations".

It follows from Yablo's two observations that mental properties are not excluded from causal relevance by their underlying neural properties. As with redness and crimson in the example about the pigeon, mental properties and neural properties do not compete for causal relevance. And so, contrary to the exclusion principle, a mental property can be causally relevant to some physical behaviour, and this despite the fact that its underpinning neural properties are causally sufficient for the behaviour.

Yablo does not explain how the concept of causal relevance is to be understood. But clearly his intention is that it be understood inclusively so as to allow both determinable and determinate properties to be causally relevant to some effect at the same time. Causal relevance, so understood, is a loose and undiscriminating concept in so far as it applies to properties irrespective of whether they contain extraneous causal information. By contrast, the concept of causation is more discriminating, Yablo says, in that it requires causes to be commensurate or proportional with their effects: a cause must be specific enough for its effect but no more specific than required. Yablo (1992: 279) imposes a constraint on causation that he calls the proportionality constraint. It is useful to employ some terminology, introduced by McGrath (1998), to describe this constraint. Let us say that a property F *screens off* a property G from another property H if and only if, for any object x, if x were F but not G, then x would still be H. Then Yablo's constraint (or at least one that is roughly equivalent to it) states that a property instance Fa is *proportional* to a property instance Gb (where it may be that b = a) if and only if the following conditions hold:

(i) If it were not the case that Fa, then it would not be the case that Gb (*contingency*);
(ii) if it were the case that Fa, then it would be the case that Gb (*adequacy*);
(iii) F screens off all its determinates from G (F is *enough* for G); and
(iv) none of F's determinables screens off F from G (F is *required* for G).

Conditions (i) and (ii) are familiar from counterfactual analyses of causation. Yablo imposes condition (iii) to eliminate properties that are not specific enough. To illustrate the point, he asks us to imagine that a safety valve connected to a boiler is very stiff so that its slow opening at a time when pressure is building up causes the boiler to explode. The valve's opening slowly is proportional to the boiler's explosion, but its opening *simpliciter* is not, because it does not screen off one of its determinates, namely the property of opening slowly, from the explosion. (It is not true that if the valve had opened but not opened slowly, the boiler would still have exploded.) He imposes (iv) to eliminate properties that are too specific. Again to illustrate the point, he asks us to suppose that Socrates can't drink the hemlock without guzzling. His drinking hemlock is proportional to his death, but his guzzling the hemlock is not, because one of its determinables, namely his drinking the hemlock, screens it off from the death. (If Socrates had drunk the hemlock without guzzling, he would still have died.)

While Yablo does not claim that the proportionality constraint is necessary for causation, he argues that it is a plausible constraint on causation in the sense that when faced with a choice between two candidate causes, normally the more proportional candidate is to be preferred. So in the example about the pigeon, for instance, it is preferable to cite the triangle's being red rather than its being crimson as the cause of the pigeon's pecking, given that the first but not the second is proportional to this effect. Likewise if a mental property and its underlying neural property are considered as candidate causes of some fairly coarse-grained bodily movement, it is often preferable to cite as the cause the mental property rather than the neural property on the grounds that it better meets the proportionality constraint. Causation is different in this respect, Yablo remarks, from causal relevance: whereas determinables and determinates do not compete for causal relevance, they do compete for the role of cause. At any rate, it would seem that the exclusion principle, whether its consequent clause is stated in terms of causal relevance or causation, is false as it applies to determinables and determinates: a determinable property can be causally relevant to some effect, and indeed a cause of it, notwithstanding the fact that one of its determinates is causally sufficient for the effect.

3. THE DETERMINABLE/DETERMINATE RELATION

Yablo's account of the determination relation and his account of the proportionality constraint on causation are useful in providing a framework for discussing the exclusion principle. However, in the end they do not, in my view, provide the basis for a successful refutation of the principle. In this section I outline some reasons for being sceptical about his claim that mental properties are related to their underlying neural properties as determinables to determinates; and about his claim that causes satisfy a proportionality constraint of the kind he describes.

To evaluate Yablo's claim that neural properties are determinates of mental properties we need a better understanding of the determination relation. His account of this relation is incomplete, as it states only necessary and not sufficient conditions. One defect of the stated conditions is that they do not rule out the possibility of a property F determining the disjunctive property F v G, or the conjunctive property F & G determining the property F. But it has traditionally been thought that F is not a determinate of F v G and that F & G is not a determinate of F (see W. E. Johnson 1921; A. Prior 1949). So we need a more complete account of the determination relation that will, at very least, rule out these possibilities.

The best account I know of is that given by Eric Funkhouser (2006). The central insight of this paper is that determinates are more specific than their determinables with respect to a limited number of features or dimensions. These *determination dimensions*, as Funkhouser calls them, are the fundamental dimensions of variation between determinates of a common determinable. For example, the determination dimensions for colour are hue, brightness, and saturation, with these representing the minimally sufficient criteria for distinguishing all colours from one another. In addition to their values along determination dimensions, determinables and determinates also have what Funkhouser calls non-determinable necessities. These are the features that each determinate of a determinable must have. For instance, all triangles must be three-sided, closed, plane figures and every determinate of the property triangular must have these features. But because every triangle must have these features, different determinates of the property triangular cannot differ with respect to these non-determinable necessities. So, in summary, determinates of the same determinable have exact similarity in non-determinable necessities, but differ with respect to their values along their determination dimensions.

In many cases, the n-determination dimensions of a determinable and its determinates can be represented as the axes of a n-dimensional space. For example, the determination dimensions of colour—hue, brightness, and saturation—can be represented as the axes of a three-dimensional space. Funkhouser calls the n-dimensional space associated with a property its *property space*. So the property space for colour is the entire three-dimensional space defined by the axes representing values for hue, brightness, and saturation. The property space for a specific colour, say red, is a subregion of this space. A point in this subregion corresponds to a specific shade of red, say Coca Cola red. Such a specific shade of red corresponds to what Funkhouser calls a *superdeterminate*—a property that does not have any determinate. Any point in a property space represents a superdeterminate of some higher-level determinable.

With a restriction to cases where determinables are associated with property spaces, Funkhouser proposes the following analysis of the determination relation:

> Property F *determines* property G if and only if (i) F and G have the same determination dimensions; and (ii) F and G have the same non-determinable necessities; and (iii) the property space of F is a proper subset of the property space of G.

It is easy to see that these conditions rule out the possibility of F determining F v G and F & G determining F. For example, the property of being red and square cannot be a determinate of being red since these properties have different determination dimensions. Red has the determination dimensions of hue, brightness, and saturation, and squareness has no place among them. More informally, an object's being red and square is not a more specific way of its being red.

If the determination relation is understood according to Funkhouser's analysis, are mental properties determined by the neural properties that realize them? Funkhouser himself considers this question, answering it in the negative. The main reason that he gives for his negative answer—and in this he seems correct to me—is that the mental properties and neural properties do not have the same determination dimensions. Consider, for example, a mental property like believing and consider the different ways in which one belief can differ from another. It seems that there are two principal determination dimensions for beliefs: content and degree of confidence. Beliefs may differ from one another because they have different contents: the belief that it is going to rain is different from the belief that the sun will shine. Then again beliefs with the same content may differ because they are held with different degrees of confidence: the belief that the sun will shine that is held with degree of confidence 50% is different from the belief that the sun will shine that is held with degree of confidence 90%. It does not seem that realization by neural property is an intuitive dimension of variation among beliefs. Or consider another kind of mental property such as pain. Pains can differ with respect to their bodily location and their phenomenological characteristics—whether they are sharp or dull, long or short, throbbing or aching, and so on. Again it does not seem that the manner of realization by neural property is a natural dimension of variation among pains. We should not, in any case, automatically think that the way in which a property is materially constituted will play a role in its determination dimensions. We do not regard two objects as having different kinds of squareness because one is made of wood and other made of steel. Correspondingly, we should not automatically regard two people as having two kinds of beliefs because the beliefs are neurally realized in different ways.

This argument is not completely conclusive because it is generally agreed that settling the determination dimensions of a determinable property is not a purely *a priori* matter. Accordingly, it may possibly be established by *a posteriori* investigation that the intuitive determination dimensions of beliefs and pains are in fact aligned with the natural dimensions of variation in the neural properties that realize them. If this is an empirical possibility, then the natural dimensions of variation in the neural properties may play a role in the determination dimensions of the corresponding mental states. There is, however, an argument that suggests that this possibility is very unlikely. (See Ehring 2003; Funkhouser 2006.) The argument runs that, whatever determination dimensions we settle on for a mental property like belief, we will be able to locate a superdeterminate in the associated property space—perhaps the belief that the sun will shine, held with degree of confidence 90%—and in all likelihood this superdeterminate will be capable of multiple realization by different neural properties. If this is the case, it shows that the realizing neural properties have an extra dimension of variation not possessed by the mental property in question. In other words, the determination dimensions of mental properties do not align precisely with those of the neural properties that realize them. That the determination dimensions of the two kinds of properties differ makes it implausible to think that neural properties are determinates of mental properties.

Let us turn now to another important part of Yablo's critique of the exclusion principle—his proportionality constraint on causation. Tim Crane (Chapter 10 in this volume) argues that the constraint is metaphysically misguided in allowing determinables to be causes; and misguided precisely because a proper metaphysical account of causation would allow only superdeterminates to be causes. I do not subscribe to this kind of criticism since I think that the kind of metaphysical concept of causation it embraces is so remote from any concept of causation that is used in everyday or scientific practice.

My criticism of Yablo's proportionality constraint is based on rather different grounds. First, the proportionality constraint, as formulated, is of limited application, since it makes essential use of the determination relation in conditions (iii) and (iv). Consequently, if one is not convinced that neural properties are determinates of mental properties, the constraint is of no use to one in determining whether mental properties can cause some effect when their neural realizers are sufficient for the effect.

Secondly, the conditions of the proportionality constraint are not sufficiently clear that they always yield a determinate answer to the question whether one property is a cause of another. For example, suppose that the pigeon of Yablo's example had been trained to peck at reddish things, including pink and orange objects as well as red objects. Presented with a red object, the pigeon pecks it. The problem is that the counterfactuals involved in conditions (i) and (iv) of the proportionality constraint are hard to evaluate in this case: if the triangle had not been red, would the pigeon have pecked? If the triangle had been coloured but not red, would she have pecked? On the one hand, if the closest worlds in which the triangle was coloured but not red are ones in which it is still a reddish colour like pink or orange, then the pigeon would have pecked. On the other hand, if the closest worlds are ones in which the triangle is not reddish at all, but rather some other colour like blue or green, then the pigeon would not have pecked. Yablo does not specify a similarity relation between possible worlds to be used in evaluating his counterfactuals and that is what is required to answer these questions.

Thirdly, even if a similarity relation is specified, it is not so clear that conditions (iii) and (iv) would be required in the proportionality constraint. For instance, Yablo argues for condition (iv) on the grounds that it eliminates candidate causes that are too specific: in his example, Socrates' drinking the hemlock satisfies condition (iv) but Socrates' guzzling the hemlock does not. However, if the right similarity relation is supplied for the counterfactuals, condition (i) is sufficient by itself to eliminate the overly specific candidate. For example, if one assumes that the closest worlds in which Socrates does not guzzle the hemlock are worlds in which he nonetheless drinks the hemlock in a non-guzzling manner, then the counterfactual "If Socrates had not guzzled the hemlock, he would not died" comes out false, so disqualifying this overly specific candidate cause. So a solution to the second problem mentioned above may, in effect, simplify the formulation of the constraint so as to make conditions (iii) and (iv) redundant. This would call into question whether the causal judgements apparently licensed by the proportionality constraint have anything to do with the determinable/determinate relation.

4. THE CONTRASTIVE CHARACTER OF CAUSATION

Yablo justifies the constraint that causes should be proportional to their effects on the basis of the dictum that causes should make a difference to their effects. While I believe that this dictum is correct, I do not think that it justifies the proportionality constraint exactly as Yablo formulates it. I suggest that the dictum implies that variation in cause is associated with variation in the effect; and that the best way to articulate the dictum is to reconstruct causal claims as claims about relationships between variables. On this understanding, causal claims tell us about how changes in the value of the causal variable are related to changes in the value of the effect variable.

A broad consensus has emerged among a group of philosophers of causation (Hitchcock 2001; Pearl 2000; and Woodward 2003) about how to capture the idea that a cause makes a difference to its effects within the framework of variables and values. In setting out this framework, it will help to impose some simplifying restrictions. Let us restrict our attention to deterministic systems that do not involve processes of pre-emption and overdetermination, which bring in complications that are not germane to our discussion.

This framework recognizes two kinds of causal relations—causal relations between variables and causal relations between values of variables. It is tempting to see this distinction as mapping onto the familiar philosophical distinction between property or type-level causation and event or token-level causation. But in fact this is not correct. It has to be kept in mind that a value of a variable is not an event or a particular occurrence, but a property like the variable itself: having mass and having a mass of 10 grams are both properties that can be instantiated by objects. (Indeed the relationship between a variable and its values is the relationship between a determinable and its determinate.) This means that both property or type-level causation and event or token-level causation can be represented in terms of causal relations between the values of variables. Property or type-level causal claims are easily translated into claims about causal relationships between the values of certain variables. For example, the claim "Arsenic poisoning causes death" can be reconstructed as a claim about the relationship between a binary variable **AP**, which takes the value 1 if any arsenic poisoning occurs and 0 if not, and a binary variable **D**, which takes the value 1 if a death occurs and 0 if not. The claim is reconstructed as saying that **AP** = 1 causes **D** = 1. It is straightforward to reconstruct event or token-level causal claims in a similar manner. For example, the event causal claim "Jones' suffering arsenic poisoning caused his death" can be translated as making a similar claim about the relationship between the values of the binary variables **AP** and **D**, but in this case the variables must be understood in terms of particular occurrences: **AP** takes the value 1 if Jones suffered arsenic poisoning and 0 if not, and **D** takes the value 1 if he died and 0 if not. The fact that this framework translates type- and token-causal claims in the same way implies the existence of structural isomorphisms between the two kinds of causation, an implication that is very contentious but beyond the scope of our discussion.

As remarked, the central idea of this framework is that a cause makes a difference to its effects in the sense that changing the value of the cause variable leads to a change in the value of the effect variable. The following account of causal relations between values of variables spells out this idea:

> **X** = x *causes* **Y** = y (relative to a particular system of kind S) if and only if (i) the actual values of **X** and **Y** are x and y, respectively; and (ii) there are contextually determined values of these variables, call them x* and y* respectively, such that if an intervention were to occur in the systems of this kind to change the value of x to the different value x*, then **Y** would change from y to the different value y*.

Some features of this account deserve special mention.

First, the notion of an intervention plays a crucial role in this kind of account, though it will not be so important for our discussion. Roughly speaking, an intervention on the variable X (with respect to variable Y) is an idealized manipulation that sets the value of X by a causal process that is independent of all other possible causes of Y. It is important that interventions have this feature to ensure that the changes in Y variable are due solely to the changes in the X variable and not to changes in some other variable associated with X, e.g. a variable that causes both X and Y. An intervention so characterized is clearly a causal notion, and advocates of this framework openly acknowledge that this kind of account should not be understood as a reductive account that attempts to reduce the causal concept to simpler, non-causal concepts. Despite its non-reductive character, this type of account is extremely illuminating about the nature and structure of causal concepts. (For more on this see Woodward (2003: chapter 2).)

This kind of account of causation is sometimes framed in terms of counterfactuals. For example, the following condition framed in terms of counterfactuals has roughly the same content as the condition above:

> $X = x$ *causes* $Y = y$ (relative to a kind of system S) if and only if (i) the actual values of X and Y are x and y, respectively; and (ii) there are contextually determined values of X and Y, call them x^* and y^* respectively, such that the counterfactuals are true:
>
> If it were the case that $X = x$, then it would be the case that $Y = y$;
> If it were the case that $X = x^*$, then it would be the case that $Y = y^*$.

The counterfactuals in this condition are given a particular interpretation. The most similar worlds in which the antecedents are true are ones in which the past history of the system is preserved but the antecedent is realized by an intervention. The notion of an intervention plays the role in this framework that the notion of a miracle plays in Lewis's framework. There is no presumption in this framework that when an antecedent is true the set of closest antecedent-worlds is restricted to the actual world. (For more on the 'interventionist' interpretation of these counterfactuals see Woodward (2003: chapter 3).)

Thirdly, and most importantly for our discussion, the account implies that causation is essentially contrastive in character. It says that statements describing causal relations between values of variables such as "$X = x$ caused $Y = y$" are elliptical for statements describing causal relations between contrasts such as "$X = x$ rather than $X = x^*$ caused $Y = y$ rather than $Y = y^*$". More particularly, it anchors these contrasts to certain baseline or default values, x^* and y^*. Sometimes the default values are made explicit, but more often they have to be retrieved from the context.

What reason is there for thinking that causal statements have a contrastive structure? One reason is that the contrastive structure is sometimes made explicit in a causal statement such as "Socrates' drinking the hemlock rather than guzzling it caused him to die rather than live". Another reason is that a number of linguistic devices—e.g. contrastive focus—are best understood as having the function of indicating the contrastive structure of causal statements. If someone asserts a statement like "Giving the patient *100 mg* of penicillin cured him", the contrastive focus serves to highlight the fact that only certain dosages within a range of possible dosages were causally effective. It suggests that we should take the cause variable to be a quantitative variable, which can take various values such as 0, 50 mg, 100 mg, 200 mg, and so on; and that the causal statement is to be understood as saying something along the lines "Giving the patient 100 mg of the drug rather than some other dosage in the given range caused the patient's recovery rather than non-recovery".

An important feature of this account is that it says that the contrast cases for the cause and effect variables are determined by context. The contextual rule for determining the contrast case for a binary variable is simple: it is just the non-actual value of the variable. But for many-valued variables where there can be more than one non-actual value, the contextual rule is to select the value that is considered to be the normal value of the variable. In the example above where the cause variable is many-valued, the causal statement might be interpreted as saying something like "Giving 100 mg rather than *usual* dose of 50 mg caused the patient's recovery rather than non-recovery". But with most causal statements asserted in everyday contexts, whether they are property or event causal statements, the variables are simple binary variables and the contrast cases will be simply the values that represent the absence of the property or the non-occurrence of the event.

The implicit contrastive structure of causal statements is easily overlooked because the surface form of causal statements does not always reveal it. But the implicit contrastive structure plays a central role in the truth-conditions of causal statements; and so has implications for the assessment of truth-values of such statements. For instance, in a situation in which a patient recovers if and only if he is given 100 mg or more of penicillin, it would be false to assert "Giving a dose of 200 mg caused his recovery" even if indeed the patient was given this dose and did recover. For when the statement is construed as involving binary variables, the statement must be understood as saying that giving the patient 200 mg rather than a different dose made the difference between recovery and non-recovery. (Even if the cause variable is not binary, the same problem can arise.) This is false simply because an intervention that set the dose at 100 mg rather than 200 mg would still produce recovery. In this connection, it is important to note that the account states that causes are difference-makers and not just causally sufficient conditions. Giving the patient 200 mg was causally sufficient for recovery but it did not make the difference in the sense required. This feature of the account will play an important role in our account of how mental states can be causally relevant to behaviour even when their underlying neural states are causally sufficient.

5. APPLICATION TO THE EXCLUSION PROBLEM

Let us return to Yablo's example about the pigeon, which he claims demonstrates the falsity of the exclusion principle. Recall that there are two rival causal judgements we can make about the example:

Red: The triangle's being red caused the pigeon to peck.

Crimson: The triangle's being crimson caused the pigeon to peck.

Yablo argues that if we are concerned with causation rather than the weaker notion of causal relevance, then our judgements should conform to the proportionality constraint, which requires that causes should be specific enough but no more specific than is required to make the difference to their effects. In this case, the causal judgement *Red* satisfies the proportionality constraint and the judgement *Crimson* does not. Accordingly, we have our counterexample to the exclusion principle in virtue of the fact that the crimson of the triangle is causally sufficient for the pigeon's pecking, but it does not exclude the redness of the triangle from being causally relevant or even from being the cause of the pecking.

I agree with Yablo that his example demonstrates the falsity of the exclusion principle, as it is traditionally formulated. However, I think that the contrastive account of causation provides a better explanation of our causal judgements about the example than his proportionality constraint. A first step in applying the contrastive account to the example is to determine the relevant variables and the relevant contrasts. Let us suppose that all the variables are binary variables that take the value 1 if the relevant property is present and 0 if the property is absent; and that accordingly, the contrast case for each variable will simply be the non-actual value of the variable. In this case, the rival causal judgements can be taken to have the same content as the following judgements:

Red′: The triangle's being red rather than not red made the difference to the pigeon's pecking rather than not pecking.

Crimson′: The triangle's being crimson rather than not crimson made the difference to the pigeon's pecking rather than not pecking.

The first judgement is true: given the triangle's redness, the pigeon pecked, but if the triangle had been a different colour altogether, she would not have pecked. On the other hand, the second judgement is false: given the crimson of the triangle the pigeon pecked, but if the triangle had been non-crimson, say scarlet, the pigeon would still have pecked. So the intuitively correct verdict about these judgements falls out as a consequence of the contrastive character of causation.

Indeed the contrastive account given above provides a good explanation of the examples that Yablo employs to motivate the conditions of his proportionality constraint. The *enough* condition (iii) is supposed to ensure that the cause is specified in sufficient relevant detail. But this is captured by the contrastive nature of our causal judgements: the valve's opening slowly rather than speedily made the difference to the boiler's explosion rather than non-explosion, whereas the valve's opening rather than not opening did not. The *required* condition (iv) is supposed to ensure that the cause is specified with no more detail than is necessary. Again, the contrastive account has the same effect: Socrates' drinking hemlock rather than not drinking it made the difference with respect to his dying rather than not dying; his guzzling rather than not guzzling the hemlock did not make the difference. The fact that these causal judgements can be spelled out in terms of counterfactuals suggests that the extra conditions (iii) and (iv) that Yablo imposes in addition to the counterfactual conditions (i) and (ii) are not necessary to capture the central idea that causes should be proportional or commensurate to their effects.

How does all of this apply to the case of mental causation? Let us consider a schematic example in which we are considering whether an agent's having a mental property M causes his display of physical behaviour B; where M can be realized by a number of (mutually exclusive) neural properties $N_1, \ldots, N_n$, each of which is causally sufficient for the behaviour B; but where M on the given occasion is realized by the neural property N_i. Here we have two rival causal judgements:

> *M as cause*: having M rather than not having M made the difference to displaying B rather than not displaying B.
>
> *N_i as cause*: having N_i rather than not having N_i made the difference to displaying B rather than not displaying B.

Which of these two rival causal judgements is vindicated depends on the details of properties M, B, and N_i. But assume that B is a coarse-grained behavioural property such as waving one's arm, M is another coarse-grained property such as intending to attract the attention of a taxi driver, and N_i is a neural property fine-grained enough to act as a realizer of the mental property M. Then it would be reasonable to think that the first causal judgement is true and the second false. The crucial reason for thinking this is that it is reasonable to judge that the agent in question would not have displayed the behaviour B if he had not had the mental property M, but might have displayed it if he had not had the property N_i. (Note that this is not the judgement that he *would* have displayed it if he had not had property N_i—merely that he *might* have displayed it.) This judgement presupposes that the set of closest worlds in which the neural property N_i is not instantiated includes at least some worlds where other neural realizers of M are instantiated. At any rate, a causal judgement in favour of the mental property M, as opposed to N_i, as the cause of B would constitute a counterexample to the exclusion principle, applied to the case of mental causation.

Notice that this causal judgement, which falsifies the exclusion principle, does not require us to settle whether or not neural properties determine mental properties. The causal judgement depends simply on which contrast—the contrast between M and not-M or the contrast between N_i and not-N_i—makes the difference between the display or non-display of the behaviour property B. And indeed the judgement holds good regardless of whether or not mental properties are determined by neural properties. In this respect, the contrastive account of causation enables us to sidestep the whole issue of whether neural properties determine mental properties or stand in some different relation to them.

6. THE EXCLUSION PRINCIPLE REFORMULATED

We have seen there is good reason to think that the exclusion principle, as it is traditionally formulated, is false. A conspicuous feature of this traditional formulation is that it is couched in terms of causal sufficiency: it states that a property that is causally sufficient for some effect excludes all other properties from being causally relevant or efficacious with respect to the effect. But one might ask: "Why talk here of causal sufficiency rather than causation?" James Woodward (Chapter 12 in this volume) has commented that this reference to nomological sufficiency betrays the influence of the deductive-nomological model of explanation. There are, to be sure, several features of the traditional formulation of the exclusion argument that depend on assuming that causes are nomologically sufficient for their effects. This is very problematic in view of the fact that this assumption is known to be unsatisfactory in many ways.

Naturally enough, this raises the question: "What happens if we reformulate the exclusion principle, replacing the reference to nomological sufficiency in the antecedent clause with reference to causation proper?" Let us consider the following version of the principle, where the reference to causation is understood in terms of the contrastive account given above:

> *Exclusion principle reformulated*: If property F *causes* property G, then no property F* distinct from F *causes* G.

Is this principle true or false? I am uncertain about the answer to this question. In order to have some chance of being true, the principle would need, at the very least, to be qualified so that it states that no two properties F and F*, *instantiated at the same time*, could cause the same instance of G, since there is every reason to think that different properties, instantiated at different times, can cause the same instance of property G. However, instead of pursuing the question of the truth-value of this general principle, I shall focus on two specific instances of the principle that are central to the exclusion problem:

Neural-excludes-mental principle: If a neural property N causes a physical behavioural property B, then no mental property that supervenes on N causes property B.

Mental-excludes-neural principle: If a mental property M causes a physical behavioural property B, then no neural property N that realizes M causes property B.

I aim to show that the contrastive theory of causation implies the truth of both these specific principles.

The examples discussed in the last section provide some insight into why the specific principles might be true. The examples suggest that if a contrast is explicable in terms of a coarse-grained variable, it is unlikely to be explicable in terms of a fine-grained variable, and vice versa. For example, if we can explain why a person displays some behaviour rather than not displaying it in terms of the fact that he was in one mental state rather than another, then it seems unlikely that we can also explain this contrast in terms of his brain being in one neural state rather than another, assuming of course that the relevant mental states are distinct from neural states. However, we can replace this impressionistic argument with rigorous arguments for each of the specific principles, with the arguments being slightly different in the two cases.

Take the principle *neural-excludes-mental* first. Let us consider the principle in terms of a schematic example about a randomly selected subject with a mental property M. The mental property M has several physically possible neural realizers, N_1 and N_2, but in this case M is realized by N_1. Let us also suppose that the agent's being in N_1 rather than not being in N_1 has caused him to display a physical behavioural property B rather than not display B. We want to know whether the fact that N_1 makes a difference to B excludes M from making a difference to B, according to the contrastive theory of causation. The situation of the schematic example is represented in Fig. 11.1, which depicts the set of possible worlds.

There are several features of the diagram requiring explanation. The mental property M is represented by the binary variable **M** that takes the value 1 when the mental property M is present and 0 when absent. The neural properties N_1, N_2, N_3, N_4, and the behavioural property B are represented in a similar way by binary variables.

The inner rectangle represents the set of possible worlds which Frank Jackson (1998) calls the minimal physical duplicates of the actual world: these worlds contain only the physical properties and relations that are instantiated in the actual world. (Lewis (1986) calls these the non-alien worlds.) Lewis and Jackson argue very plausibly, in my view, that this set of worlds should be the base set for the specification of physicalist supervenience or realization theses. The set of

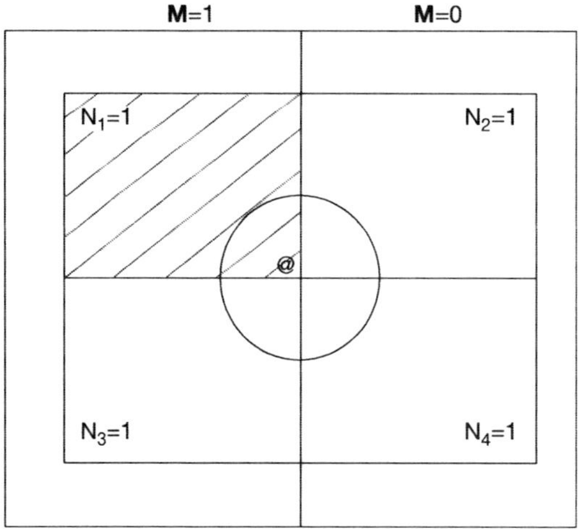

Fig. 11.1

minimal physical duplicates of the actual world is partitioned by the four neural variables $\mathbf{N_1} = 1, \mathbf{N_2} = 1, \mathbf{N_3} = 1, \mathbf{N_4} = 1$ to represent the fact that $\mathbf{N_1} = 1$ and $\mathbf{N_2} = 1$ realize $\mathbf{M} = 1$ and $\mathbf{N_3} = 1$ and $\mathbf{N_4} = 1$ realize $\mathbf{M} = 0$. So the figure depicts the fact that any worlds in this set that differ with respect to the mental property M must differ in a neural property N_i; and that any worlds in the set that agree with respect to a neural property N_i must agree with respect to the mental property M. The fact that the set of minimal physical duplicate worlds does not exhaust the entire space of possible worlds is intended to indicate that the mental property can be realized in non-physical ways.

The shaded region represents the worlds in which $\mathbf{B} = 1$ holds and the unshaded region the worlds in which $\mathbf{B} = 0$ holds. The symbol '@' denotes the actual world. It is easy to see that at the actual world it is true that $\mathbf{M} = 1, \mathbf{N_1} = 1$, and $\mathbf{B} = 1$.

The sphere within the inner rectangle represents the set of worlds that are the most similar worlds to the actual world for the purposes of the evaluation of non-backtracking counterfactuals. In orthodox semantics for counterfactuals it is assumed that this set just consists of the actual world. However, for the reasons given in section 4, I assume that when we evaluate non-backtracking counterfactuals, the set of closest worlds contains other worlds besides the actual world: in other words, I assume that other worlds may be as similar in causal respects to the actual world as the actual world is to itself. I have assumed that the set of closest worlds is included in the set of minimal physical duplicate worlds. This seems a reasonable assumption, but nothing essential to the argument below depends on this. I have also assumed that we need to go no further out from the set of closest worlds to find the closest antecedent-worlds in which

$\mathbf{N_1} = 1, \mathbf{N_2} = 1, \mathbf{N_3} = 1$, and $\mathbf{N_4} = 1$ are true. Again this seems a reasonable assumption but nothing essential to the argument below depends on it. Finally, note that in the closest worlds in which $\mathbf{N_1} = 0$, then either $\mathbf{N_2} = 1$ or $\mathbf{N_3} = 1$ or $\mathbf{N_4} = 1$ must be true.

Now the figure represents the fact that the contrast between $\mathbf{N_1} = 1$ and $\mathbf{N_1} = 0$ makes it the case that $\mathbf{B} = 1$ rather $\mathbf{B} = 0$ by virtue of showing that the following counterfactuals are true:

(a) $(\mathbf{N_1} = 1 \;\Box\!\!\rightarrow \mathbf{B} = 1)$ & $(\mathbf{N_1} = 0 \;\Box\!\!\rightarrow \mathbf{B} = 0)$

The question which we now need to settle is this: Is it possible, consistently with these facts, for the contrast between $\mathbf{M} = 1$ and $\mathbf{M} = 0$ to make it the case that $\mathbf{B} = 1$ rather than $\mathbf{B} = 0$? In other words, is it possible for both of the following counterfactuals to be true:

(b) $(\mathbf{M} = 1 \;\Box\!\!\rightarrow \mathbf{B} = 1)$ & $(\mathbf{M} = 0 \;\Box\!\!\rightarrow \mathbf{B} = 0)$?

It is easily shown that the first counterfactual of (b) must be false. For it follows from the fact that all the closest $\mathbf{N_1} = 0$ worlds are $\mathbf{B} = 0$ worlds that some of the closest $\mathbf{M} = 1$ worlds are not $\mathbf{B} = 1$ worlds. Hence, the figure demonstrates that the conditions which make it true that the contrast between $\mathbf{N_1} = 1$ and $\mathbf{N_1} = 0$ accounts for the difference between $\mathbf{B} = 1$ and $\mathbf{B} = 0$ render it impossible for the contrast between $\mathbf{M} = 1$ and $\mathbf{M} = 0$ to account for this difference as well. In other words, the figure demonstrates quite simply that the counterfactual dependence between $\mathbf{N_1} = 1$ and $\mathbf{B} = 1$ rules out the counterfactual dependence between $\mathbf{M} = 1$ and $\mathbf{B} = 1$, which requires the truth of both counterfactual conjuncts in (b).

Let us now consider the converse principle—the *mental-excludes-neural* principle. Fig. 11.2 represents a schematic example like the one above. The conventions of representation are the same as before. In this example we will assume that the contrast in the values of the mental variable **M** accounts for the contrast in the behavioural variable **B**. This figure represents this by making the counterfactuals in the conjunction (b) above true. The question we now need to ask is this: Is the counterfactual dependence between $\mathbf{M} = 1$ and $\mathbf{B} = 1$ compatible with existence of a counterfactual dependence between $\mathbf{N_1} = 1$ and $\mathbf{B} = 1$, assuming once more that in the randomly selected individual the mental property M is actually realized by the neural property N_1?

The answer seems to be a straightforward "No", as the second counterfactual in the conjunction (a) above is false. The fact that all the closest worlds that make it true that $\mathbf{M} = 1$ are $\mathbf{B} = 1$ worlds implies that not all the closest worlds in which $\mathbf{N_1} = 0$ are $\mathbf{B} = 0$ worlds: in particular, the closest worlds in which it is true that $\mathbf{N_3} = 1$ are $\mathbf{B} = 1$ worlds so falsifying the counterfactual $\mathbf{N_1} = 0 \;\Box\!\!\rightarrow \mathbf{B} = 0$. Once more we can see that the conditions required for a difference-making relation between $\mathbf{M} = 1$ and $\mathbf{B} = 1$ are incompatible with the conditions required for a difference-making relation between $\mathbf{N_1} = 1$ and $\mathbf{B} = 1$.

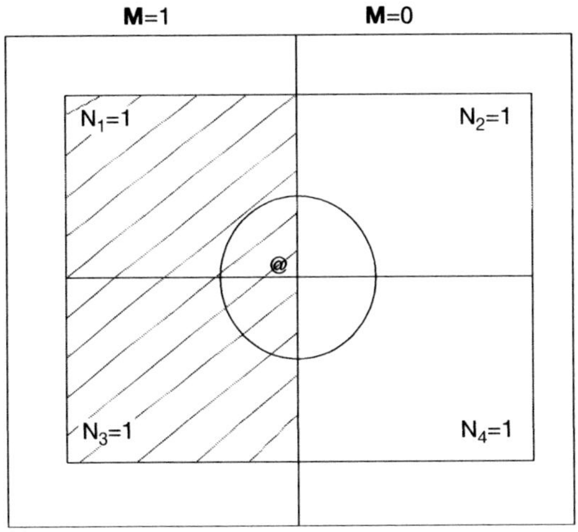

Fig. 11.2

So we have established that the two specific exclusion principles are true. By substituting "causation" for "causal sufficiency" in the antecedent of these specific instances of the exclusion principle, we have transformed them into truths. How does all of this affect the exclusion argument? Does this mean that we are now compelled to accept the conclusion of the exclusion argument after all?

7. THE EXCLUSION ARGUMENT RE-EVALUATED

In the light of the preceding discussion, let us revisit the exclusion argument to consider whether we are now committed to accepting its conclusion.

Recall that the argument begins with the initial supposition, entertained for the purposes of *reductio*, that a mental property M causes a physical behavioural property B. The argument invokes the causal closure principle to posit the existence of physical property P that is causally sufficient for B; and then appeals to the exclusion principle, in its original formulation, to conclude that the mental property B is excluded from causal relevance by the physical property B. As we have seen already, this version of the argument is defective, as the exclusion principle, in its original formulation, is false.

Nonetheless, our discussion in the last section has supported a reformulated exclusion principle to the effect that a mental property and its underlying neural realizer property cannot both be difference-making causes of the same physical behavioural property. This suggests that a new version of the exclusion argument could be formulated if we had reason to believe a strengthened formulation of the causal closure principle along the following lines:

> *Causal closure of the physical reformulated*: For every physical property G, there is a physical property F that is a difference-making cause of G.

This differs from the original formulation in that it replaces the reference to the existence of a physical property F that is causally sufficient for G with a reference to the existence of a physical property F that is a difference-making cause of G. As we have seen, a difference-making cause must satisfy stronger conditions than a merely causally sufficient condition; and so this principle is stronger than the original principle.

Let us consider how a reformulated exclusion argument might work. Again it would start with the supposition that some mental property M causes a behavioural property B. However, we do not have to entertain this as an idle supposition without any support or warrant. Let us suppose that we conduct careful experimentation to determine whether this property really does make a difference to the behavioural property. Perhaps we conduct controlled experiments, randomly assigning people to treatment and control groups, and intervening so as to ensure that the members of the treatment group have the mental property M and members of the control group do not. If we were to find that the members of the treatment group displayed property B and members of the control group did not, we would have very good evidence in support of this causal claim. Now continuing with the exclusion argument, we might appeal to the strengthened causal closure principle to posit the existence of a physical property P that is not just causally sufficient for B but is a difference-making cause of B. But exactly how plausible would this appeal be? We know from the discussion of the last section that M and a neural property that realizes it cannot both be difference-making causes of B. So our epistemic situation is one in which we have to decide between the well-confirmed hypothesis that M is the cause of B and the purely conjectural hypothesis that there exists some physical property P that is a difference-making cause of B. It would not be irrational under these circumstances to favour the first hypothesis over the second, concluding that the strengthened causal closure principle is false in this case. (Of course, consistently with thinking that M is the cause of B, we can still suppose that there exists a physical property that is causally sufficient for B. We have not found any reason to reject the causal closure of the physical, as originally formulated.)

So, acceptance of the new version of the exclusion principle does not automatically compel us to accept the conclusion of the exclusion argument to the effect that mental properties do not cause physical properties. However, the plausibility of the new exclusion principle does mean that the critical spotlight needs to be shifted to the other crucial principle of a reformulated version of argument—the strengthened causal closure principle. I have sketched a possible epistemic situation—indeed, one that is reasonably common—in which it would be rational to stick to the belief that a mental property is a difference-making of some physical property and reject the belief in the strengthened causal closure principle.

REFERENCES

Ehring, Douglas. 2003. "Part–Whole Physicalism and Mental Causation", *Synthese*, 136, 359–88.

Funkhouser, Eric. 2006. "The Determinable–Determinate Relation", *Noûs*, 40, 548–69.

Hitchcock, Christopher. 2001. "The Intransitivity of Causation Revealed in Equations and Graphs", *Journal of Philosophy*, 98, 273–99.

Jackson, Frank. 1998. *From Metaphysics to Ethics: A Defence of Conceptual Analysis*. Oxford: Oxford University Press.

Johnson, W. E. 1921. *Logic*, vol. i. Cambridge: Cambridge University Press.

Kim, Jaegwon. 1989. "Mechanism, Purpose, and Explanatory Exclusion", *Philosophical Perspectives*, 3, 77–108.

—— 1998. *Mind in a Physical World*. Cambridge, MA: MIT Press.

—— 2005. *Physicalism, or Something Near Enough*. Princeton: Princeton University Press.

Lewis, David. 1983. "New Work for a Theory of Universals", *Australasian Journal of Philosophy*, 61, 343–77.

McGrath, Matthew. 1998. "Proportionality and Mental Causation: A Fit?", *Philosophical Perspectives*, 12, 167–76.

Menzies, Peter. 2003. "The Causal Efficacy of Mental States", in S. Walter and H. Heckmann (eds.), *Physicalism and Mental Causation*. Imprint Academic, 195–223.

—— 2007. "Mental Causation on the Program Model", in Geoffrey Brennan, Robert Goodin, and Michael Smith (eds.), *The Common Mind: Essays in Honour of Philip Pettit*. Oxford: Oxford University Press.

Pearl, Judea. 2000. *Causality: Models, Reasoning, and Inference*. Cambridge: Cambridge University Press.

Prior, A. 1949. "I. Determinables, Determinates, and Determinants", *Mind*, 58, 1–20.

Woodward, James. 2003. *Making Things Happen: A Theory of Causal Explanation*. Oxford: Oxford University Press.

Yablo, Stephen. 1992. "Mental Causation", *Philosophical Review*, 101, 245–80.

12

Mental Causation and Neural Mechanisms

James Woodward

Issues about the causal role of the mental—about whether mental states (beliefs, desires, intentions and so on) can cause or figure in causal explanations of other mental states or behavior, about what it even means to attribute causal efficacy to a mental state, and about how claims about mental causation/explanation fit with (or fail to fit with or are undermined by) claims about causation by neural mechanisms—have been matters of intense debate within the philosophical literature over the past decade. Some philosophers argue that generally accepted claims about what makes a relationship causal and about the relationship between mind and body yield the conclusion that mental states cannot cause anything—that the mental is entirely causally inert or epiphenomenal. The arguments for this conclusion are largely metaphysical and *quasi-apriori* in the sense that the conclusion is supposed to follow from the combination of very general and presumably uncontroversial empirical assumptions about the relationships between the mental and the physical (the causal closure of physics and the absence of systematic causal over-determination of mental states by both mental and physical causes) together with assumptions about what is involved in mental causation. Other philosophers have found this conclusion literally incredible and have sought to identify flaws in the arguments that seem to support it. However, no particular counterargument has won general acceptance.

In this paper, I propose to examine these issues within the framework of the account of causation and causal explanation worked out in my recent book, *Making Things Happen* (*MTH*). One of my themes will be that many of the standard arguments for the causal inertness of the mental rest on mistaken assumptions about what it is for a relationship to be causal, and about what is involved in providing a causal explanation. These mistaken assumptions involve an inter-related complex of ideas, described below: a conception of causation according to which a cause is simply a condition (or

Thanks to Chris Hitchcock, John Heil, Jakob Hohwy, Jesper Kallestrup, Philip Pettit, David Robb, and Jiji Zhang for helpful comments on earlier drafts.

a conjunct in a condition) which is nomologically sufficient for its effect, and the closely associated deductive-nomological (*DN*) conception of explanation according to which explaining an outcome is simply a matter of exhibiting a nomologically sufficient condition for it. Given these assumptions, it is indeed hard to understand how there can be such a thing as mental causation. However, the account of causation defended in *MTH* undercuts these assumptions and in doing so, allows us to reach a better understanding of what is involved in mental causation and of the real empirical issues surrounding this notion.

My discussion is organized as follows: Section 1 sets out my general framework for understanding causation and causal explanation. Sections 2–6 then discuss and criticize several arguments, including the so-called causal exclusion argument, that attempt to show that mental causal claims and claims that attribute causal efficacy to neural structure are always in competition with each other, with the former being undercut or "pre-empted" by the latter. The conclusion of this section is that these arguments present no barrier to attributing casual efficacy to the mental. Section 7 then comments very briefly on what I take to be the real empirical issues raised by claims of mental causation which have to do with the extent to which such claims are stable or insensitive to the details of their neural realization.

1.

MTH defends a *manipulationist* or *interventionist* account of causation: causal (as opposed to merely correlational) relationships are relationships that are potentially exploitable for purposes of manipulation and control. As an illustration of what this means, consider the well known correlation between attendance at a private (that is, non-government run) secondary school in the contemporary U.S. and scholastic achievement: students who attend private schools tend to score higher on various measures of scholastic achievement than students who attend public schools. This correlation raises the question of whether private school attendance *causes* superior scholastic achievement or whether instead the relationship between these two variables is merely correlational, with the correlation between them due to the causal influence of some other variable(s). To take only the most obvious possibilities, it may be that parents with higher SES are more likely to send their children to private schools and that SES (socio-economic status) also directly causes scholastic achievement. Or it may be that parents who send their children to private schools tend to value educational achievement more and these values directly influence their children's performance. If we let P be a variable measuring whether a child attends public or private school, S a variable measuring scholastic achievement, and E and A be variables measuring, respectively, parents' social economic status and attitudes toward education, these possibilities might be represented as shown in Fig. 12.1, with an arrow from X to Y meaning that X causes Y.

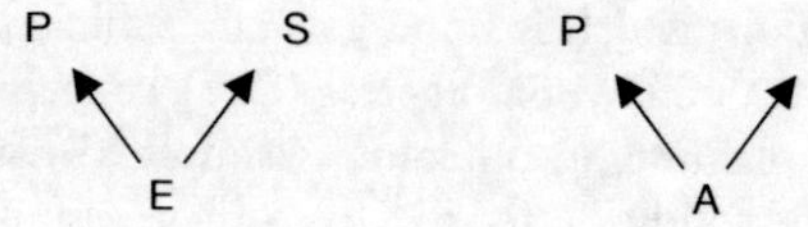

Fig. 12.1

On a manipulationist conception of cause, the question of whether *P* causes *S* is identified with the question of whether *S* would change under some suitable manipulation of *P*. If *P* causes *S*, then other things being equal, this will be a good or effective strategy. If on the other hand, if *P* and *S* are merely correlated as in Fig. 12.1, changing the school the child attends should have no effect on achievement. Instead changing SES or parental attitudes would be an effective strategy for affecting achievement.

How might one determine whether *S* would change under a suitable manipulation of *P* and what does "suitable" mean in this context? One possibility would be to perform a randomized experiment: children in the population of interest are randomly assigned to one of two groups, one of which is sent to private schools and the other to public schools. One then looks to see whether there is a correlation between *P* and *S*. The effect of the randomization (it is assumed) is to remove any systematic difference between the two groups with respect to parental SES, attitudes, or indeed any other factors that might influence *S* independently of *P*. Any remaining correlation between *P* and *S* should thus be attributable to the causal influence of *P* on *S*. If Fig. 12.1 represents the correct causal structure there should be no correlation between *P* and *S* under any such intervention on *P*.

A natural way of representing such a randomized experiment, due to Spirtes, Glymour and Scheines, 2000 and Pearl, 2000 is to think of the experimental manipulation of *P* (represented by means of a variable *I* for intervention) as accomplishing the following. It breaks or removes arrows directed into the variable intervened on while preserving all the other arrows in the graph, including any arrows directed out of the variable intervened on. Thus an intervention on *P* in the structure in Fig. 12.1 replaces it with the structure shown in Fig. 12.2.

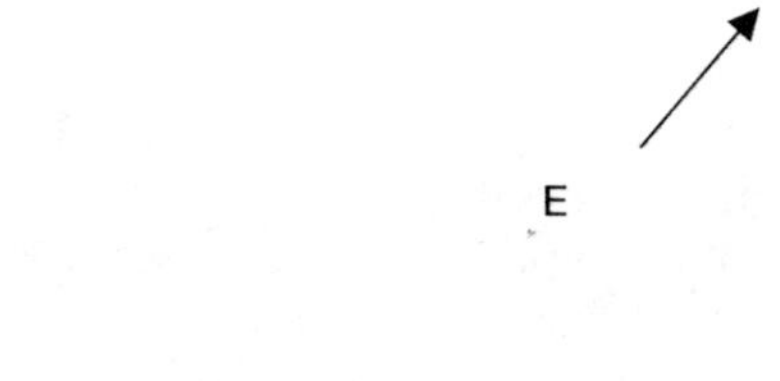

Fig. 12.2

On the other hand if, say, the correct causal structure is one in which it is true *both* that E is a common cause of P and S *and* that P causes S (i.e. the correlation between P and S is due to both of these factors) then the result of intervening on P is to replace the structure shown in Fig. 12.3*a* with that shown in Fig. 12.3*b*.

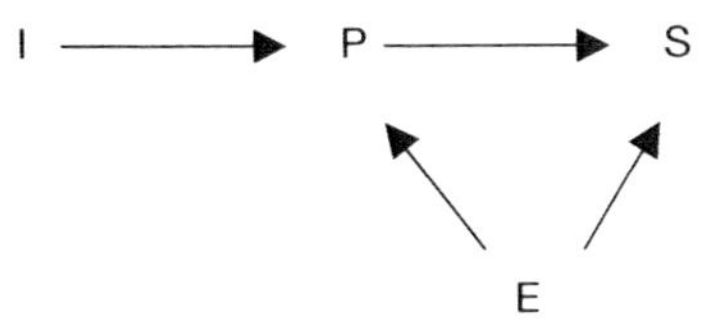

Fig. 12.3*a*

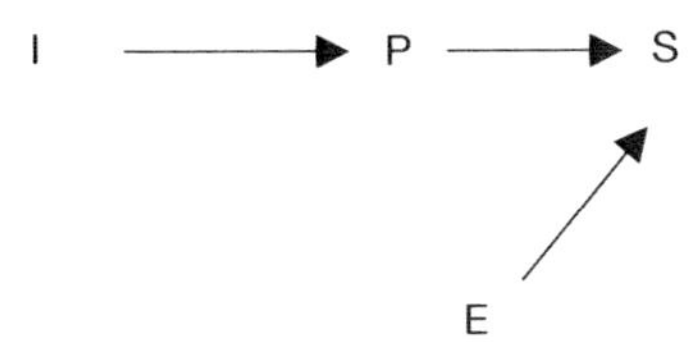

Fig. 12.3*b*

In this case there *will* be a change in S under an intervention on P, reflecting the fact that (unlike the situation represented in Fig. 12.1) P makes a causal contribution to S that is independent of, or in addition to, the contribution made by E.

Note that if we want to do an experiment of this sort to determine whether P causes S it is crucial to the logic of the experiment that the intervention not itself cause or be correlated with other causes of S that are independent of P. For example, if Fig. 12.1 is the correct structure, an alternative way of manipulating P (besides what is represented by Fig. 12.2) would be to manipulate E (perhaps we give parents a very large cash grant). This manipulation of E would change the value of P in the population (since E causes P), but it would (obviously) not be a good experimental design for determining whether P causes S since it confounds any effect of P on S with the effect of changing E on S. Instead, what we want is that, among other desiderata, the experimental manipulation be such that the variation in P it introduces is uncorrelated with or independent of other possible causes of its putative effect S (except of course for those other possible causes that lie on any causal route (should one exist) from P to S). An experimental manipulation of P that has this feature and also features that rule out other confounding possibilities is what we mean by an *intervention*.

Giving a precise characterization of the notion of an intervention turns out to be non-trivial and the reader is referred to *MTH*, chapter 3 for details. For the purposes of this essay, it will be enough to stick with the intuitive conception just illustrated: think of an intervention on one variable *X* with respect to a second variable *Y* as an idealized experimental manipulation of *X* which is well designed for the purpose of determining whether *X* causes *Y*, in the sense that it excludes various confounding possibilities such as those illustrated above. As we shall see, in contexts (including discussions of mental causation) in which values of some variables supervene on others, the issue of what counts as such a confounding possibility requires some careful thought—this is addressed below, especially in Section 6.

Given this notion, we may use it to give an interventionist characterization of what it is for a variable *X* to cause or be causally relevant to a second variable *Y*. (I will use "cause" and "causally relevant" interchangeably and in a generic sense according to which *X* causes *Y* if it is either positively or negatively relevant or of mixed relevance for *Y*.)

> (**M**) *X* causes *Y* if and only if there are background circumstances *B* such that if some (single) intervention that changes the value of *X* (and no other variable) were to occur in *B*, then *Y* would change.[1]

(**M**) obviously requires some explication. First, note that it relates *variables*, which as Woodward, 2003 explains, are the natural candidates for the relata of causal claims within an interventionist framework. A variable is simply a property, quantity etc., which is capable of taking two or more "values". Philosophers often focus on causal claims relating types of events, and we can think of these relata as two-valued, with the values in question corresponding to the presence or absence of this type of event. For example, we may think of the claim that short circuits cause fires as relating variables which take values corresponding to <short circuit present, short circuit absent>, and <fire present, fire absent>. However, some variables such as pressure or mass may take many different values.

The reference to background conditions is added to accommodate the familiar fact that it may be that it is only under certain conditions, not specified in the description of *X* itself, that interventions on *X* are associated with changes in *Y*. Thus, for example, according to **M**, short circuits cause fires as long as it is true that in some background circumstances (having to do with the presence of oxygen etc.) interventions that change whether a short circuit occurs are associated with changes in whether a fire occurs (or in the probability of fire).

Next, note that the formulation **M** relates *changes* in *X* (due to an intervention) to *changes* in *Y* (or in the probability distribution of *Y*). Focusing first on the

[1] Purely for reasons of expository convenience, I will assume that the systems with which we are dealing in this paper are deterministic, so that there is always a determinate answer to the question of how if at all *Y* would change under an intervention on *X*. However, **M** may be readily extended to stochastic systems by talking about whether a change in the probability distribution of *Y* would occur under an intervention *X*. I don't think that anything important will turn in what follows to this restriction to deterministic systems.

case in which the causal claim relates changes in the value of X to the changes in the value of Y, I take this to imply that there is a pattern of association between X and Y such that each of these variables can take at least two different values ($X = x, x'$ with $x \neq x'$, $Y = y, y'$ with $y \neq y'$) such that one (e.g., x) of these values of X (when produced by an intervention) is associated with one (y) of the values of Y and a different value x' of X (when produced by an intervention) is associated with a different value y' of Y. That is, X causes Y if and only if there are distinct values of X and Y meeting the conditions just described and background circumstances B in which two counterfactuals of the following form are true:

(**M***)
(M1*) If an intervention that sets $X = x$ were to occur in B, then $Y = y$.
(M2*) If an intervention that sets $X = x'$ were to occur in B, then $Y = y'$.

When M1* and M2* hold, I will say that a change in the value of X from $X = x$ to $X = x'$ (where $x \neq x'$) in background circumstances B *causes a change* in the value of Y from $Y = y$ to $Y = y'$ (and vice versa).

For reasons of space I cannot provide a complete explication or defense of (**M**) (or the closely related **M***) here. Instead I draw attention to just a few features that will be important to our subsequent discussion. First, **M** is intended as a characterization of what is sometimes called *type* as opposed to *token* or actual causation. That is, **M** is intended as an explication of the notion of cause that figures in claims like "attendance at private school causes improved scholastic achievement" (alternatively: "a change in attendance from public to private school causes a change in scholastic achievement from better to worse") or "smoking causes lung cancer" as opposed to such token claims as "Smith's attendance at private school in 1990 caused his scholastic achievement in the same year to improve" or "Jones' smoking caused his lung cancer". As *MTH* shows, the interventionist account can also be used to capture a notion of token causation, but with the exception of some remarks about pre-emption and redundancy in Section 6, my focus in this essay will be entirely on type causal notions of the sort captured by **M** and on type causal claims about mental causation. The reason for this focus is that I take issues about the causal role of the mental to be in the first instance issues about type casual claims involving mental states—whether beliefs, desires, intentions cause other mental states or behavior. If such claims about mental causation are never true, then presumably it is also never true that, e.g., some particular token mental state of Jones caused some bit of his behavior. The latter token claims also, however, raise some distinctive issues of their own that for the purposes of this essay are simply distractions.

Second, although (**M**) takes causal claims to have implications for the results of interventions and vice versa, **M** does not claim (and it is obviously false that) the only way to *tell* whether X causes Y is to experimentally intervene on X and see what happens to Y. Plainly one can sometimes learn about causal relationships by means of inference from passive, non-experimental observations—for example, by the use of various causal modeling techniques. What (**M**) implies is that to the extent that the output of such techniques provide accurate descriptions of causal relationships, they should correctly describe how effect variables would respond to hypothetical experiments in which interventions occur on cause variables.

As the previous paragraph makes explicit, (**M**) embodies a counterfactual account of causation in the sense that it links the claim that X causes Y to a claim about what would happen to Y if, perhaps contrary to actual fact, an intervention on X were to occur—what I will call an *interventionist counterfactual.* As *MTH* explains in more detail, the conditions that characterize the notion of an intervention do roughly the same work as the similarity metric in Lewis's version of a counterfactual theory of causation: given an appropriately characterized notion of an intervention, the counterfactuals that figure in **M** will be non-backtracking, the joint effects of a common cause will not be counterfactually dependent on one another when dependence is understood in terms of interventionist counterfactuals, and other standard counter-examples to counterfactual accounts of causation will be blocked.

I assume that interventionist counterfactuals and the causal claims associated with them can be true even if the interventions that figure in their antecedents cannot in fact be carried out by human beings because of practical or other sorts of limitations. However, I also assume that if a candidate causal claim is associated with interventions that are impossible for (or lack any clear sense because of) logical, conceptual or perhaps metaphysical reasons, then that causal claim is itself illegitimate or ill-defined. In other words, I take it to be an implication of **M** that a legitimate causal claim should have an intelligible interpretation in terms of counterfactuals the antecedents of which are coherent or make sense.

As an illustration, the claim that an asteroid impact caused the extinction of the dinosaurs can be understood within an interventionist framework as a claim about what would have happened to the dinosaurs if an intervention had occurred to prevent such an asteroid impact during the relevant time period. In this case we have both (i) a reasonably clear conception of what such an intervention would involve and (ii) principled ways of determining what would happen if such an intervention were to occur. By contrast, neither (i) nor (ii) hold if we are asked to consider hypothetical interventions that make it the case that $2 + 2 \neq 4$ or that the same object is at the same time both pure gold and pure aluminum or that transform human beings into houseflies. Causal claims that require for their explication claims about what would happen under such interventions ("$2 + 2 = 4$ causes it to be the case that . . .") are thus unclear or at least have no legitimate role in empirical inquiry. This idea—that the counterfactuals that are relevant to the explication of causal claims must have a clear interventionist interpretation—will play an important role below.

A closely related idea, to which I will also appeal, is that genuinely competing or rival causal claims must make different predictions about what would happen under some possible intervention or interventions, where the interventions in question are again such that we have some coherent conception of what it would be like for them to occur. Thus if we have two apparently competing claims, the first contending some mental state is causally inert and the other contending that it causes some outcome, it must be possible to specify some set of (coherent, well-defined) interventions such that the two claims make competing predictions about what would happen under those interventions. If we cannot associate such an interventionist interpretation with one or both of the claims, the claim(s) in question lack a clear sense and if they fail to make different predictions about what would happen under such interventions, they are not genuine competitors.

Note that **M** characterizes a rather weak and non-specific notion of "cause": for X to cause Y all that is required is that there be some change in X such that when this is produced by an intervention in some background circumstances, it is associated with a change in Y or in its probability distribution. One reason for formulating **M** in this way (rather than, say, in terms of the claim that *all* changes in X must be associated with changes in Y) is that many causal claims (including claims involving mental or psychological causation) exhibit threshold effects: X may cause Y even though some changes in the value of X are not associated with any changes in Y, as long as some other changes in X are associated with such changes—see example (1.1) below. Ideally, of course, we would like to know much more than this: we'd like to know exactly which changes in X are associated with exactly which changes in Y and in what background circumstances. Within the interventionist account such information is spelled out in terms of more fine-grained interventionist counterfactuals specifying in a detailed way how Y changes under various interventions that change the value of X.

Next, let me make explicit a consequence of the fact that (**M**) relates changes in the value of X to changes in the value of Y: as the formulation in terms of **M*** underscores, (**M**) implies that for X to count as a cause of Y, there must be at least two different values of X, x and x', and at least two different values of Y, y and y' such that under an intervention that changes the value of X from x to x', the value of Y changes from y to y'. This captures the intuition that whatever else a cause is, it must *make a difference* to its effect: to say that a cause makes a difference to its effect implies that there must be at least two possible states, corresponding to the cause being present or the cause being absent or to the cause being in one state rather than another state such that which of these is realized is associated with some change or difference in the state of the effect (the difference between the effect being present or absent etc.).[2] Causal claims thus

[2] I have glossed over a number of issues here. For a discussion of how this difference-making conception of causation can accommodate examples involving over-determination etc. see Woodward, 2003, chapter 2. The idea that causes must be difference-makers does not by itself exclude the possibility that causes must also satisfy other conditions that can't be captured in

have built into them the feature that philosophers call *contrastive focus* or "rather than" structure: when we make the structure of a causal claim explicit, we see that the real content of the claim is something like this: it is the contrast between X's taking some value x and its taking some different value x' that causes the contrast between Y's taking value y and value y' (or alternatively it is the fact that $X = x$ rather than $X = x'$ which causes Y to be y rather than y' or the change from $X = x$ to $X = x'$ that causes the change from $Y = y$ to $Y = y'$). The causal claim that it is the contrast between $X = x$ rather than $X = x'$ that causes the contrast between $Y = y$ rather than $Y = y'$ is thus a different causal claim, with a different content, from a causal claim involving a different contrast in the values of X such as the claim that $X = x$ rather than $X = x''$ (where $x'' \neq x'$) accounts for the contrast between $Y = y$ rather than $Y = y''$.

We noted above that there are many cases in which some changes in the value of a candidate cause variable X will be associated with changes in the value of a candidate effect variable Y, but other changes in which X will not be associated with changes in Y. Making the contrastive focus of a causal claim explicit is a natural way of representing such facts. When the contrastive focus of a causal claim is not made explicit, there may or may not be a natural default specification of the contrast situation which corresponds to the cause being different or absent. As an illustration of the first possibility, if the claim of interest is that short circuits cause fires, the natural default contrast (if this is not explicitly specified) is a situation in which no short circuits of any kind and no alternative causes of fire are present—this (rather than a situation in which, e.g., no short circuit occurs but some other source of fire is present) is taken to be the situation that corresponds to the "absence" of short circuits. That is, the claim is naturally interpreted as the claim that the contrast between the presence of a short circuit and a contrasting situation in which no short circuits or other causes of fire are present (or a change from one of these situations to another) causes the contrast between (or a change from) an outcome in which some fire is present and a contrasting situation in which no fires occur. On the other hand, in many cases in which the cause variable is quantitative or capable of taking a number of values (rather than just two—present and absent) and no contrastive state is explicitly specified, there may be many different possible candidates for this state and different outcomes associated with each. In such cases, the causal claim may be ambiguous unless we make clear what contrastive focus is intended.

Whether or not there is a natural default, a causal claim will be defective to the extent that it suggests that some contrast or difference in the value of the cause variable is associated with changes in the effect variable when this is not the case or if it fails to make explicit which changes in the cause variable are

difference-making terms, such as those emphasized in causal process accounts. For discussion, see Woodward, 2003, chapter 8 and p. 244 below.

associated with which changes in the effect variable (as would be the case, for example, if there is no obvious default and the contrastive focus is not specified). In some cases of this sort, it may seem most natural to think of this defect as a matter of the causal claim being false and in other cases, more natural to think of the claim as true but misleading or as failing to covey information that it should convey. For our purposes, it often will not matter much which of these alternative assessments is adopted.

As an illustration, consider a platform that will collapse if and only if a weight greater than 1000 kg is placed on it. If it is claimed that (1.1) it is the fact that the weight on the platform was greater than 1000 kg that causes the platform to collapse, this is naturally interpreted as the claim that it is the contrast between the weight being greater than rather than less than 1000 kg that caused the platform to collapse—a claim that is correct in the specified circumstances. That is, the weight's being less than 1000 kg is the natural default for the absence of the cause when no explicit contrast is specified.

Suppose that in these same circumstances, it was instead claimed that (1.2) the weight's being 1600 kg causes the collapse. According to (**M**), this claim is also true since there is some intervention (namely one that changes the weight to below 1000 kg) that would be associated with a change in the effect. Nonetheless there is an obvious sense in which (1.2) is potentially misleading since it is naturally interpreted as suggesting that it is the contrast between the weight being 1600 kg rather than some different (presumably lesser) weight that accounts for the collapse and this is not true for many weights that are different from 1600 kg. At the very least (1.2) is deficient, in comparison with (1.1), in failing to communicate information about the conditions under which the platform would not have collapsed. Put in terms of **M***, (1.2) does not tell us which changes in the weight cause changes in whether the platform collapses (or not). This observation will turn out to be important in connection with claims about mental causation.

Finally, note that according to (**M**), if no changes (produced by interventions) in the value of X are associated with changes in the value of Y, then X does not cause Y. Instead, X is causally irrelevant or causally inert with respect to Y. Put slightly differently, if we understand causal (ir)relevance in the manner just suggested (X is causally relevant to Y if and only if there is at least one change in the value of X such that if it were produced by an intervention, there would be a change in the value of Y), there is no such thing as a cause of Y that is not causally relevant to Y. Equally, if X is causally relevant to Y, then X causes Y. Bona fide causal claims *always* have relevance claims built into them. I stress this point because some influential writers on mental causation seem to assume (more or less explicitly) that there is a notion of causation or causal efficacy according to which X can cause Y without being causally relevant (in the sense just defined) to Y or, alternatively, that X can be causally relevant to Y, without its being true that X causes Y.

So far I have been talking about causation. What does *causal explanation* involve on an interventionist conception? Some philosophers distinguish very sharply between providing a casual explanation of an outcome (hereafter the *explanandum* outcome) and making true claims about the causes of that outcome. I agree that these are different activities, but see them as very closely related. On my view, providing a causal explanation of an outcome requires making true claims about its causes. Of course, typically, there will be many different true causal claims one may make about an outcome of interest. Some of these true causal claims will be superior to others from the point of view of explanation—superior because they are, e.g. more general or provide more information about the conditions under which alternatives to the explanandum outcome occur. (See below for illustrations.) But these more general etc. causal claims are still just ordinary causal claims that must (if interventionism is correct) possess the sorts of features set out in **M**—they are not some special sort of causal claim with special features that play a role in causal explanation but not in other kinds of causal ascription. In my view, there is thus a connection between features of our explanatory practice involving mental events and the truth of causal claims about the mental in the following sense: *if* various features of our practice of giving causal explanations involving mental events are correct or well founded, then the causal claims figuring in those explanations must be true.

With this as background, let me flesh out the interventionist conception of causal explanation a bit: we may think of this as embodying a *what-if-things-had-been-different* conception of explanation: we explain an outcome by identifying conditions under which the explanandum-outcome would have been different, that is, information about changes that might be used to manipulate or control the outcome. More generally, successful causal explanation consists in the exhibition of patterns of dependency (as expressed by interventionist counterfactuals) between the factors cited in the explanans and the explanandum—factors that are such that changes in them produced by interventions are systematically associated with changes in the explanandum outcome. Other things being equal, causal explanations will be better to the extent that the cited patterns of dependency are detailed, complete, and accurate in the sense of identifying all and only those factors such that changes in them (when produced by interventions) are associated with changes in the explanandum phenomenon. In other words, good explanations should both *include* information about all factors which are such that changes in them are associated with some change in the explanandum-phenomenon of interest and *not include* factors such that no changes in them are associated with changes in the explanandum-phenomenon (such factors are causally or explanatorily irrelevant to the explandandum-phenomenon).

How does this conception of causal explanation compare with the well-known deductive-nomological (*DN*) model of explanation, according to which we explain an explanandum by deriving it from a "law" and other true statements (typically about "initial conditions") and in this sense exhibiting a nomologically sufficient condition for it? One crucial difference,[3] which is of central importance in the mental causation/explanation debate, is that the *DN* model does *not* impose the requirement that a successful explanation answer a what-if-things—had-been-different question. This is the source of a number of well-known counterexamples to the *DN* model. Consider the following derivations, due to Wesley Salmon (1984):

All men who take birth control pills fail to get pregnant
Jones is a man who takes birth control pills
Jones fails to get pregnant

All samples of hexed salt dissolve in water
This is a sample of hexed salt
This dissolves in water

In both cases, the derivations are sound and the generalizations in them satisfy the criteria for lawfulness found in the philosophical literature. Nonetheless, the derivations don't seem explanatory. In both cases, the underlying defect seems the same: the derivations cite conditions that, although nomologically sufficient for their explananda, are not causally relevant (in the sense captured by (**M**)) to those explananda. That is, we judge that the above explanations are defective *because* they cite conditions that are not causes of (or causally relevant to) the outcomes they purport to explain. For example, changes in whether Jones takes birth control pills (when produced by interventions) are not associated with changes in whether he gets pregnant, and, in accordance with (**M**), this is reflected in our judgment that taking birth control pills does not cause and is not causally relevant to Jones' failure to get pregnant. Similarly, changes in whether the salt is hexed or not (when produced by interventions) are not associated with changes in whether it dissolves and this is what accounts for our judgment that the hexing does not cause and is not causally relevant to the dissolving. The causal irrelevance of Jones' taking birth control pills and the hexing of the salt to these outcomes is also reflected in the fact that explanations that appeal to these factors do not provide answers to what-if-things-had-been-different questions about these outcomes. As these examples illustrate, citing a nomologically sufficient condition for some outcome is *not* the same thing as answering a what-if-things-had-been-different question with respect to that outcome. Similarly, contrary to what a number of philosophers of mind seem to suppose, a condition that is linked by law to an outcome is *not* necessarily a condition which causes or is causally relevant (in the sense of cause and causal relevance captured by (**M**)) to that outcome.

A parallel observation applies to accounts of causation which take C to be a cause of E if and only if C is a nomologically sufficient condition for E

[3] Another difference, discussed in more detail in *MTH* is that, unlike the *DN* model, the interventionist account does not require that a successful explanation cite laws; instead citing an appropriately *invariant* relationship is enough.

(or what we might loosely call a "part" or "conjunct" in such a condition). The hexing of the salt is nomologically sufficient for its dissolution when placed in water but does not cause this dissolution and Jones' taking birth control pills is (we assume) nomologically sufficient for but does not cause his failure to get pregnant. In both cases, (**M**) elucidates the basis for these judgments: the conditions cited as causes are not such that any interventions on them are associated with changes in their putative effects.

Let me conclude this section with some brief remarks about an issue that will be a source of concern to a number of readers. The account sketched above links causal claims and explanations to the truth of certain interventionist counterfactuals. A common contention is that counterfactuals cannot be "barely true"—instead they require "truth makers" that presumably must be specified in non-counterfactual terms. "Laws" are the usual candidates for such truth makers. For a variety of reasons I am skeptical about this contention, but, as nearly as I can see, nothing will turn in what follows on what we take the truth makers for counterfactuals to be. What matters for the arguments that follow is whether causal claims and explanations are related to interventionist counterfactuals in the way that I have claimed—any account of the truth conditions for counterfactuals that is consistent with these relationships will be acceptable for the purposes of this essay.

That having been said, there is a certain tempting but plainly mistaken inference that we need to be careful to avoid. The inference goes something like this: counterfactuals require laws as truth makers; therefore, any account of causation in terms of counterfactuals is committed to an account according to which all that is involved in one item, property etc. *A* causing or being causally relevant to another *B* is that *A* be linked by law to *B*. In other words, the inference is from the claim that the laws are the truth makers for counterfactuals (and causal claims) to the conclusion that a nomological sufficiency account of causation and causal relevance is adequate.

The problem with this inference is that even if laws are required as truth makers for counterfactuals, this does not settle the question of *which* counterfactuals matter for the characterization of causation and causal relevance—in particular, it does not show that the *only* counterfactual that matters is the counterfactual linking the occurrence of the cause to the occurrence of the effect. The interventionist account of causation claims that for it to be true that (C) *A*s cause *B*s, then (among other things) a counterfactual (F) specifying that *B* would be different or be absent under some intervention that changes *A* or causes it to be absent must be true. The fact—if it is a fact—that there is some law (L) specifying that *A* or *A* in conjunction with other factors *K* is nomologically sufficient for *B*, does not settle the question of whether the counterfactual (F) is true: As described above, (L) is not in itself a truth maker for the counterfactual (F), even though (L) is a truth maker for other counterfactuals that matter for the truth of (C) such as (F*) "If *A* were to occur as a result of an intervention in *K*, then *B* would occur".

Of course if the contention about counterfactuals requiring laws as their truth makers is correct, then (F) will also have some law as its truth maker but this observation does not undermine the claim that (F) and not just (F*) is relevant to the truth of the claim that *As* cause *Bs*.

2.

What are the implications of the framework described in Section 1 for the status of "mental causation"? Prima-facie, it seems to support the claim that mental states can be causes. We do after all seem to regularly (and successfully) intervene to change the mental states of others and perhaps our own mental states as well and these changes in turn sometimes seem to be regularly associated with changes in other mental states and in behavior. Indeed, this seems to be what successful persuasion and deception are all about—in persuasion I manipulate your beliefs and desires by providing you with information or material inducements, typically with the goal in mind that these changes will in turn lead to further changes that I desire in your mental state or behavior. On an interventionist conception of cause, this is all that is required for mental causation—nothing more metaphysically portentous is needed. That is, all that is required for changes in a mental state M_1 to cause changes in a second mental state M_2 (or in behavior B) is that it be true that under some intervention that changes M_1, M_2 (or B) will change. Common sense certainly supposes that episodes like these are very widespread.

Moreover, mental causation in the interventionist sense doesn't seem confined to such contexts. Many experiments in psychology and the social sciences are naturally regarded as involving, among other things, successful attempts by the experimenters to manipulate subject's beliefs by giving them verbal instructions (about e.g., what the experimental task is, what they will be rewarded for doing etc.), where the goal of the experiment is to discover how these changes are systematically associated with changes in subjects' behavior. Similarly, it is very natural to interpret many experiments (in, e.g. social psychology and experimental economics) involving *interactions* between people as investigations of, among other things, how changes in subject's beliefs about one another's beliefs and desires cause changes in behavior. For example, changes in my beliefs about how likely you are to cooperate in an iterated prisoner's dilemma or trust game will cause changes in my behavior toward you, changes in responder's beliefs about the alternatives available to the proposer in an ultimatum game will cause changes in the probability of responder rejecting the proposer's offer and so on. Even experimental demonstrations that show that certain beliefs do not, contrary to what subjects and others expect, causally influence subject's behavior (as with experiments that show a position effect in the choice among identical consumer items and that subsequent reason giving is confabulation) seem to require some conception of what would be evidence for a causal influence of belief on behavior—it is the failure to find such evidence that shows the belief to have no causal influence. There would be no point in performing the experiment if beliefs could never, as a matter of principle, causally influence behavior.

3.

Although the notion of mental causation thus seems, at least on the surface, unproblematic from an interventionist perspective, the philosophical literature is full of arguments to the contrary—arguments that purport to show that mental states or properties cannot (ever) cause other mental states or behavior. In what follows I want to explore some of these arguments. I will begin at a relatively general and intuitive level and then consider some more precise arguments.

One motivation for skepticism about assigning any causal role to the mental derives from the assumption that mental states are "multiply realizable"[4] by different neural or physical states, combined with the thought that there is a general preference for detailed or fine-grained or more micro level causal claims/explanations (in this case claims at some physical or neural level) over less fine-grained, more macro (e.g mental or psychological) claims. Suppose that my intention I to reach for a grape on some particular occasion is followed by my reaching for that grape. (Call this behavior R.) Assume (as is standard) that I has neural/physical "realization" N_1 (on this particular occasion), but that this same type of intention I might also have had a number of other possible realizations N_2, N_3,. . . etc. where the description of each of these realizations contains a great deal more fine-grained detailed information than the description that just adverts to I. If, furthermore, N_1 is by itself (nomologically) sufficient for the occurrence of R, given the rest of the condition of my brain, why isn't it at least preferable and perhaps mandatory to think of N_1 as causing or causally explaining R? And once we do this, what causal or explanatory role can I play?

To explore the cogency of this reasoning, let us consider some other examples involving a choice between more or less fine-grained causal information.

[4] The thesis that mental states are (or can be) multiply realized by different neural states is received wisdom in philosophy of mind and in part just for ease of exposition I will adopt this terminology in what follows. It is important to emphasize, however, that this thesis is unclear in a number of crucial respects, as recent discussion (e.g., Shapiro, 2000) has emphasized. I will also add that although it is often claimed that if mental states are multiply realizable, then this rules out the possibility of any theory according to which types of mental states or mental properties are identical with types of physical states or properties, this is simply a non-sequitur. As emphasized below, there is nothing in the idea of multiple realizability per se that rules out the possibility that all of the different realizers share some common physical structure at an abstract level of description. For example, different realizations of the same intention may share some aggregate feature that is a function of firing rates exhibited by a group of neurons, just as the same temperature may be realized by a variety of molecular configurations, all of which possess the same average kinetic energy. To the extent this is so, it may (depending on the details of the case) be legitimate to identify the upper level property (intention, temperature, etc.) with this abstract physical property.

3.1) Suppose that a mole of ideal gas at temperature T_1 and pressure P_1 at time t_1 is confined to a container of fixed volume V. The temperature of the gas is then increased to T_2 by the application of a heat source and the gas is allowed to reach a new equilibrium at time t_2 where its pressure is found to have increased to P_2. One strategy (the *macroscopic* strategy) for explaining (or exhibiting the causes of) the new pressure is to appeal to the ideal gas law $PV = nRT$ which describes the relationship between the macroscopic variables pressure, temperature and volume. According to this law, when the temperature is increased to T_2 and the volume remains fixed, the new pressure at equilibrium must increase to $P_2 = nRT_2/V$.

Now contrast this with the following (entirely impractical) *microscopic* strategy for explaining the behavior of the gas: one notes the exact position and momentum of each of the 6×10^{23} molecules making up the gas. Call this configuration G_1. From G_1, the details of how the temperature source contributes to the kinetic energy of each of the individual molecules and knowledge of the exact laws governing the interactions between each of these molecules, one traces the trajectory of each gas molecule through time, eventually ending up with the exact position and momentum of each molecule making up the gas at time t_2. This molecular configuration, G_2, communicates a net force per unit area to the surface of the container which is just the new pressure P_2.

This microscopic strategy is obviously impossible to carry out: among other difficulties, we cannot determine the positions and momentum of the individual molecules with the required exactness and the 6×10^{23} body problem of their interaction is of course computationally intractable. But the inadequacies of this strategy do not just have to do with our epistemic limitations. There is a more fundamental difficulty: while the strategy succeeds in tracing the particular trajectories of individual molecules that in fact led on this particular occasion to the macroscopic outcome P_2, it omits important causally relevant information: that there are a very large number of *other* molecular trajectories, compatible with the macroscopic conditions satisfied by the gas (its temperature, volume, and pressure at t_1 and its new temperature at t_2) that would lead to the same macroscopic outcome—that is, the new pressure P_2. In fact, one may show that for all except a very small set of initial conditions (a set of measure zero) for the molecules of the gas that satisfy these macroscopic conditions, the trajectories of the individual molecules will be such that the gas will exert pressure P_2 at t_2. There is thus an important respect in which the micro-explanation is overly specific, given that what we want to explain is why the gas ends up exerting pressure P_2 rather than some alternative pressure P_3. Just giving the micro-explanation, without further elucidation, doesn't convey the information that almost all trajectories compatible with the initial conditions to which the gas is subject would have produced the same result. Indeed, on one natural interpretation, the micro-explanation misleadingly suggests that the fact that the gas ends up exerting pressure P_2 depends in some way on the particular set of molecular trajectories and collisions leading from G_1 to G_2 that actually occurred and this of course is false. By contrast, the macroscopic strategy does not have this limitation. From the point of view of this paper little turns on whether we regard the claim that the new pressure is caused by the evolution from G_1 to G_2 as false, or as true but misleading (or defective from the point of view of explanation) in some way. What matters is that the macroscopic strategy conveys causally relevant information that is omitted by the microscopic strategy.

We can express these observations in terms of the ideas about contrastive focus and role of tracing dependency relationships in causal explanation described in Section 1. When one asks for a causal explanation of why the gas is in some macroscopic state—e.g. that of exerting pressure P_2, this is most naturally understood as a request for an explanation of why the gas is in that macroscopic state rather than other alternative *macroscopic* states—why it has pressure P_2 rather than some alternative pressure(s) P_i different from P_2. The microscopic explanation simply doesn't answer this question, since as stated it tells us nothing about the conditions under which such a macroscopic alternative to P_2 would have occurred. By contrast the macroscopic explanation that appeals to the macroscopic state of the gas and the ideal gas law does provide such information, since it allows us to see that if, for example, the new temperature of the gas had been T_3 rather than T_2, the gas would have evolved to new pressure $P_3 = nRT_3/V$. This is not to say that the micro-explanation is entirely unexplanatory—for example, if for some reason we were interested in explaining why the gas ends up at the new equilibrium in the exact molecular configuration G_2 rather than the alternative exact molecular configuration G_3, the exact configuration of the molecules at their starting point G_1 and the details of their subsequent evolution would be highly relevant. But most often, this is not what we are interested in. In the more usual case, where the intended explanandum involves a macro-contrast, the more fine-grained and microscopic explanation is not automatically better.

We can also relate these points directly to some of the foundational issues in the theory of explanation canvassed above. If we hold that to explain an outcome is simply to provide a nomologically sufficient condition for its occurrence, then it will be natural to conclude that the micro-explanation provides a fully satisfactory explanation for why the gas exerts pressure P_2, for this explanation certainly provides a nomologically sufficient condition for this explanandum. Suppose, however, that one holds instead, as suggested in Section 1, that something more or different is required of a good causal explanation—that it answer a what-if-things-had-been-different question or identify conditions such that under changes in those conditions some alternative to the explanandum would be realized and that more generally causal explanation is a matter of tracing dependency relationships and accounting for contrasts. Then, assuming that the explanandum in which we are interested is why the gas exerts pressure P_2, the micro-explanation leaves out something of importance that is provided by a more macroscopic explanation. In other words, under the right conditions, the interventionist conception favors causal claims and explanations involving more macroscopic variables. This suggests that to the extent that the relationship between some candidate mental cause claim (e.g. that *I* causes *R* in the example above) and the underlying physical/neural physiological realizations of the candidate cause (N_1) and its effect are like the relationship between on the one hand, pressure, volume, and temperature, and, on the other hand, some particular molecular configuration that realizes these variables, the upper level, mental cause claim may be preferable to the claim framed in terms of its neuro-physiological realization N_1. More weakly, it seems plainly wrong-headed to think that the microscopic causal claims that appeal to the exact molecular configuration in the case of the gas or to the details of the neuro-physiological realization N_1 somehow compete with the more macroscopic causal claims and "exclude" these in the sense of showing them to be false. I will return to this idea below.

3.2) To further explore this point, consider the following example, derived from Yablo (1992). A pigeon has been trained to peck at a target when and only when presented with a red stimulus (that is a stimulus of any shade of red). Suppose that on a series of occasions the pigeon is presented with a stimulus that is a particular shade of scarlet and in each case pecks at the target. Consider the following two causal claims/causal explanations:

(3.2.1) The presentation of scarlet targets causes the pigeon to peck
(3.2.2) The presentation of red targets causes the pigeon to peck.

If we adhere to the characterization in **M**, then both (3.2.1) and (3.2.2) are true, since in both cases there is an intervention (namely one that changes the color of the target from scarlet to a non-red color) that will change whether the pigeon pecks. Nonetheless, as Yablo argues, there is an obvious sense in which (3.2.1), like the micro-explanation of the behavior of the ideal gas, seems inappropriately specific or insufficiently general, in comparison with (3.2.2). Or at least, to make a much weaker claim, it does not seem plausible that (3.2.1) should be judged superior to (3.2.2) just on the grounds of its greater specificity. Even if we accept (3.2.1) as a true causal claim, it seems misguided to regard it as in competition with (3.2.2) in the sense that acceptance of the former requires us to regard the latter as false. The basis for these assessments again falls naturally out of the interventionist account of causation and explanation described above. What we are usually interested in when we ask for a causal explanation or cause of the pigeon's pecking is something that accounts for why it pecks rather than alternatively not pecking at all. There is relevant information about the conditions under which both pecking and not pecking will occur that is conveyed by (3.2.2) but not by (3.2.1) when both are given their natural default reading. The default reading of (3.2.2) with its contrastive focus made explicit is:

(3.2.2*) The contrast between the targets being red rather than not red causes the contrast between the pigeon's pecking rather than not pecking.

(3.2.2*) thus tells us for example, that if the target had been some other shade of red besides scarlet the pigeon still would have pecked and that for the pigeon not to peck we must produce a target that is not red at all. By contrast, the default reading of (3.2.1) is:

(3.2.1*) The contrast between the targets being scarlet rather than not scarlet causes the contrast between the pigeon's pecking rather than not pecking.

In my idiolect, it is most natural to interpret (3.2.1/3.2.1*) as claiming that the pigeon will not peck if the target is not scarlet (but still red). On this interpretation, (3.2.1) is false. Even if we find this default interpretation uncharitable, it remains true that (3.2.1) tells us less than we would like to know about the full range of conditions under which the pigeon will peck or not peck.[5] It is again true that, under the imagined conditions, the presentation of the scarlet target is nomologically sufficient (given the way that the philosophy of mind literature understands the notion of "law") for the pigeon to peck, but this just illustrates the point that there seems more to successful explanation or informative casual claims than the provision of nomologically sufficient conditions.

It is also worth noting the obvious point that under a different experimental set-up in which the pigeon was instead trained to peck only in response to the target's being scarlet, these assessments would be reversed. This again underscores the point that on their most natural interpretation (3.2.1) and (3.2.2) have different implications about the manipulability relationships or the patterns of counterfactual dependency that hold in the situation of interest: (3.2.1) claims that we can manipulate whether the pigeon pecks by changing the target from red to not-red, while (3.2.2) claims that merely changing whether the target is scarlet will do this. If this is correct, there can be no general preference for (3.2.2) over (3.2.1) simply on grounds of its greater specificity—the appropriateness of each will depend on such facts as whether the pigeon pecks in response to non-scarlet shades of red.

3.3) Finally, suppose (cf. Jackson and Pettit, 2004, p. 172) that John coughs just as the conductor is about to begin his performance and the conductor becomes irritated.

Consider the following two claims

(3.3.1) John's coughing caused/causally explains the conductor's becoming irritated

(3.3.2) Someone's coughing caused/causally explains the conductor's becoming irritated.

[5] In part for this reason, I don't find it useful to worry, as many commentators do, about whether, within a Lewis-style semantics, the "closest" possible world in which the target is not scarlet is one in which it is or is not red. First, the claim that the non-red world is closest seems unmotivated, given Lewis's official similarity metric. More fundamentally, even if we interpret (3.2.1) according to this standard of closeness, it still is defective in comparison with (3.2.2) in failing to convey the information that the pigeon would peck if the target was non-scarlet but red.

A general preference for more detailed causal claims/explanations suggests that (3.3.1) is automatically preferable to (3.3.2). Again, however, it is natural to associate these with different contrastive claims. (3.3.1) naturally suggests that the conductor's irritation is specifically the result of *John's* coughing: that the contrast between the actual situation in which John coughs and an alternative in which someone else coughs is responsible for the conductor's irritation. (Imagine that the conductor is generally unflappable and undisturbed by coughing but has a particular animus toward John, who he correctly believes is trying to disrupt his performance.) That is, the conductor would not have become irritated if anyone else had coughed. By contrast, (3.3.2) does suggest that the conductor would have become irritated as long as there was coughing by anyone. Which of these claims is correct obviously depends on the empirical facts of the situation—again there are no grounds for supposing that the more specific (3.3.1) is automatically preferable on *apriori* grounds to the less specific (3.3.2).

At a number of points above I have framed my contentions about the superiority of the less specific causal claims in terms of their providing better (causal) explanations, since this seems to me to be the most natural way of putting matters. But while my argument involves an appeal to what is sometimes called "explanatory practice" (Robb and Heil, 2007), let me re-iterate that the notion of explanation to which I am appealing requires the *truth* of the causal claims that figure in those explanations. That is, my contention throughout is that the less specific causal claims are true (if they were not, we could not appeal to them to explain) and that regardless of what we may think about the truth of the more specific claims, they at least don't exclude the truth of the less specific claims. Thus, on my view, someone who accepts that it is correct to appeal to (3.2.2) to causally explain the pigeon's pecking cannot at the same time hold that (3.2.2) is false or that its truth is excluded by the truth of (3.2.1).

What do these examples have to do with mental causation? My completely unoriginal suggestion is that claims about mental or psychological causation will be true when the relationship between mental states and their underlying realizations are relevantly like the relationships between the more macro or less specific causal claims and their underlying, more specific realizations in the examples described above.[6]

[6] Stephen Yablo (1992) holds that the relationship between mental states and their neural realizations is just the relationship between determinables and their determinates—that is, it is just like the relationship between red and scarlet. Peter Menzies (Chapter 11 in this volume), following Funkhouser, 2006 rejects this claim. My use of Yablo's example in 3.2 is not meant to endorse his general claim that the relationship between the mental and the physical is the relationship between determinable and determinate. This example as well as the others above are just meant to illustrate a range of cases in which causal claims that are less specific and which omit detail are not automatically excluded by or ruled out by other more specific causal claims and to motivate the contention that same may be true of causal claims about the mental. My assumption is that there are many different kinds of cases in which more specific causes fail to exclude less specific causes, some but not all of which are naturally conceptualized in terms of the relationship between determinables and

As a simple illustration, consider some research concerning the neural coding of intention to reach carried out by Richard Andersen and colleagues at Caltech (Musallam et al., 2004). These researchers recorded from individual neurons using arrays of electrodes implanted in the PRR (parietal reach region) of the posterior parietal cortex in macaque monkeys. Previous research had suggested that this region encodes what Musallam et al. call intentions to reach for specific target—that is higher order plans or goals to reach toward one target or goal rather than another (e.g. an apple at a specific location rather than an orange at some other location) rather than more specific instructions concerning the exact limb trajectory to be followed in reaching toward the target—the latter information being represented elsewhere in motor areas.

Andersen was able to develop a program which systematically related variations in aggregate features of the recorded signals to variations in intentions to reach for specific goals, as revealed in reaching movements and which indeed allowed for accurate forecasting of reaching behavior from these signals. His eventual hope is that paralysed subjects will be able to control the goals toward which prosthetic limbs are directed by forming different intentions, which would then be decoded, the resulting neural signals directing the limb. From an interventionist perspective, this is about as clear a case of mental causation as one could imagine, since the subject uses the formation of one intention rather than another to manipulate the position of the limb.

The signals that are recorded (and which do seem to encode different intentions up to some reasonable degree of resolution) are an aggregate of the firing rates (spikes/second) over a temporal period from a number of individual neurons. Like all accounts of neural coding, this inevitably involves discarding or abstracting away from various features of the behavior of individual neurons. In particular, since it is the aggregate behavior of a large group of neurons that is taken to encode differences in intention, there will be some individual variation in neuronal behavior that is consistent with relevant sameness of the aggregate profile. Moreover, the assumption, shared with most accounts of neural coding, that the crucial variable is firing rate implies that variations in the behavior of neurons that are consistent with their having the same firing rate, such as variations in the temporal course of their firing, will be irrelevant to which intention is represented. The picture that emerges is thus that there is some range of variation in the behavior of individual neurons which is consistent with the holding of the same intention, while some other range of variation in the behavior of individual neurons (associated with a different aggregate firing rate) will be associated with a different intention. In this sense the same intention may be multiply realized in somewhat different patterns of neuronal activity.

determinates. For example, the relationship between the average value of a quantity and the particular realizations of that quantity is also arguably not the relationship between a determinable and a determinate (at least according to the Menzies/Funkhouser account of what that relationship is).

Suppose then that on some specific occasion t a monkey forms an intention I_1 to reach for a particular goal—call this action R_1. Suppose N_{11} is the particular (token) pattern of firing in the relevant set of neurons that realizes or encodes the intention I_1 on this particular occasion. Assume also that there are other token patterns of neural firing, N_{12}, N_{13} that realize the same intention I_1 on other occasions, so that I_1 is multiply realized by N_{11}, N_{12}, etc. The preference for micro or fine-grained causation that we are considering recommends that we should regard N_{11} as the real cause of R_1 on occasion t. But this seems wrong for the same reason that it seems wrong to say that it is the scarlet color of the target that causes the pigeon to peck in circumstances in which the pigeon will peck at any red target and wrong to say that it is the specific molecular configuration G_1 rather than the fact that the temperature of the gas has been increased to T_2 which is responsible for its new pressure P_2. Just as with these two examples, the causal claim/causal explanation that appeals to N_{11} to explain R_1 seems overly specific. It fails to convey a relevant pattern of dependence: that there are some alternatives to N_{11} (namely, N_{12} and N_{13}) that would have led to the same reaching behavior R_1 and other alternatives (those that realize some different intention I_2, associated with reaching for a different goal) that would not have led to R_1. Put slightly differently, Andersen's concern in this example is in finding the cause of variations in reach toward different goal objects—why the monkey exhibits reaching behavior R_1 rather than different reaching behavior R_2. According to the interventionist account, to do this, he needs to identify states or conditions, variations in which, when produced by interventions, would be correlated with changes from R_1 to R_2. Ex hypothesi, merely citing N_{11} does not accomplish this, since it tells us nothing about the conditions under which alternatives to R_1 would be realized. By way of contrast, appealing to the fact that the monkey's intention is I_1 rather than some alternative intention I_2 does accomplish this, assuming (as we have been all along) that there is a stable relationship between the occurrence of I_1 (however realized) and R_1 and that under I_2 some alternative to R_1 (reaching toward a different goal) would have occurred.

Note that there is nothing about this argument that relies on the specifically *mental* (however this is understood) character of I_1 in establishing its explanatory credentials with respect to R_1. The argument would proceed in the same way if we instead appealed to neural or physically characterized facts about the aggregate profile—call this A_1—of the firing rates that realize or correspond to I_1. In other words, insofar as this aggregate profile A_1 corresponds to the different ways N_{11}, N_{12}, N_{13} of realizing I_1, and A_1 leads to R_1 and A_1 contrasts with whatever aggregate profile of neural activity A_2 corresponds to the different intention I_2, it will be equally appropriate to cite A_1 as causing or figuring in the causal explanation for the monkey's exhibiting R_1.

This of course raises the question of how we should conceive of the relationship between I_1 and A_1—are these identical or do they bear some other relationship to one another? We will explore some aspects of this issue in Section 6 below. Here I confine myself to the following observation: insofar as A_1 and I_1 enter into exactly the same manipulability or dependency relationships with respect to R_1, it is natural (from an interventionist point of view) to think of them as involving the same rather than competing causal claims with respect to R_1. That is, for it to be the case that the claim that (3.4) I_1 causes R_1 and the claim that (3.5) A_1 causes R_1 to be competing claims about the causes of R_1 (in the sense that at best one of (3.4–3.5) can be correct) it must be the case that they make inconsistent predictions about what would happen to R_1 under some possible set of interventions.[7] Prima facie, at least, (3.4) and (3.5) do not do this. If this appearance is correct, they are not competing causal claims in any sense that requires us to choose between them. Hence, whatever view we take about the relationship between I_1 and A_1 must be consistent with this fact.

4.

In this section I want to add some clarifications to the argument in Section 3 and also to place the argument in a more general context. First, some philosophers[8] have argued, with respect to set-ups of the sort under discussion, as follows: (4.1) If the realizer N_{11} of I_1 that actually occurred had not occurred, then some other alternative realizer of I_1—say N_{12}—would have occurred instead and would have caused R_1. They take this to support the claim that I_1 causes (or at least plays some causal role in the occurrence of) R_1. This is *not* the argument made above and I see no reason to accept the counterfactual (4.1).[9] The argument

[7] We should of course distinguish between the question of whether two causal claims are inconsistent and whether they are different—the latter requires only that they make different claims about what happens under some interventions. It is not clear, however, that (3.4) and (3.5) are different in this sense.

[8] See Lepore and Loewer, 1987. A somewhat similar argument seems to be suggested in Yablo, 1992, as Bennett, 2003 notes, and it may be that Jackson and Pettit have something similar in mind when they speak of a higher level property "programming" for its realizer—if one realizer does not occur, the "program" ensures that another will. The argument may seem particularly natural within Lewis's framework : it may seem tempting to argue that if N_{11} actually occurs, then among those worlds in which N_{11} does not occur, those in which some alternative realizer of I_1 occurs are closer to the actual world then those in which the neural realizer of some different intention from I_1 occurs. I take no stand on whether Lewis's theory licenses this sort of inference but a little thought will show that making it leads one into difficulties.

[9] Within an interventionist framework, the above argument (and (4.1)) would only be correct if some back-up mechanism were in place that somehow ensured that if N_{11} is not realized, some specific alternative to N_{11} (like N_{12}) that leads to R would occur instead, and that it is not the case that some different alternative N_{21} that does not lead to R would occur. In other words, it is assumed that the causal structure is like one in which a rifleman shoots a victim but if he hadn't, a second, back-up rifleman would have done so. (The analogue to (4.1) would be true in such a case.) But no such back-up mechanism is stipulated to be present in the original example involving (4.1). Moreover if such a mechanism were present, then it *would* be appropriate to cite the first rifleman's shot (and by analogy N_{11}) as causing R_1 which is just the result proponents of this argument want to avoid.

that I give above is that we can conclude that I_1 causes R_1 because of the truth of various interventionist counterfactuals linking the occurrence of I_1 to R_1 and the occurrence of alternatives to I_1 to alternatives to R_1. This argument does not depend upon any claims about what would have happened if N_{11} had not occurred, although it does of course depend on claims about what would have happened if I_1 had not occurred.

Next some remarks about the role played by considerations having to do with supervenience and multiple realizability in the arguments just described: in the examples considered in Section 3, upper level properties that are causally relevant to other level properties supervene on and are multiply realized by lower level properties. It is important to realize, however, that what establishes a role for the upper level property—again let's call it M_1—in the causation of a second upper level property M_2 is not just the multiple realizability of M_1 and M_2 per se (and not even the conjunction of multiple realizability with the existence of laws that in some way link realizers of M_1 to realizers of M_2). Instead, what is required is the combination of the right sort of multiple realizability with the existence of a relationship between M_1 and M_2 such that different values of M_1 are systematically associated with different values of M_2 and where this relationship is stable or invariant under some range of variations in different lower level realizations of those properties, when these are produced by interventions. In other words, what is required is the existence of a relationship that both involves a dependency between the upper level variables (different values of M_1, produced by interventions map into different values of M_2) and that is realization independent in the sense that it continues to stably hold for a range of different realizers of these values of M_1 and M_2. It is the presence of this sort of *realization independent dependency relationship* (hereafter *RIDR*) that ensures that interventions that change M_1 are stably associated with changes in M_2—hence that M_1 causes M_2.[10]

[10] The claim that such a *RIDR* exists is thus importantly different from (and stronger than) the usual claims about "multiple realizability" in the philosophy of mind literature. Consider the gas law $PV = nRT$ which is *RIDR* involving temperature, pressure and volume that holds for a ideal gas. In this case, there is a range of variation in the microstates compatible with, say, the temperature having the value it does such that the gas law holds for almost all of these. Further, the variations in question actually do occur—indeed, they are equally likely to occur—and the gas behaves in the same way regardless of which variant is realized. The "multiple realizability" emphasized in the philosophy of mind literature is different in that (i) the focus is just on logical rather than real causal possibility (the generalizations of common sense psychology are multiply realizable because it is logically possible they might be realized in silicon or in the minds of extra-terrestrials but of course there is no evidence that they are so realized) and (ii) often at least, there is no serious attempt made to argue that in humans, these generalizations would continue to hold in some range of actual or realistically possible variations in or perturbations of neural organization. In other words, it is compatible with the philosophy of mind conception of multiple realizability that the same psychological generalizations might be multiply realizabile in humans and extra-terrestrials but highly sensitive to the precise details of realization in both—if you change or perturb the realizers even a little bit, the generalizations will no longer hold. The gas law is not like this.

To illustrate the significance of this point consider the following example. An ordinary, fair roulette wheel (the operation of which is deterministic at a micro level) is spun by a croupier C. C has a set of possible hand movements B_i for putting the wheel in motion—he can start the wheel at one of a number of positions and he can spin the wheel with more or less force or momentum. Even if the B_i are finely grained from a macroscopic point of view (e.g. they correspond to the maximally fine movements that C can distinguish or control), each B_i will be multiply realized by a range of different exact positions and momenta for the wheel. Similarly, whether the ball ends up in a red or black slot will be multiply realized.

If the wheel is fair, C will be unable to control or manipulate, by employing one set of hand movements B_j rather than another set B_k, whether the ball will land in a red slot or a black slot—indeed he will be unable to even influence the probability of this happening. For all the different possible B_i, the probability of red will be the same—one half. Consider those occasions on which C pushes the wheel with the specific motion B_k and on which the ball ends in a red slot R. On each of these occasions B_k and R presumably will have different micro-realizations and, moreover, for each such micro-realization of B_k, there will be a law linking it to the micro-realization of R that occurs. (Remember this is a deterministic system.) However, within an interventionist framework, it is *not* true that

(4.2) Imposing motion B_k on the wheel causes the ball to fall in a red slot.

The reason for this is two-fold. First, there are no stable upper level relationships of the form

(4.3) If C pushes the wheel with motion B_i, the ball will land in a red slot.

Instead, when C employs B_i, (for any value of i) whether the ball ends up in a red or black slot depends on the specific micro-realization of B_i that is imposed: generalizations of form (4.3) are not realization independent. Second, there *are* stable generalizations of the form

(4.4) If C pushes the wheel with motion B_i, the probability the ball will land in a red slot is p.

That is, motions of type B_i do endow the ball with a stable probability of landing in the red slot. However, all alternative possible motions also endow the ball with the same probability of landing in red—thus, there are no interventions on the B_i that make a difference for where the ball ends up or for the probability of where it ends up. In other words, the relationship between C's behavior and the final position of the ball is not what we called a *RIDR*, and this is so despite the fact that both of these are "multiply realized". The reason for this has to do with the character of the underlying physics governing the wheel—what matters is not just the existence of some set of deterministic laws linking the initial conditions of the wheel to the outcome but rather very specific features of these laws and how they relate to the macroscopic predicates used to characterize the behavior of the wheel.[11]

In each of the examples considered in Section 3, we in effect assumed that we were dealing with systems that (with respect to the relationships of interest) did not behave like the roulette wheel. For example, in the case of the gas, we assumed *both* that all (or more strictly virtually all) of the different microstates that realize the same temperature T_2 will have the same stable effect on other macroscopic variables like the new pressure measurement P_2 *and* that there are alternatives to T_2—e.g., alternative temperature T_3 such that all the different micro-realizations of T_3 lead to different pressure measurements P_3. (In fact, both these claims are roughly true, as an empirical matter, and statistical mechanics gives us some insight into why they are true.) Similarly, in the discussion of Andersen's research, we assumed that all of the different possible neural realizations of the intention I_1 led stably (assuming the right background circumstances) to the same behavior R_1, and that the neural realizations of the appropriately different intention I_2 would lead to different behavior R_2.

As we have seen, discussions of the causal role of mental and other upper level properties have tended to focus on whether it follows just from considerations having to do with multiple realizability (and the absence of type identities) that such properties are causally inert. I have argued that this conclusion does not follow. However, undercutting this conclusion certainly does not by itself vindicate claims about the causal efficacy of upper level properties, including mental properties. We also need to ask, in connection with each upper level causal claim, whether the additional requirements embodied in *RIDR* are likely to be satisfied. This is a non-trivial empirical question that must be answered on a case by case basis: it is certainly not obvious that the answer to this question is "yes" for many claims of mental causation. I will return briefly to this issue in Section 7 below.

Finally, the general form of the solution described in Section 3 to the problem of how mental properties can play a causal role is not original with me. Broadly similar proposals have been advanced by Yablo (1992) and by Jackson and Pettit (2004*b*), among others. Yablo describes his proposal in terms of the requirement that causes fit with or be "proportional" to their effects—that they be just "enough" for their effects, neither omitting too much relevant

[11] Very roughly, the dynamics of this system are such that it exhibits extremely sensitive dependence on initial conditions—initial states of the position and momentum of the wheel that are very, very close to each other map onto to very different final positions of the ball (whether it ends up in a red or black slot) and moreover, for an appropriately chosen partition of the phase space into small contiguous regions, the volume of the regions that are mapped into each of these outcomes is equal or approximately so within each cell of the partition. Thus for any distribution of initial conditions that C is able to impose—any choice of B_i—there will be a probability for red equal to one half in repeated trials.

detail nor containing too much irrelevant detail. In this terminology, I_1 fits with (or is proportional to) R_1 in a way that N_{11} does (is) not, since the latter involves too much irrelevant detail. However, Yablo's treatment relies heavily on essentialist metaphysics in explaining what is involved in a cause being proportional to its effect. I think that this essentialist metaphysics is not necessary and that the intuition behind the requirement of proportionality need only appeal to the considerations invoked in Section 1—an interventionist account of causation, contrastive focus and so on. Roughly speaking, a cause variable will be "proportional" to an effect variable when the pattern of dependence of all alternative possible states of the effect on alternative possible states of the cause is exhibited and there are no additional "irrelevant distinctions" among alternative states of the cause variable—irrelevant in the sense that these alternatives are not associated with differences in the effect variable.[12]

Jackson and Pettit's discussion of mental causation in their (2004*b*) is organized around their account of "program explanation" and an associated notion of causal relevance (which they also associate with "instrumental effectiveness"—see below). A mental state such as the belief that p is causally relevant to some effect A if "variations in how [this mental state] is realized remains consistent with invariance in the appearance of the effect [A, of this mental state]" (2004, p. 2). If we interpret this characterization of what it is for a mental state to cause or be causally relevant to an outcome along interventionist, *RIDR* lines (that is, that different interventions on the same mental state that involve different realizers of this state lead to the same effect and that the realizations of different mental states, also produced by interventions, lead to different effects), then the characterization will be essentially the same as (or at least very close to) the characterization offered above. However, Jackson and Pettit also distinguish sharply between causal relevance and what they call *causal efficacy* where "a casually efficacious property with regard to an effect is a property in virtue of whose instantiation, at least in part, the effect occurs". They associate causal efficacy with the notion of causal "production" and suggest that "relations of causal efficacy" may be "restricted to certain properties of fundamental physics" (2004*b*, p. 61) and perhaps that "causal efficacy is a relation between forces" (2004*b*, p. 61 n. 25). Causal relevance is thus a broader notion than causal efficacy: causally efficacious properties are causally relevant but a property can be causally relevant or instrumentally effective without being efficacious. According to Jackson and Pettit, this is true of mental states; they are causally relevant to behavior but not in themselves causally efficacious in producing behavior. Instead

[12] For additional discussion of Yablo's proportionality constraint, see Menzies (Chapter 11 in this volume). Reformulating the idea along the grounds I suggest also has the advantage that it would not be so closely tied to the details of Yablo's treatment of the determinable–determinate relationship. Added in proof: Philip Pettit has also drawn my attention to Jackson's and his (2004*a*) in which less emphasis is placed on the notion of causal efficacy and more on the idea that mental states are causally relevant to behavior in virtue of programming for causally efficacious states.

it is the particular physical realization of the mental state on a given occasion which is causally efficacious in producing behavior. They write:

no matter how the notion of causal efficacy is understood, it is distinct from the notion of instrumental effectiveness. A property will count as instrumentally effective *vis-à-vis* a particular effect, if it would have been a good tactic for producing the effect to realize that property. But such effectiveness does not entail efficacy: it does not mean that the effect occurred in virtue of the instantiation of the property. (2004, p. 120)

Jackson and Pettit suggest that mental states like beliefs do not themselves produce behavior but instead "program" for the production of behavior in the sense that they "(non causally) ensure that no matter how it is realized, things will be arranged at the neural and more basic levels, so that behavior is more or less reliably bound to appear" (2004, p. 2).

This distinction between causal efficacy and relevance and the associated idea that explanations that appeal to beliefs provide only information about relevance but not efficacy relations provides a natural opening for critics such as Kim, 1998. Kim claims that a true vindication of the causal status of the mental requires showing that mental states are causally efficacious rather than merely causally relevant; since Pettit and Jackson concede that on their approach mental states are not causally efficacious in producing behavior, they are, according to Kim, really epiphenomenalists about the mental (Kim, 1998, p. 75).

Many other philosophers similarly distinguish between causal relevance and what they suppose to be a stronger notion of causal efficacy (although with a different understanding of the latter notion than Jackson and Pettit), and also contend, like Kim, that showing that mental states are causes requires showing that they are causally efficacious in this stronger sense rather than merely causal relevant to their effects. Often (and confusingly[13]), however, what is meant by "efficacy" seems to amount simply to nomological sufficiency: *a*'s being *F* is causally efficacious in making it the case that *b* is *G* if and only if *a*'s possession of *F* is nomologically sufficient for *b*'s possession of *G*. Consider the following view, which Robb and Heil, 2007 ascribe to Jerry Fodor:

On Fodor's view, mental properties can be relevant to behavior in a stronger sense [than the sense captured by counterfactual accounts of causal relevance, like the interventionist account], a sense in which they are *sufficient* for their effects and in this way "make a difference". Fodor spells out this sufficiency in terms of laws: a property makes a difference if "it's a property in virtue of the instantiation of which the occurrence of one event is nomologically sufficient for the occurrence of another".

There is of course nothing to prevent someone from introducing "causal efficacy" as a technical term which is simply defined or stipulated to be identical

[13] Confusingly, because on this understanding of causal efficacy, it is not a (logically) stronger notion than causal relevance (when this is understood along interventionist lines) since a condition can be causally efficacious for an outcome without being causally relevant to it—see below.

with nomological sufficiency. However, we need to realize that this notion is very far removed from the various notions of causation or causal explanation that are commonly used in either ordinary life or in science. Instead, the commonly used causal notions all embody in some way or other the requirement that causes must be relevant (where relevance is understood along the interventionist or counterfactual lines described above) to their effects. (This is reflected in our reluctance to accept the judgment that the fact that hexing salt is causally efficacious in producing dissolution in water despite the fact that the former is nomologically sufficient for the latter.) Moreover, contrary to the view that Robb and Heil attribute to Fodor, it is wrong to equate the idea of a cause's making a difference to its effect with the idea that the cause is nomologically sufficient for the effect. The claim that a cause "makes a difference" to an effect requires that some claim be true about how the effect would be absent or different if the cause were absent or different—the whole idea of a cause as a difference-maker must embody some idea about the cause being one way rather than another making a difference to the effect. The idea of nomological sufficiency says nothing about this: it is a claim about what would happen if the cause were present but says nothing about what would happen if the cause were absent or different. Nothing in the idea of nomological sufficiency taken in itself requires that causes be difference-makers (this is the point of the Salmon counterexamples to the *DN* model discussed in Section 3) and to the extent that difference-making is crucial to the notion of causation, causal efficacy (understood as nomological sufficiency) seems to leave out something central to any legitimate notion of causation. Moreover, it isn't, as it were, just a linguistic or conceptual accident that our current notion(s) of cause is (are) tied in this way to the requirement that causes should be difference-makers or relevant to their effects in what Robb and Heil call the counterfactual sense—there are good reasons related to the goals of inquiry for this requirement.

One way of bringing out this last point is to consider what research like that conducted by Musallam et al. would look like if its focus or goal were simply the identification of conditions that are causally efficacious (in the sense of nomological sufficiency) in the production of reaching behavior. If this were the goal, it would be acceptable to cite the entire state of the whole brain (or any part of it that includes the PRR as a proper part) during the time immediately preceding the behavior of interest, for this will assuredly be a nomologically sufficient condition for the behavior, if anything is. Of course, neither Andersen nor any other neuroscientist does this. Andersen's goal, as he puts it, is to identify "intention specific" neurons—that is to identify the specific neurons variations in the state of which correlate with the monkey's intentions and which hence are responsible for or make a difference for the monkey's behavior. Then, among these neurons he wants to identify those specific features of their behavior (whether this has to do with some aggregate function of spike rate or whatever) which encode different intentions. Other states of the monkey's brain in, e.g. occipital cortex that don't covary with changes in the monkey's intentions are irrelevant to this task and hence are ignored. This concern with neural specificity falls naturally out of a concern with causal relevance or difference-making but is lost if we focus just on the identification of nomologically sufficient conditions for behavior.

It seems clear that part of the motivation for introducing a notion of causal efficacy or production that is distinct from the notion of causal relevance (or instrumental effectiveness) derives from the idea that information about causal relevance relationships and relationships relevant to manipulation or "instrumental effectiveness" reflects a metaphysically thin, weak, or insubstantial notion of cause and casual explanation. Thus Kim, in the course of commenting on Jackson and Pettit's claim that explanations that appeal to mental states involve causal relevance but not causal efficacy, says that this involves "giving up on mental causation and a robust notion of mental causal explanation" and substituting for it "a looser and weaker model of explanatory relevance" that is not (properly speaking) causal at all (Kim, 1998, p. 75). A similar thought that causal relevance, understood along interventionist lines, involves only a "weak" notion of causation is reflected in the passage from Robb and Heil quoted above. Those who invoke the notion of causal efficacy are thus motivated by the thought that this is a "stronger" or metaphysically richer notion—a notion with more "push" or "umph" than mere causal relevance. The contrary view which is embodied in the interventionist account is that all there is to our various notions of causation is captured by interventionist counterfactuals and information about manipulability relationships—there is no distinct, richer notion of cause of the sort that Robb and Heil, and Jackson and Pettit gesture at. If so, it is of course not a ground for complaint or concern that mental states fail to be causally efficacious in this stronger sense.

I have already recorded my grounds for skepticism that nomological sufficiency is a good candidate for this "richer" notion of cause. What about Jackson and Pettit's association of causal efficacy with relationships that figure in fundamental physics? It is unclear exactly how to interpret this suggestion, but if what it means is that the only true claims about causal efficacy are those that explicitly invoke fundamental physical force laws or other relevant notions from fundamental physics, then, as they themselves explicitly recognize, most causal claims in most areas of science are not true claims about causal efficacy. For example, as they note, even neurally realistic computational models in neurobiology will not be claims about the causal efficacy of one neural state in producing another, and ingesting arsenic will not be causally efficacious in producing death—instead these are mere claims about casual relevance.[14] An additional, quite general

[14] Of course it is also true that on this conception of causal efficacy, one doesn't require anything like the causal exclusion argument to reach the conclusion that mental properties are not causally efficacious: this conclusion follows immediately just from the fact that mental cause claims do not

problem is that, at least according to a number of philosophers of physics, causal notions (of any kind) do not play a fundamental or foundational role in fundamental physics—indeed, in some respects fundamental physical theories are quite resistant to causal interpretation. To the extent that this assessment is correct, it will be a mistake to locate the ground or basis for a metaphysically rich notion of cause in basic physics.[15]

In view of these observations it is natural to wonder whether vindication of the idea that mental states can be causes really requires showing that they are causes in some stronger sense that goes beyond causal relevance. If mental states have the same status qua causes of behavior as arsenic ingestion has qua cause of death, why isn't that causation enough? Indeed, although it is of course an empirical question what ordinary people (or scientists) have in mind when they invoke the notion of mental causation, it is far from clear that either group thinks that mental causation requires anything more than the instrumental effectiveness of the mental. Consider again a paralysed subject who is able to move a prosthetic limb (or a cursor on a screen) merely by thinking or by forming the right intention. Would most lay people and scientists think that this sort of "instrumental efficacy" is insufficient for true mental causation, with something metaphysically richer being required in addition? I suspect not. Certainly if we ask why we should *care* about whether there is mental causation, this looks very much like an issue about instrumental effectiveness: the concern is that we are deluded in our common sense belief that our intentions, desires, beliefs play a role in controlling our mental life and behavior, that we can change our behavior by changing these, that we can manipulate the mental states and behavior of others by changing other mental states of theirs and so on. This concern is adequately addressed by showing that mental states are causes in the sense captured by the interventionist account. We are thus left with the possibility that the only people who think that vindicating the claim that mental states are causes requires

cite fundamental physical forces. In other words, on this conception, the mental would be causally inefficacious even if the exclusion argument is entirely bogus.

[15] For an influential recent statement of this sort of skepticism about the role of causal notions in physics, see Norton, 2007. Woodward, 2007 defends the view that causal notions are most at home and apply most naturally in so-called special sciences like biology and the behavioral and social sciences, as well as in common sense contexts, rather than in fundamental physics. It is also worth observing in this connection that while many philosophers seem to find "physical" accounts of causation appealing (because they are thought to capture the "umph" aspect of causation) it has proved very difficult to formulate such theories in even a roughly acceptable way. For example, by far the best worked out version of such a theory is the Salmon (1984)/Dowe (2000) physical process theory and this faces huge internal difficulties, has at best a very limited range of application, and generates lots of counterintuitive consequences—see, e.g. Woodward, 2003, chapter 8. So while philosophers of mind may find it natural and intuitive to suppose that there must be a notion of cause that goes beyond mere causal relevance (understood in terms of interventionist counterfactuals), this does not mean that we presently have a workable account of this notion. To the extent that we don't have such an account, this is another reason for not regarding mental causal claims as lacking something important that is supplied by a more robust physical notion of causation.

showing that they are causes in a richer, more metaphysical sense are certain philosophers of mind.

5.

The Causal Exclusion Problem: So far I have focused on trying to provide intuitive motivation for the claim that lower level causal claims (involving, e.g., physical or neural properties) do not always undercut or render superfluous more upper level (e.g. mental) causal claims. I turn now to an examination of a more specific argument, the so-called causal exclusion argument (or problem), which is probably the most widely discussed attempt in the literature to motivate the claim that unless mental and physical properties are type-identical, it follows from various uncontroversial empirical premises that mental states are causally inert. There are a number of versions of this argument in the literature; I will focus on a version of the argument due to Kim. Kim's claim is this:

> Causal efficacy of mental properties is inconsistent with the joint acceptance of the following four claims: (i) physical causal closure, (ii) causal exclusion, (iii) mind–body supervenience, (iv) mental/physical property dualism—the claim that mental properties are irreducible to physical properties. (Kim, 2005)

The physical closure principle (i) claims that "if a physical event has a cause at t, then it has a physical cause at t". The principle of causal exclusion (ii) states that "if an event e has a sufficient cause c at t, no event at t distinct from c can be a cause of e (unless this is a genuine case of causal over-determination)". Principle (iv) is supposed to follow from the thesis that mental properties are multiply realizable by physical properties; hence mental properties cannot be identified with any particular physical property. The causal exclusion argument then goes as follows (I lightly paraphrase from Kim, 2005, pp. 39 ff):

(1) Assume, for the sake of argument that some mental property M causes a distinct mental property M*
(2) Since the mental is supervenient on the physical, M* will have some physical property P* as its supervenience base and similarly M will have some physical property P as its supervenience base
(3) Then M causes M* by causing its supervenience base P*
(4) P causes P*
(5) M $\neq$ P (this is simply the claim (iv) above that mental and physical properties are not identical)
(6) Both P and M cause P* (from (3) and (4))
(7) By the causal exclusion principle (ii) this must be a case of causal overdetermination.
(8) It is enormously implausible that most or all cases of mental causation involve overdetermination

> Therefore (9) the claim (1) that M causes M* must be rejected. As Kim puts it, "The putative mental case, M, is excluded by the physical cause P. That is, P, not M is a cause of M*" (Kim, 2005 p. 43)

I assume that (i) physical closure is uncontroversial and relatedly, that premise (4) above is as well. Moreover (8) also seems prima facie convincing, at least if over-determination is taken in its standard sense—that is, as involving two independent causes, each sufficient for the same effect, as when two riflemen shoot a victim simultaneously, with each shot being causally sufficient for death.[16] Kim's justification for (3) is as follows:.

> (1) and (2) [above] together give rise to a tension when we consider the question "Why is M* instantiated on this occasion? What is responsible for, and explains, the fact that M* occurs on this occasion?" For there are two seemingly exclusionary answers: (a) "Because M caused M* to instantiate on this occasion," and (b) "Because P*, a supervenience base of M*, is instantiated on this occasion." . . .: Given that P* is present on this occasion, M* would be there no matter what happened before; as M*'s supervenience base, the instantiation of P* at *t* in and of itself necessitates M*'s occurrence at *t*. This would be true even if M*'s putative cause, M, had not occurred—*unless, that is, the occurrence of M had something to do with the occurrence of P* on this occasion.* This last observation points to a simple and natural way of dissipating the tension created by (a) and (b): (3) M caused M* *by* causing its supervenience base P*. (Kim, 2005, pp. 39–40)

Put more informally, the argument is simply that if we allow mental states or properties to be causes, we end up with too many causes: *P* must cause *P** because of the causal closure of the physical and *P** must be by itself sufficient for *M** since *M** supervenes on *P**. Also, on the seemingly unavoidable principle that causal sufficiency is "transmitted through" the supervenience relation, *P* must also be causally sufficient for *M**. But then it would appear that "all of the causal work" required to produce *M** has already been done by *P* (and *P**) and there is "no work left over" for *M* to do in causing *M**. So *M* is rendered causally superfluous or inert by the physical causes *P* and *P**.

Kim claims that the picture of the relationship between the mental and physical that emerges from the exclusion argument is this:

> P is a cause of P*, with M and M* supervening respectively on P and P*. There is a single underlying causal process in this picture, and this process connects two physical properties, P and P*. The correlations between M and M* and between M and P* are by no means accidental or coincidental; they are lawful and counterfactual-sustaining regularities arising out of M's and M*'s supervenience on the causally linked P and P*. These observed correlations give us an impression of causation; however, that is only an appearance, and there is no more causation here than between two successive shadows cast by a moving ear or two succession symptoms of a developing pathology. This is a simple and elegant picture, metaphysically speaking, but it will prompt howls of protest

[16] For additional discussion See section 6 below.

from those who think that it has given away something very special and precious, namely the causal efficacy of our minds. (2005, p. 21)

Robb and Heil, 2007 give the following, slightly different formulation of the exclusion argument:

How could functional properties make a causal difference? Suppose being in pain is a matter of being in a particular functional state. That is, being in pain is a matter of possessing a particular functional property, *F*. *F* is realized in your case by, say, some neurological property, *N*. Now, *N* is unproblematically relevant to producing various behavioral effects. *N* is relevant to your reaching for aspirin, say. But then what causal work is left for *F* to do? It seems to be causally idle, "screened off" by the work of *N*. This version of the problem of mental causation has appeared in various guises: . . . It is called the exclusion problem because it looks as if the physical properties that realize mental properties exclude the latter from causal relevance.[17]

If my discussion in Section 3 is correct, there must be something wrong with this whole line of reasoning. After all, in the pigeon example, the target's property of being red supervenes on but is not identical with the property of its being scarlet. However, it seems clearly misguided to conclude from this that any role for the redness of the target in causing the pigeon's pecking is "excluded" or pre-empted by the causal activity of the scarlet. Similarly for the other examples in Section 3. One way of diagnosing what is wrong with the argument focuses on its apparent[18] reliance on the assumption (A) that *C*'s causing *E* (or *C*'s being causally relevant to *E*) is to be understood in terms of *C*'s being a sufficient condition of some kind ("nomologically" or "causally sufficient") for *E*. Kim is right that once one makes this assumption and combines it with property dualism (5 above), one faces a major problem in finding a causal role for the mental, for the obvious reason that if some state or event *M* has a mental cause M^* (and hence M^* is, according to (A), causally sufficient for *M*), then since there is also a physically sufficient condition *P* (on which *M* supervenes) for M^* which is not identical with M^*, there must be two distinct sets of causally sufficient conditions (hence according to (A) two sets of causes) for whatever happens—one mental and the other physical. Moreover, the physically sufficient conditions must, given supervenience, be causally sufficient for whatever happens mentally, assuming (as we did above and as seems uncontroversial) that if a condition is

17 Since Robb and Heil frame their discussion around the issue of the causal role of *functional* properties, let me note for the sake of completeness that there may well be special problems in combining a purely functionalist construal of the mental with the assumption that such properties are causally relevant. (This essay does not explore this question.) However, the claims that Robb and Heil go on to make in the quoted passage do not seem to turn on the property *F*'s having a distinctively functional interpretation. It is just the fact that *F* is realized by *N* that is claimed to create problems.

18 I say "apparent reliance" because although discussions of the exclusion problem in the philosophy of mind literature make free use of terms like "causally sufficient" and "causally relevant" these are usually illustrated by means of examples rather than explicitly defined. As a result it is not always clear what is assumed when such terms are used.

causally sufficient for some property it is also causally sufficient for whatever supervenes on that property.[19] It is thus hard to see what possible role there could be for mental causation, barring some apparently unintuitive systematic over-determination? It would seem that physical causation already supplies all of the sufficient conditions (and hence all of the causation) that are (is) needed. By definition, a sufficient condition does not require anything "more" to do its work.

As explained in Section 3, I think that the crucial mistake in this reasoning is the failure to recognize the way in which the notions of causation, causal relevance and the notion of a sufficient condition are related to one another: causation requires casual relevance, *C*'s being causally relevant to *E* is not just a matter of *C*'s being a sufficient condition for *E* and *C*'s being sufficient for *E* does not "exclude" some other factor *K* (distinct from *C*) from causing or being causally relevant to *E*, even in the absence of causal over-determination of *E*. Although ingesting birth control pills is "sufficient" for Mr. Jones' failure to get pregnant, ingestion does not cause Jones' non-pregnancy and does not exclude its being true that Jones' lack of a female reproductive system causes his non-pregnancy. Similarly, although the target's being scarlet is (in at least one obvious sense) sufficient for the pigeon's pecking, this does not exclude its being true that the target's being red is causally relevant to the contrast between pecking and not pecking in a way in which the target's being scarlet is not.

6.

A More General Perspective. Rather than further belaboring these points, I instead want to use the interventionist framework to explore the more general issue of how different views we might adopt about the relationship between the mental and the physical interact with and constrain the causal status of the mental. Among other things, this will give us an additional perspective on what is wrong with the causal exclusion argument. In what follows, I will represent the relationship between mental events and the neural events that realize them by means of a double headed vertical arrow $\Updownarrow$ and the existence of an ordinary causal relationship from X to Y by means of an arrow from X to Y: $X \to Y$.

The general set up with which we will be concerned thus can be represented as shown in Fig. 12.4.

[19] Although this assumption seems unavoidable if we think of causation in terms of one condition being sufficient for another, note that the corresponding principle framed in terms of causation understood along interventionist lines is far from obvious and may well be false. That is, as the examples in Section 3 show, it is not all clear that if P causes P^* and M^* supervenes on P^*, then P causes M^*.

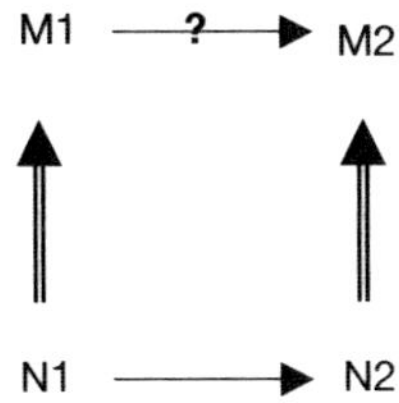

Fig. 12.4

M_1 and M_2 are mental states and N_1 and N_2 are the neural states that realize them, which we allow to be disjunctive to accommodate MRT. Assume it is uncontroversial that, as indicated in the diagram, N_1 causes N_2. The question that will interest us is the following: Under what conditions, if any, and for what interpretation of the supervenience relation $\Uparrow$, are we justified in drawing an $\rightarrow$ from M_1 to M_2 or from M_1 to N_2—that is in regarding M_1 as a cause of these variables?

Suppose, for starters, that $\Uparrow$ represents an ordinary causal relationship—that is, mental states are caused by their neural realizations, which are thus distinct from them. This is a minority position in the philosophical literature, but is adopted (under some interpretation of "cause") by at least one prominent figure—John Searle. By the rules given in Section 1, if M_1 causes M_2, it should be possible to carry out an intervention I on M_1 and this intervention I should break the causal relationship between M_1 and N_1. If, under such an intervention, M_2 changes, then M_1 causes M_2. (Cf. Fig. 12.5.) However, this is not a coherent scenario from the point of view of most philosophers of mind, including anyone who thinks that the mental is supervenient on the physical. First, according to the supervenience thesis, the relationship between M_1 and N_1 is unbreakable. According to the interventionist account, if N_1 causes M_1, then an intervention on M_1 should change M_1 while leaving N_1 unchanged. However, this violates supervenience since it involves a change in mental state with no corresponding change in realizing neural state. In addition, if the value of M_2 changes under some intervention on M_1 (as it must if M_1 causes M_2), the relationship between M_2 and its supervenience base N_2 would also be disrupted, which is again contrary to the supervenience thesis.

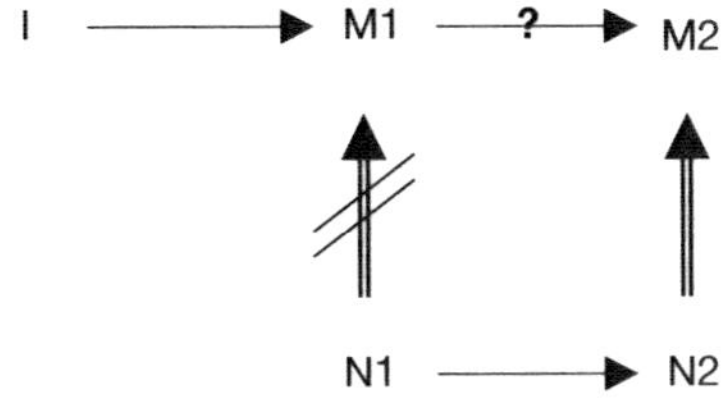

Fig. 12.5

Can we get around this problem by supposing that M_1 does not cause M_2 directly but only via N_2, as in Fig. 12.6?

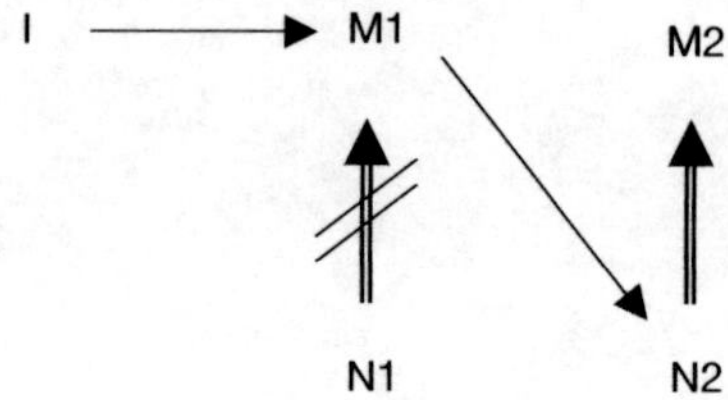

Fig. 12.6

No. This still requires that an intervention on M_1 change M_1 independently of N_1 which, as we have seen, violates supervenience. In addition, this scenario would involve breaking the arrow from N_1 to N_2 or at least making the value of N_2 depend on M_1 as well as N_1, violating the causal closure of the physical. So it looks like there is no acceptable interpretation ⇑ of as "causes".

Note that in assessing the causal role of M_1 with respect to M_2 under a scenario in which the supervenience relationship between N_1 *and* M_1 is interpreted as "causes", we asked about the truth of the following counterfactual:

(C) What would happen to M_2 if we were to vary M_1 by means of an intervention while holding N_1 fixed?

(C) makes perfectly good sense (and *is* the appropriate counterfactual to use for determining whether M_1 causes M_2) *if* the relationship between N_1 and M_1 is causal. The reason for this is that under this interpretation of the supervenience relation, N_1 is an alternative cause of M_2 in addition to M_1 and this alternative cause is correlated with M_1, since N_1 causes M_1 and, moreover, N_1 affects M_2 via a route that does not go through M_1. (This is because N_1 causes N_2 which in turn causes M_2.) In general, as we have seen (cf. Section 1), if X and Y are candidates for causes of Z which are correlated and which affect Z if at all by independent routes, and we wish to assess the causal influence of X on Z, we must control or correct for the causal influence of Y on Z. Thus, in particular, in assessing the causal influence that M_1 by itself has on M_2, we must "control" for the correlated alternative cause N_1 of M_2. We do this within the interventionist framework by "breaking" the causal relationship between M_1 and N_1 and then varying M_1 independently of N_1 by intervening on M_1. In just the same way, in the scenario in which parental SES (E) was (or was suspected of being) a common cause of school attendance P and scholastic achievement S, we test for whether there is a causal relationship from P to S by intervening to vary P while holding E fixed and noting whether there is any change in S. It is much more dubious, however, that on *other* (non-causal) interpretations of the supervenience relationship, use of counterfactuals like C are sensible or appropriate for assessing the causal influence of M_1 on M_2.[20]

Suppose, for example, that the supervenience relationship corresponds to something like "type identity". Then presumably everyone would agree that the counterfactual question (C) makes no sense or at least is inappropriate for capturing the causal influence of M_1 on M_2. On this interpretation of the supervenience relationship, M_1 just *is* N_1 differently described and the antecedent of the counterfactual (C) has no coherent "interventionist" interpretation. Put slightly differently, if M_1 and N_1 are identical, then to carry out an intervention on M_1 is also to carry out the very same intervention on N_1, so that there is no possibility of crediting M_1 and N_1 with different effects under this intervention. To attempt to use (C) in this sort of case as a test for whether M_1 is causally inert with respect to M_2 is to illegitimately import a test which would be appropriate if N_1 were a cause of M_1 into the very different situation in which N_1 is not a cause of but is rather identical with M_1.

A similar conclusion seems warranted for at least some interpretations of the supervenience relationship that do not involve type identity—e.g., when the relationship is that of a determinate property to a determinable property. Consider once more the example of the pigeon trained to respond to red and presented with a particular shade of scarlet (see Fig. 12.7):

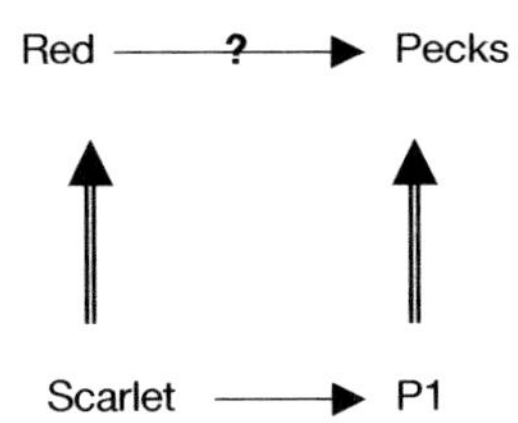

Fig. 12.7

Here Red supervenes on Scarlet and Pecks supervenes on P_1 which (we may suppose) is some lower level description which "realizes" pecking on this particular occasion. It seems clear that it would be inappropriate to employ the following C-like counterfactual question to assess the causal influence of Red on Pecking:

(6.1) If (a) an intervention were to occur that changes the target from Red to not Red while the target remains fixed at scarlet, would (b) the response change from pecking to not pecking?

[20] For some very similar arguments about when it is reasonable to assess whether M_1 causes M_2 by considering what would happen if one were to vary M_1 while holding fixed certain other variables such as N_1, see Shapiro and Sober, forthcoming. The remarks that follow are much indebted to their discussion.

The reason why this question is inappropriate for determining whether Red causes Pecking is again that the antecedent (a) in (6.1) describes a situation that for conceptual reasons cannot be realized by any intervention or combination of interventions—again this is a counterfactual whose antecedent lacks a coherent interventionist interpretation. Assuming that scarlet is a particular shade of red, it is not possible (for conceptual or semantic reasons having to do with the relationship between scarlet and red) to intervene to change the color of a scarlet target from red to not red, while at the same time retaining the scarlet color of the target. As in the previous case, it would be a mistake to infer from this impossibility that changing of the color from red to not red is causally inert with respect to pecking, and that the real cause of the pecking is the lower level, more specific property scarlet.

This last example shows that the cases in which it is inappropriate to apply a counterfactual test like (C) are not confined to cases in which the upper level property and the property on which it supervenes are identical: other sorts of relationships can make the test inappropriate as well. Does this same conclusion then hold whenever one property supervenes on another, including when a mental property supervenes on its physical realizer? Obviously, this depends on exactly how the supervenience relationship is understood. Those who invoke the notion of supervenience, particularly in the context of the mind–brain relationship, often think of this relationship as embodying a very strong kind of necessity—e.g. "metaphysical necessity", whatever that may be. That is, it is claimed that it is metaphysically impossible for two subjects to differ with respect to their mental properties while sharing the same physical properties. To the extent that this or some comparably strong notion such as logical or conceptual impossibility is intended, a scenario in which we imagine intervening to change M_1 while holding the value of N_1 fixed again seems inappropriate for assessing the causal efficacy or inertness of M_1.[21]

Before leaving the exclusion argument, there are several other features of Kim's discussion that are worth examining. Consider first his contention that granting

[21] I don't intend by these remarks to advocate an uncritical attitude toward all the various notions of supervenience that have figured in discussions of the relationship between the mental and the physical. In fact, I think that many of these notions are full of obscurities. I claim only that to the extent that the mental supervenes on the physical in accord with some well-defined or well-behaved notion of supervenience, the counterfactual test C is inappropriate for assessing the causal influence of the mental. If a candidate notion of supervenience seems to license this test as appropriate, this is a reason for being skeptical of that notion. I will add that on one interpretation of Kim's arguments, they are not directed so much at the clam that mental states can be causes but are rather designed to show that (many) proponents of supervenience and multiple realization (understood as something distinct from type identity) have failed to explain in a principled way what the rules are for combining supervenience claims and causal claims.

the premises of the exclusion argument, it follows that mental causation is "epiphenomenal"—that the relationship between one mental state and another is like the relationship between the successive positions of a shadow cast by a physical body or like successive images in a mirror. In these two cases, the successive positions of the shadow and the successive images exert no causal influence on each other; instead these are effects of the successive states of some physical object, with the earlier state P_1 of the object exerting a causal influence on the later state P_2 (see Fig. 12.8)

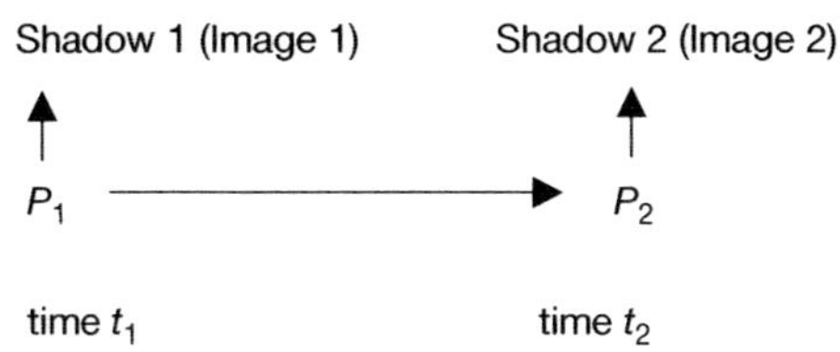

Fig. 12.8

where each of the arrows represents an ordinary causal relationship.

Does Fig. 12.8 represent a good analogy for the relationship between the mental and the physical?[22] A causal structure of the sort portrayed in Fig. 12.8 makes distinctive predictions about what would happen under various interventions. Suppose we were to intervene on the state of shadow 1, while leaving the state of the body P_1 undisturbed. If Fig. 12.8 correctly describes the causal structure with which we are dealing, there should be no change in the state of shadow 2. (Operationally, this might be done by partly blocking the light source that helps to create shadow 1 at time t_1 in such a way that this shadow is altered but P_1 is unchanged. If the block is then removed at t_2 (i.e., if there is no separate intervention on shadow 2), there should be no corresponding change in the state of shadow 2.) On the other hand, if we were to intervene to alter the state of the physical object P_1, there should be, according to Fig. 12.8, a corresponding change in both P_2 and shadow 2.

If the relationships described in Fig. 12.8 are like the relationship between the mental and physical (that is, if mental states are epiphenomenal and causally inert with respect to each other in the way that the successive states of a shadow are, with all of real causal action occurring at the physical level, as portrayed in Fig. 12.9) then a parallel set of claims about what would happen under interventions should hold in this case as well.

[22] Essentially the same argument is also given in Shapiro and Sober, forthcoming.

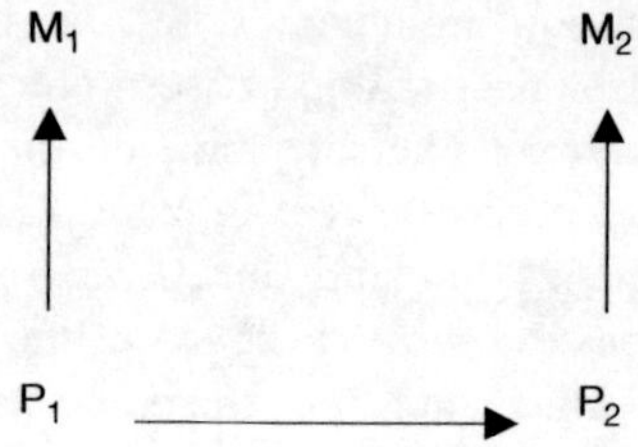

Fig. 12.9

That is, in Fig. 12.9, (i) it should be possible to intervene to change M_1 independently of P_1 and the result of any such intervention should be that there is no change in M_2, while (ii) there should be interventions that change P_1, independently of M_1, and which change P_2 (and M_2). But, as we have already seen, anyone who holds that the mental supervenes on the physical (including both supporters and critics of the exclusion argument), agrees that (i) doesn't hold, since it is impossible to intervene to change M_1 independently of P_1. So, at least within an interventionist framework, it is misguided to think that the supervenience of the mental on the physical implies that the relationship between mental states is like the relationship between the successive positions of a shadow; on the contrary, supervenience is inconsistent with such a construal.

Similar objections apply to some of the other ways in which Kim and others describe (or consider describing) the relationship between mental and physical. As we have seen, many philosophers worry that if there are mental causes, then this would require a bizarre and implausible kind of causal over-determination—the physical states that realize the causal effects of mental states would be caused both by mental states and by physical states.

To assess the appropriateness of this description, consider a paradigmatic case of causal over-determination: two riflemen each shoot separate bullets that simultaneously strike the heart of a victim, killing him, where each bullet by itself, in the absence of the other, would have caused victim's death. Although I lack the space for detailed discussion, within an interventionist framework, the presence of this sort of causal over-determination is signaled by the truth of a group of counterfactuals, given the usual interventionist interpretation: (a) (b) If bullet one (two) had not hit the victim but bullet two (one) had struck his heart, victim still would have died. (c) If neither bullet had struck victim, he would not have died. It is crucial to this analysis that the two shooters affect the victim by means of separate or independent causal mechanisms or processes—it is this that makes it sensible to talk about what would happen to the victim if one of these processes had not occurred, but the other had.

For example, in the scenario as described, it makes sense to suppose that one of the rifleman shoots (this shot resulting from an intervention) while the second doesn't or that the second bullet is deflected in flight. But an analogous account does not apply to the alleged over-determination by both mental and physical causes—again, assuming a well-behaved supervenience relationship, it is impossible that the physical cause be present but the putative mental cause that supervenes on it be absent. Thus the counterfactuals that give sense to the over-determination present in the rifleman case lack any clear sense in the cases in which there is a worry about the possibility of mental/physical over-determination.[23]

A similar point holds for Kim's claim that given the premises of the exclusion argument, physical causes "pre-empt" any mental causes. In a paradigmatic case of pre-emption, rifleman one fires first, his bullet striking and killing the victim, who is already dead by the time he is hit by the bullet from rifleman two, which would have killed the victim in the absence of the bullet from rifleman one. Again within an interventionist framework, certain counterfactuals will hold that allow us to make sense of what this pre-emption involves. For example, holding fixed the path and time of the first bullet, the victim's death is not counterfactually dependent on whether the second rifleman fires.[24] Again the analogues to these counterfactuals have impossible or incoherent antecedents when mental/physical supervenience holds, suggesting that whatever may be the correct way to conceive of the causal role of the mental under such supervenience, "pre-emption" of the mental by the physical is not the right picture.

In all three sets of claims about the causal status of the mental (that mental states are epiphenomenal, that they are pre-empted, that they are potentially at least, over-determining causes), causal descriptions are used that make perfectly good sense in some situations. However, the features of these situations that warrant the use of these descriptions are not present in contexts in which mental states are supervenient on physical states. I conclude that all three descriptions are inappropriate in the latter contexts.

7.

In Section 4, I observed that within an interventionist framework causation between upper level properties requires that there be dependency relationships

[23] For a more detailed treatment of this sort of over-determination within an interventionist framework, see Woodward, 2003, chapter 2.

[24] For a more detailed treatment of such pre-emption cases, again see Woodward, 2003, chapter 2.

between those properties that exhibit some degree of stability under different lower level realizations of those properties. Whether and to what extent such stability is present is an empirical question that depends both on the upper level relationship and the nature of their realizers and the generalizations governing them. I want to conclude this essay by suggesting that to the extent there are issues about the reality and extent of mental causation, these have to do with such empirical consideration, rather than with the very general arguments for the causal inertness of the mental discussed in Sections 3–5.

Consider again the relationship (7.1) between the push communicated to the roulette wheel and the color on which the ball lands and the relationship (7.2) between the pressure, volume and temperature of a good approximation to an ideal gas. These represent two extremes: (7.1) is extremely sensitive to the exact micro details of how the push is implemented while for virtually micro-realizations of its macroscopic variables (7.2) will continue to hold. The question of whether various candidates for mental causal relationships are bona-fide causal relationships seems to me to come down, in substantial measure, to whether the relationships in question are more like (7.1) or more like (7.2).

In some cases, the assumption that we are dealing with dependency relationships between mental states that exhibit some substantial degree of realization independence seems fairly plausible. For example, while the assumption (made above) that relationship between intention and motor action is completely insensitive to the way in which the intention is realized neurally—that is, that intention I_1 always leads to R_1 regardless of how I_1 is realized—is almost certainly an idealization, it is not implausible that this is roughly true: that most or a very substantial range of realizations of I_1 lead to R_1 and that the same is true for many other intentions and behaviors. If this were not so, there would be no reason to expect any coherent relationship between intentions and simple motor actions. A similar conclusion holds for many cases involving chains of reasoning, plans, and learning procedures: it is hard to see how we could usefully employ these at all if they did not have some substantial degree of realization dependence. As observed in Section 2, our ability to manipulate the mental state and behavior of others also suggests some degree of realization dependence for some relationships between mental states and between mental states and behavior.

On the other hand, it seems entirely possible (perhaps likely) that some commonly employed generalizations about the mental are not even approximately realization independent because, e.g., the concepts in terms of which they are framed lump together more specific realizers that are causally quite heterogeneous, with the generalization in question holding for some of these but not others. For example, to the extent that there are different fear systems, with very different characteristics, it may well be that many candidate generalizations linking "fear", taken as a general category or variable, to behaviorial changes are in fact highly unstable: it may be that to formulate stable relationships we have to descend to the level of more specific fear systems (e.g. we need to talk about specific nuclei in the amygdala and specific pathways in and out of these) and then consider specific manipulations of these.[25] More radically, it may be that to find stable relationships we have to talk about systems and properties that are even more micro and biochemically specific—levels of specific neurotransmitters, variations in receptors for these and so on.

REFERENCES

Bennett, K. (2003). "Why the Exclusion Problem Seems Intractable and How, Just Maybe, to Tract It", *Noûs* 37/3, pp. 471–97.

Blair, J., Mitchell, D., and Blair K. (2005). *The Psychopath: Emotion and the Brain.* Malden, MA: Blackwell.

Dowe, P. (2000). *Physical Causation.* Cambridge: Cambridge University Press.

Funkhouser, E. (2006). "The Determinable-Determinate Relationship", *Noûs* 40, 548–69.

Jackson, F., and Pettit, P. (2004*a*). "Program Explanation: A General Perspective", in Jackson, Pettit and Smith, *Mind, Morality, and Explanation: Selected Collaborations.* Oxford: Oxford University Press, 119–30.

—— —— (2004*b*). "Causation in the Philosophy of Mind", in Jackson, Pettit and Smith, *Mind, Morality, and Explanation: Selected Collaborations.* Oxford: Oxford University Press, 45–68.

—— —— and Smith, M. (2004). "Introduction", in Jackson, Pettit and Smith, *Mind, Morality, and Explanation: Selected Collaborations.* Oxford: Oxford University Press, 1–10.

Kim, J. (1998). *Mind in a Physical World: An Essay on the Mind-Body Problem and Mental Causation.* Cambridge, MA: MIT Press.

—— (2005). *Physicalism or Something Near Enough.* Princeton: Princeton University Press.

Lepore, E. and Loewer, B. (1987). "Mind Matters", *Journal of Philosophy* 84: 630–42.

Musallam, S., Corneil, B. Greger, B., Scherberger, H., and Andersen, R. (2004). "Cognitive Control Signals for Neural Prostethics", *Science* 305: 258–62.

Norton, J. (2007). "Causation as Folk Science", in H. Price and R. Corry (eds.), *Causation, Physics and the Constitution of Reality: Russell's Republic Revisited.* Oxford: Oxford University Press.

Pearl, J. (2000). *Causality: Models, Reasoning, and Inference.* Cambridge: Cambridge University Press.

Robb, D. and Heil, J. (2007). "Mental Causation", Stanford Encyclopedia of Philosophy. http://plato.stanford.edu (accessed 24 June 2007).

[25] For an argument that something like this is the case for generalizations linking the behavior of psychopaths to deficits in their "fear systems" and to a general lack of fearfulness, see Blair et al., 2005.

Salmon, W. (1984). *Scientific Explanation and the Causal Structure of the World*. Princeton: Princeton University Press.

Shapiro, L. (2000). "Multiple Realizations", *Journal of Philosophy*, 97: 635–54.

—— and Sober, E. (forthcoming). "Epiphenomenalism: The Do's and the Don'ts", in G. Wolters and P. Machamer (eds.), *Studies in Causality: Historical and Contemporary*. Pittsburgh: University of Pittsburgh Press.

Spirtes, P., Glymour, C. and Scheines, R. (2000). *Causation, Prediction, and Search*. Cambridge, MA: MIT Press.

Woodward, J. (2003). *Making Things Happen: A Theory of Causal Explanation*. New York: Oxford University Press.

—— (2007). "Causation with a Human Face", in H. Price and R. Corry (eds.), *Causation, Physics and the Constitution of Reality: Russell's Republic Revisited*. Oxford: Oxford University Press.

Yablo, S. (1992). "Mental Causation", *Philosophical Review* 101: 245–80.

13

Distinctions in Distinction

Daniel Stoljar

PUZZLE

According to a standard view in contemporary metaphysics, there are no necessary connections between distinct properties. But according to a standard view in philosophy of mind there *are* necessary connections between distinct properties. In short, we have a puzzle: standard metaphysics is inconsistent with standard philosophy of mind.

By 'a standard view in contemporary metaphysics' I mean, of course, Hume's dictum that there are no necessary connections between distinct existences. I don't mean the historical Hume; whether the historical Hume held Hume's dictum I am sure is a controversial issue, and will not concern us. What will concern us rather is the idea that contemporary metaphysicians such as David Lewis and David Armstrong discuss and attribute to Hume (see, e.g., Lewis 1986 and Armstrong 1997). Of course Hume's dictum does not say anything explicitly about properties; it talks of existences rather than properties. But 'existences' I take it, means 'things that exist' and, if we set nominalism aside—as I will do here—properties are things that exist. Hence the Humean dictum entails as a special case that there are no necessary connections between distinct properties.

By 'a standard view in contemporary philosophy of mind' I mean a view that may itself take a number of forms. One particularly clear version of the view,

I presented versions of this chapter to a conference on mental causation at Macquarie University organized by Alex Miller, and a conference on the special sciences at Aarhus University organized by Jakob Hohwy. I am grateful for the many very good comments I received from the participants at both conferences and from others with whom I have discussed this material; particular thanks to Suzy Bliss, who commented on the paper at Macquarie, Karen Bennett, David Chalmers, Jordi Fernandez, Derk Pereboom, Ted Sider, and Jessica Wilson. Bennett (Chapter 14 in this volume) reaches conclusions about dualism similar to those I reach, but in a complementary way, while unpublished work by Jessica Wilson covers some similar ground on Hume's dictum. Thanks also to David Sanford who sent me some very detailed comments on the paper—too late alas to be properly incorporated. Finally, special thanks to Jakob Hohwy and Jesper Kallestrup for their help in preparing the paper for publication.

and the one I will mostly focus on, starts from the claim that psychological properties are second-order properties, i.e. properties expressed by predicates containing a quantifier over other properties. On this view, if Smith is in pain, Smith instantiates the property of *having some property or other that plays a certain role*—often abbreviated to the pain role. This second-order view of psychological properties is attractive for at least two reasons. First, it permits an easy explanation of multiple realizability: if Smith is a Martian, the first-order property that plays the pain role might be one thing; if Smith is a monotreme, the first-order property might be something else; and so on. Second, it permits a formulation of physicalism often described as 'non-reductive'. It is physicalist, in so far as the total physical facts about Smith will or might metaphysically necessitate that he has some property that plays the pain role; and it is non-reductive, in so far as the psychological properties on such a construal are distinct from the physical properties that necessitate them, at least if the physical properties in question are all of them first-order properties. It is in its connection to non-reductive physicalism that we see the second-order view in apparent conflict with Hume's dictum. The physicalist part of non-reductive physicalism says that psychological properties are *necessarily connected* to physical properties; the non-reductive part of non-reductive physicalism says they are *distinct*.

So standard metaphysics is inconsistent with standard philosophy of mind, and we have a puzzle. However, my reason for raising the puzzle is not to see *whether* it can be solved; I am certain it can. Nor is my reason to see *how* it can be solved; I am certain one may solve the puzzle by drawing distinctions in distinction, i.e. by separating out different notions doing business under the label 'distinctness'. Rather my interest in raising the puzzle is that assembling the materials for solving it has applications to *other topics* that are greatly discussed in philosophy of mind, in particular, the exclusion problem, and the problem of the distinction between non-reductive physicalism and emergentism.

We will come to applications later; first, what is the solution to the puzzle?

SOLUTION

I said that the solution to the puzzle is to draw distinctions in distinction. More particularly, there are five possible notions here, and on none of them is the puzzle on reflection as puzzling as it at first appears.

The first possibility is that 'distinct' means 'numerical distinctness,' where:

F is numerically distinct from G if and only if F is not identical to G.

This is a very natural suggestion; after all, that is what 'distinctness' *usually* means. Moreover, this interpretation makes good sense of the philosophy of mind half of the puzzle; on the second-order view, psychological properties are numerically distinct from first-order physical properties. For one thing, the psychological properties are second-order properties, while the relevant physical properties are not. But, on this interpretation, what the metaphysicians say (and so the Humean dictum itself) is false and trivially so. For consider: being red is numerically distinct from being coloured, since something could be coloured and not red; i.e. these are numerically distinct properties. Yet they are necessarily connected since being red entails being coloured. So, on that interpretation, Hume's dictum is false, and we have no puzzle.

It might be thought that being red, being coloured (etc.) are not existences in the sense at issue in Hume's dictum. Perhaps 'existence' in this context is to be restricted to ordinary physical objects rather than to properties. However, as I have already noted, 'existences' just means 'things that exist' and that is a completely general notion—*the* most general notion in fact. Moreover, if 'existence' is to be restricted to ordinary physical objects, we have no puzzle in the first place. For the philosophy of mind part of the puzzle is precisely that psychological *properties* are distinct from physical ones. If properties are not at issue in Hume's dictum, there is no puzzle.

The second possibility is that 'distinct' means (as I will say) 'weakly modally distinct', where:

> F is weakly modally distinct from G if and only if it is possible that F is instantiated and G is not *or* it is possible that G is instantiated and F is not.

Once again, this interpretation certainly makes sense of the philosophy of mind half of the puzzle. On the second-order view psychological properties are weakly modally distinct from the physical properties that necessitate them, for, while it is impossible that the relevant physical properties are instantiated without the psychological properties being instantiated, the psychological properties might perfectly well be instantiated without the physical properties. But once again, this interpretation renders Hume's dictum false: being red is weakly modally distinct from being coloured, and yet they are necessary connected.

It might be thought that 'distinct' in the context of Hume's dictum could not possibly mean 'weakly modally distinct' because the latter notion is not perfectly general. The notion of weak modal distinction as so far defined applies only to properties. But Hume's dictum is apparently very general, and so would presumably apply to items of any ontological category. However, it is not impossible that one might develop the notion so that it is perfectly general. For example, one might simply add a clause for items of different ontological categories: if physical objects are what is at issue, weak modal distinction means that it is possible that one object *exists* while another not; and if states of affairs are at issue, weak modal distinction means that it is possible that one state of affairs *obtains* while another does not; and so on. Moreover, and more important, the plausibility or otherwise of this development of the notion does not affect the basic issue. In particular, it remains true that there *are* necessary connections between weakly modally distinct *properties*, and so it is no objection to the second-order view that it is asserts that there are.

The third possibility is that 'distinct' means 'strongly modally distinct', where:

> F is strongly modally distinct from G if and only if it is possible that F is instantiated and G is not *and* it is possible that G is instantiated and F is not.

It is should be clear that strong modal distinction is just like its weak cousin except that we substitute 'and' for 'or'. In consequence, one point to make about strong modal distinction is that it is not completely general as it stands. However, since the same considerations apply here as applied above I will set this point aside. The more important point is that, unlike the previous two proposals, the suggestion that 'distinction' means what 'strong modal distinction' means makes good sense of the metaphysics part of the puzzle with which we began. On this interpretation, what Hume's dictum says is that if a property F is distinct from a property G, it is possible that F is instantiated and G is not *and vice versa.* Since the possibilities of instantiation at issue here are precisely what people have in mind when they speak of necessary connection, Hume's dictum is on this interpretation not merely true but plausibly analytic.

However, while the notion of strong modal distinction makes sense of the metaphysics half of the puzzle, it makes no sense of the philosophy of mind half. For non-reductive physicalists are not asserting that psychological properties are strongly modally distinct from the physical properties that necessitate them. On the contrary, they are asserting outright that it is *impossible* that one can have the relevant physical properties instantiated without the psychological properties instantiated. In short, if 'distinct' means 'strongly modally distinct', we again have no puzzle.

The fourth possibility is that 'distinct' means 'mereologically distinct', where:

> F is mereologically distinct from G if and only if F and G—to put it vaguely at first—share no parts or constituents.

On this interpretation, it is unclear whether Hume's dictum is true. This is for two reasons. First, it is unclear what it means to say that properties have constituents or parts. Obviously ordinary material objects have parts or constituents, and it is certainly plausible to say that if two such objects share no parts then they are distinct; so here we have a clarification of the notion of distinctness where the existences in question are material objects. But it is not clear that this account can be generalized to properties, and the reason is it is not clear that mereological notions can be extended in this direction. Take the properties of being coloured and being red. These are necessarily connected. So we could conclude from this account that they must have a part in common. But what is the *part* in common between being red and being coloured? I am not claiming that there is no answer to this question, only that it is unobvious what the answer is, and part of the reason for this is surely that it is unobvious what notion of part or constituent applies properly to properties.

The second reason it is unclear whether Hume's dictum is true when the background of 'distinctness' is interpreted as mereological distinctness is that it is unclear how one would establish that it is. What Hume's dictum says on this interpretation is that there are no necessary connections between properties that share no parts. So in particular, if you have a perfectly simple property F, i.e. a property that by definition has no parts, this property can be necessarily connected only to itself or to a property that is complex and contains F as a constituent. But whether this is true or not seems to be an open question. For example, if I said that there are necessary connections between two perfectly simple properties it is at least unclear that I would be contradicting myself. In this respect, the mereological interpretation of Hume's dictum is quite different from the strong modal distinctness interpretation. More particularly, if 'distinct' means 'mereologically distinct', neither Hume's dictum nor its negation is contradictory. But then it is unclear that it is true.

However, whether or not it is true, and whether or not we can establish that it is, the important point for us is that, on this interpretation of what the metaphysicians say, we still face no puzzle. The reason is that it is not at all clear that the non-reductive physicalist holds that psychological properties are mereologically distinct from the physical properties that necessitate them. For consider: the second-order property at issue is the property of having some property which plays the pain role, and one of the first-order properties at issue is the property that has the pain role. But then the pain role will turn up as a part or constituent both of the second-order property *and* of one of the first-order properties that necessitate it. So, whatever it means precisely to speak of mereological distinction, the second-order property view is not asserting that second-order properties are mereologically distinct from the relevant first-order properties, and we have no puzzle.

The fifth and final possibility I will consider is that 'distinct' in Hume's dictum means 'distinct in essence or nature' where:

> F is distinct in essence from G just in case the essence of F is wholly distinct from the essence of G.

The essence of a thing, as I understand it, is the totality of its essential properties. Correlatively, the essence of x is wholly distinct from the essence of y if and only if none of the essential properties of x are also essential properties of y. So what it means for one property to be distinct in essence from another is for the first to have no essential properties that the second one has. On this interpretation, what Hume's dictum means is that, between two properties that share no essential properties, there are no necessary connections either.

Is Hume's dictum on this interpretation true? The answer is once again unclear. The reason this time is not that it is hard to see how to generalize from a claim about particulars to a claim about items of any ontological category; presumably items of any ontological category may instantiate properties and so instantiate them necessarily or essentially. The reason is rather that, to make sense of the denial of Hume's dictum on this interpretation, one would have to draw a distinction between the necessary properties of a thing and its essential properties, and this distinction is very hard to draw. For example to say that F and G are necessarily connected even if they have wholly distinct essences means that the property of being necessarily connected to G is not an essential feature of F. But since that distinction is difficult to draw in a satisfying way, it is hard to see whether Hume's dictum is true.

However, regardless of whether Hume's dictum on this interpretation is true or known to be true, the important point for us is—again—that, if this is the correct interpretation of what the metaphysicians are saying, we face no puzzle. For again it is far from clear that non-reductive physicalists are saying that psychological properties and physical properties are distinct in essence and yet are necessarily connected. To be distinct in essence in the relevant sense is for none of the essential properties of the psychological properties to be also essential properties of the physical properties. But non-reductive physicalists are certainly not committed to this claim. Presumably it is part of the essence of the second-order property that it involves a particular causal role; but it may also be part of the essence of the relevant physical properties that they involve this very same causal role.

It might be denied that 'distinction in essence' means that *none* of the essential properties of F are essential properties of G. Perhaps it means only that *some* of the essential properties of F are not essential properties of G. On this view, F is distinct in essence from G just in case the set of F's essential properties does not share every member with the set of G's essential properties. On this view, moreover, Hume's dictum says that there are no necessary connections between things whose essences are partially distinct. But so interpreted Hume's dictum is false. For example, it seems to be part of the essence of a second-order property that it is second-order, but it is not part of the essence of any first-order property that it is second-order. But if that is so, we have necessary connections between properties that have numerically distinct essences.

MORAL

Our question was: what does 'distinct' mean in the puzzle with which we began? The answer we have been led to is that there are at least five possible things it could mean and that, on any of them, there is no puzzle. To that extent therefore the puzzle is solved.

On the other hand, what I have said so far is disappointingly conditional in character. We have five ways of analysing distinctness. If it is analysed in this way, something goes wrong; if it is analysed this way, something else goes wrong; and so on. But we have not said anything about what distinctness is *in fact*. Moreover, when asked what distinctness is in fact, it is quite reasonable to say that distinctness is non-identity. As I noted earlier, the most natural suggestion about what 'distinctness' means is that it means 'numerical distinctness'. From this point of view, the other relations we talked about might be perfectly fine in their way, but they are not distinctness.

I have some sympathy with this point of view, but I think it ignores an important part of our talk about distinctness. For consider Hume's dictum again. It is reasonable to suppose that philosophers who invoke Hume's dictum are getting at a particular notion of distinctness. They are not making an obvious mistake. Nor are they talking about nothing. On the other hand, the notion of distinctness that is at issue in Hume's dictum just cannot be numerical distinctness, for if it were the dictum is obviously false. So, if you think that there is an interpretation of Hume's dictum according to which it is not obviously false, and not about nothing, it must be that you think that there is a notion of distinctness that is distinct from numerical distinctness. Turning this around, since Hume's dictum can only be true if the background notion of distinctness is interpreted as strong modal distinction or mereological distinctness or distinctness in essence it follows that there is a legitimate way of talking according to which these relations deserve the name 'distinctness' even though they are not numerical distinctness.

The idea that there are a number of different notions legitimately doing business under the label 'distinctness' affords a general moral for philosophical discussion. Philosophers often assert or deny distinctness in the course of philosophical argument, using at least the following expressions:

> 'independent of', 'separate from', 'over and above', 'nothing but', 'reduced to', 'wholly distinct from', 'genuine novel', 'a special creation', 'fundamental', . . .

These are all ways of asserting or denying that one thing is distinct from one another. In the light of what we have said, however, we need to be attentive to the different notions that might be legitimately at issue here. It might be that what is at issue is mere numerical distinctness. But it might also be that what is at issue is one of the notions of distinctness that emerges from reflection on Hume's dictum, i.e. either strong modal or mereological distinctness, or distinctness in essence. So the moral I have in mind is this: be attentive to which of these notions is at issue, and in particular be attentive to the possibility that premises about (e.g.) strong modal distinctness are not taken to imply conclusions about (e.g.) numerical distinctness or vice versa.

As I will now go on to explain, I think both the exclusion argument and the problem of the distinguishing non-reductive physicalism from emergence suffer from a failure to head this moral. (For some related discussion in different domains, see Sanford 2005.) I will start with the exclusion problem.

EXCLUSION I

Traditionally the target of the exclusion argument is the traditional dualist, where by 'traditional dualist' I mean the sort of dualist who says that psychological properties are, in the terminology we have introduced, strongly modally distinct from physical properties: it is possible that psychological properties are instantiated and not physical properties, and it is possible that physical properties are instantiated and not psychological properties. Such a position says in effect that the psychological and the physical are only contingently related, but does not deny that there might be various laws connecting the psychological and the physical, so long as these laws are themselves contingent.

Against such a dualist, the exclusion argument begins with the observation—where phys is the overall physical state I am in—that the following theses are inconsistent:

(1) Being in pain causes me to wince.
(2) Being in phys causes me to wince.
(3) Being in pain is distinct from being in phys.
(4) If being in pain causes me to wince, nothing distinct from being in pain causes me to wince.

The dualist is then invited to agree that (1) and (2) are both claims that are (in the context) non-negotiable; and (4) is a principle of causation or an instance of a principle we must accept, often called 'the exclusion principle'. The conclusion is that (3)—a thesis distinctive of traditional dualism—has to go.

In setting out the argument this way, I am deliberately ignoring a number of complications. First, I am not being very careful about causal relata. One might think that it is not properties that cause strictly speaking but instantiations of properties or perhaps events. Second, I am not being very careful to distinguish direct from indirect causation: it seems quite implausible that (4) could be true if the notion of causation is understood broadly to mean 'either direct or indirect causation', for it seems clear that if A causes B and B causes C it may be that A causes C but not directly. Third, I am pretending that (4) is true outright rather than just true in general: (4), or the principle behind (4), gives the impression that genuine overdetermination—the classic example is the firing squad case—is being ruled out a priori, but since this is implausible, (4) must be a generalization that has, rather than lacks, exceptions. My reason for ignoring these complications is not that they are unimportant. It is rather that attending to them properly would needlessly distract us from what is for me the main point. For me the main point is the connection between the exclusion argument and the idea of distinctness.

For of course there *is* such a connection. In particular, the argument invokes the idea of 'distinctness' at two points: at premise (3) and at premise (4). Now, which idea of distinctness is at issue in these premises? Well, it is clear that, so long as we are targeting the traditional dualist, the notion of distinctness at issue here must be, or at least entail, strong modal distinctness. The reason is that if (3) is a thesis that the traditional dualist is committed to it must be interpreted as strong modal distinctness. Hence, (3) should be replaced with (3-sm):

(3-sm) Being in pain is strongly modally distinct from being in phys.

Likewise, if (4) is supposed to be a thesis which, together with (1) and (2) is inconsistent with (3-sm) then it had better be interpreted as involving strong modal distinctness too. Hence, (4) should be replaced with (4-sm):

(4-sm) If being in pain causes me to wince, nothing strongly modally distinct from being in pain causes me to wince.

More generally, the version of the exclusion argument that targets the traditional dualist must exploit a version of the exclusion principle—i.e. the principle behind (4)—that invokes the notion of strong modal distinctness.

Is this version of the exclusion argument sound? I am not going to attempt to answer that question in this paper. Instead I will be content to make the following two points. (a) Construed as an argument against the traditional dualist, the exclusion argument is normally taken to have a considerable persuasive power: many philosophers regard it as decisive, but even those traditional dualists who don't accept it regard it as the key challenge to their position. (b) In the light of this, we may provisionally conclude that the exclusion principle has a considerable amount of prima facie support, so long as the background notion of distinctness is strong modal distinctness. So in effect we are appealing to the persuasiveness of the version of the exclusion argument that targets the traditional dualist as a reason for thinking that the relevant version of the exclusion principle is true.

EXCLUSION II

If our discussion concerned only the traditional dualist it would be not so interesting. Few of us nowadays are traditional dualists in the sense I introduced. But Jaegwon Kim has famously suggested that the traditional dualist is not the only person who lies in the target range of the exclusion argument (see, e.g., Kim 1998 and 2005). In particular, Kim says, the argument might be similarly used against the non-reductive physicalist. This—as Kim calls it—is Descartes' Revenge.

To see how Descartes' Revenge works, look again at claims (1–4):

(1) Being in pain causes me to wince.
(2) Being in phys causes me to wince.
(3) Being in pain is distinct from being in phys.
(4) If being in pain causes me to wince, nothing distinct from being in pain causes me to wince.

Kim says that the non-reductive physicalist is similarly committed to (1–4). Of course it remains true that (1–4) present a contradiction and that (1) and (2) are in the context non-negotiable. Moreover, since (4) is an instance of the exclusion principle that seemed plausible before, the only option for the non-reductive physicalist is to give up (3). But (3) is a thesis that is distinctive of that position. And this is Descartes' Revenge: the argument that is used so effectively against the traditional dualist can be used with equal power against the non-reductive physicalist.

Is Kim's extension of the exclusion argument correct? Well, in order to figure out whether it is, we need to ask what the notion of distinctness is in the version of the exclusion argument that attacks the non-reductive physicalist. If the argument is attacking the non-reductive physicalist, it must be that in (3) the notion of distinctness means either numerical distinctness or weak modal distinctness. For as we have seen the non-reductive physicalist is not saying that psychological properties are distinct from physical properties in any of the other senses we have isolated. If we concentrate for the moment on the notion of numerical distinctness, we may say that, in the version of the exclusion argument that is directed at the non-reductive physicalist, the idea of distinctness present in (3) must be numerical distinctness. In short, (3) should be replaced with (3-n):

(3-n) Being in pain is numerically distinct from being in phys.

Moreover, if (3) invokes the idea of numerical distinctness, it must be that (4) invokes the notion of numerical distinctness too. In short, (4) should be replaced with (4-n):

(4-n) If being in pain causes me to wince, nothing numerically distinct from being in pain causes me to wince.

So, in effect the proponent of the version of the exclusion argument that is directed against the non-reductive physicalist is committed to the view that there is a version of the exclusion principle that invokes the notion of numerical distinctness.

Is this version of the exclusion argument sound? This too is a large issue. However, I think the material we have assembled permits us to make at least the following two points. First, the exclusion argument directed against the non-reductive physicalist is a *different* argument from the one directed against the traditional dualist. The argument against the traditional dualist involves the notion of strong modal distinction whereas the argument against the non-reductive physicalist involves the notion of numerical distinctness. But these notions are different. It is as if someone has made an argument about riverbanks and suggested it applies to piggybanks. Premises about riverbanks don't give you conclusions about piggybanks; similarly premises about numerical distinctness don't give you conclusions about strong modal distinction. Moreover, it is only a failure to distinguish the two notions of distinctness that gives the impression that somehow the non-reductive physicalist is in the same boat as the traditional dualist. (For a related discussion about the relation between these two arguments, see Bennett, Chapter 14 in this volume.)

Second, the argument against the nonreductive physicalist is considerably less plausible than the argument used against the traditional dualist. The reason is that there are counterexamples to the exclusion principle that invokes numerical distinctness—i.e. (3-n)—that are *not* counterexamples to the exclusion principle that invokes metaphysical distinctness—i.e. (3-sm). In consequence, the version of the exclusion principle that invokes numerical distinctness is considerably less plausible than the principle that invokes strong modal distinctness.

One such example is Yablo's pigeon, Sophie, who is trained to peck at a red card at the exclusion of others (see Yablo 1992). A red card is produced and Sophie pecks. As Yablo notes, most people would unhesitatingly say that the redness of the card is what caused Sophie to peck. But of course red cards are not just red; they are specific shades of red—scarlet say. Surely being scarlet is a property of the card that is causally sufficient to get Sophie to peck, at least in the context. But then, by the exclusion principle that invokes numerical distinctness, being red is not relevant. If this is a bad result, and we want both the red and the scarlet to be causally relevant, the exclusion principle that invokes numerical distinctness is false. By way of contrast we should note that Yablo's pigeon is no counterexample to the exclusion principle that is at issue in the version of the exclusion argument that targets the traditional dualist. Being scarlet and being red are numerically distinct but they are not strongly modally distinct. So we can agree with Yablo about the exclusion principle that invokes numerical distinctness, but still accept the plausibility of the exclusion principle that invokes strong modal distinctness. More generally, we can resist the argument against the non-reductive physicalist at the same time as endorse the argument against the traditional dualist.

The case of Yablo's pigeon might be thought to be somewhat controversial because it utilizes the distinction between determinates and determinables, and this distinction is itself controversial. However, there are different ways to make essentially the same point, ways that don't involve that distinction. Imagine we have a property F that we agree to be causally relevant in the production of some effect C. Now consider a property F* that is exactly like F except that it treats one possibility differently, and imagine also that the possibility in question is very remote in logical space. (We might imagine that there is only one relevant kind of case that they treat differently.) F and F* are not co-extensive, so they are numerically distinct. Should we say that, since F is causally relevant to C, F* is not? The exclusion principle that invokes numerical distinctness would say so. But this verdict is surely questionable. Is causal relevance really *so* discriminating as to distinguish F from F*? If we think not, then we might conclude that while (3-sm) is true, (3-n) is not true, and moreover that, while the exclusion argument against the traditional dualist is sound, the exclusion argument against the non-reductive physicalists is not.

EMERGENCE I

I have argued so far that drawing distinctions among various notions of distinction is helpful when thinking about the exclusion argument, and that in particular, it permits us to say that the exclusion argument is successful against the traditional dualist but unsuccessful against the non-reductive physicalist.

I turn now to a related topic that has also been raised by Kim, viz., the question of what the distinction is between the typical non-reductive physicalist (for example, Fodor 1974 or Horgan 1983) and the typical emergentist (for example Broad 1925). Off hand, both seem to hold the same doctrine. For both adhere to the slogan: psychological properties are distinct from physical properties but are necessitated by them. On the other hand, in the standard taxonomy of positions in philosophy of mind, the emergentist is usually thought of as a kind of dualist whereas the non-reductive physicalist is usually thought of—as the name suggests—as a kind of physicalist. So the question is: what if anything justifies the standard taxonomy?

There are two main answers to this question in the literature. The first is that nothing justifies it and in fact there is no distinction. This is Kim's view (see Kim 1993, 1998; see also Crane 2001). Kim's view is that, while many contemporary philosophers certainly *describe* themselves as physicalists, they are self-deceived. They describe themselves as physicalists, but since they hold a view that is identical to emergentism, this is just a mistake. Kim draws the moral that the only thesis that deserves the name 'physicalism' is the reductive version, i.e. the one that entails that psychological properties are numerically identical to physical properties.

The other view is that the difference between non-reductive materialism and emergentism is to be drawn in explanatory or epistemological terms, rather than metaphysical terms. Broad himself (1925, p. 59) drew the distinction in terms of deducibility, saying that the mechanist, as Broad called the physicalist, held that psychological or chemical laws are deducible from other laws. It would be natural to put Broad's view in a contemporary context by saying that the non-reductive physicalist is committed to the deducibility while the emergentist is not. If so, there is some sort of explanatory or epistemological distinction between the two positions, even if they are identical from a metaphysical point of view. (For developments of this point, see Horgan 1993.)

Neither approach to the problem of distinguishing emergentism and non-reductive physicalism is very satisfactory, however. As against the no difference view, it is difficult to shake the feeling that the standard taxonomy of positions is onto something, and that there is some sort of distinction between the position of Broad and that of Fodor. As against the epistemic or explanatory view, it is difficult to shake the feeling that the distinction between the emergentist and the non-reductive physicalist is a matter of metaphysics, and not a matter of explanation or epistemology. After all, many contemporary philosophers hold that you cannot deduce psychological facts from physical facts, even if those facts are strictly identical. In view of the commitment to the identity of psychological and physical facts such philosophers are physicalists by anyone's lights; in fact, they are *reductive* physicalists. But in view of their commitment to a failure of deducibility they would be counted—mistakenly counted—as emergentists by the criterion Broad introduced.

If we are not to distinguish emergentism from non-reductive physicalism by appealing to some sort of epistemic criterion, and if we are convinced that there *is* some distinction, how might we proceed? There are a number of possibilities here; see, e.g., Pereboom 2002 and Kallestrup 2006. However, what I want to propose is that matters look much clearer if we take advantage of the idea that there are different notions of distinctness at issue here. We have already seen that both the emergentist and the non-reductive physicalist adhere to the slogan 'psychological properties are distinct from physical properties but are necessitated by them'. What does 'distinct' mean in this slogan? As I understand matters, what the emergentist means is, not numerical distinctness, but distinctness of some other sort, say mereological distinctness or distinctness in essence. In contrast what the non-reductive physicalist means is, not mereological distinctness or distinctness in essence, but numerical distinctness. So the difference between emergentism and non-reductive physicalism lies in what notion of 'distinctness' is in play: the emergentist is saying that physical properties necessitate psychological properties and yet are mereologially distinct from them, or distinct in essence from them; the non-reductive physicalist is saying only that physical properties necessitate psychological properties and yet are numerically distinct from them.

It might be thought that drawing the distinction between emergentism and non-reductive physicalism in this way is objectionable because it appeals to notions that are themselves unclear, i.e. notions such as mereological distinctness or distinctness in essence. However, I think it is possible to finesse this point rather than confront it directly. For, even if the relevant notion of distinctness is unclear, it remains the case that a distinction between these two positions may be coherently drawn. Suppose we say that Broad-necessitation is the necessitation that holds between psychological facts and physical facts when the second necessitates the first and the second is mereologically distinct from the first (or distinct in essence—but I will ignore that possibility for the moment). Either the notion of Broad-necessitation is clear (or sufficiently clear) or it is not. If it is, then the non-reductive physicalist may perfectly well deny it, while the emergentist may perfectly well assert it. That is, the emergentist can say that psychological facts are Broad-necessitated by physical facts, while the non-reductive physicalist can say that psychological facts are necessitated but not Broad-necessitated by physical facts. On this interpretation of what they are saying, the two positions are clearly distinct—assuming of course that the notion of Broad necessitation is sufficiently clear. On the other hand, if the notion of Broad necessitation is not sufficiently clear, the distinction between physicalism and emergentism may be drawn in a slightly different way, viz., that the emergentist holds the unclear doctrine that the psychological facts are Broad-necessitated by, while the physicalists hold the perfectly clear doctrine that the psychological facts are necessitated by the physical facts. Whether the notion of Broad-necessitation is clear or not, therefore, we have a distinction between emergentism and non-reductive physicalism.

Alternatively, it might be replied that my discussion both in this section and indeed throughout the paper relies on a characterization of non-reductive physicalism that is overly simple. As I noted at the outset, I am operating here with the view that psychological properties are second-order properties and so are numerically distinct from the physical properties that necessitate them. But real-life non-reductive physicalists such as Fodor and Davidson hold positions that are harder to interpret than this (see Fodor 1974 and Davidson 1970). This is particularly true of Davidson whose position officially eschews properties outright in favor of a nominalist ontology of events. So one might suspect that while the points I have made hold good if one has a certain sort of non-reductive physicalist in mind, it is unclear that the point generalizes to other sorts.

Now, interpreting the positions of Davidson and Fodor in detail is beyond the scope of this paper, so I will not attempt that here. Instead I will confront this problem by insisting that the interpretative issues are of secondary importance to the analytic question with which I am mainly concerned. What is important for me here is not so much the position of this or that philosopher, but rather that there are at least three positions that are not outright contradictory. According to the first, psychological properties are not necessitated by physical properties and yet are strongly modally distinct from them—this is the position I have called traditional dualism. According to the second, psychological properties are necessitated by physical properties and yet are numerically distinct from them—this is the position I have called non-reductive physicalism. According to the third, psychological properties are necessitated by physical properties and yet are mereologically distinct from them—this is the position I offered the emergentist in the previous discussion. Regardless of the question of which philosophers holds what view, there is no doubt here that these are distinct positions. In that sense, therefore, there is no doubt that non-reductive physicalists will be able to distinguish themselves from emergentists.

EMERGENCE II

We have distinguished three views: emergentism, traditional dualism, and non-reductive physicalism. And earlier we distinguished the version of the exclusion argument that targets the traditional dualist from a version that targets the non-reductive physicalist. The natural question at this point is this: is there a version of the exclusion argument that targets the emergentist? I will close by briefly considering this question.

A proponent of this version of the argument would again focus on the inconsistency of (1–4):

(1) Being in pain causes me to wince.
(2) Being in phys causes me to wince.
(3) Being in pain is distinct from being in phys.
(4) If being in pain causes me to wince, nothing distinct from being in pain causes me to wince.

Like the traditional dualist and the non-reductive physicalist, the emergentist is invited to agree by a proponent of this argument that (1) and (2) are claims which are (in the context) non-negotiable, while (4) is a principle of causation that we know on more or less a priori grounds to be true. But from this it follows that (3)—a claim distinctive of emergentism—needs to be given up.

Is this extension of the exclusion argument sound? Well, in order to figure out whether it is, we would need to ask what notion of distinctness is in play. If the argument is attacking the emergentist, it must be that in (3) 'distinct' means mereological distinctness (or distinctness in essence, but as before we may ignore this). In short, (3) should be replaced with (3-e):

(3-e) Being in pain is mereologically distinct from being in phys.

Moreover, if (3) is to be understood as (3-e), it must be that (4) should be replaced with (4-e):

(4-e) If being in pain causes me to wince, nothing mereologically distinct from being in pain causes me to wince.

So, in effect the proponent of the version of the exclusion argument that is directed against the emergentist is committed to the view that there is a version of the exclusion principle that invokes the notion of mereological distinctness.

Is this version of the argument sound? Once again, this is a large issue. However, I think the materials we have assembled permit us to at least make the following two points. First, it is clearly no good for a proponent of *this* version of the exclusion argument to complain that emergentism is unclear. As we have seen, the unclarity in emergentism derives from the notion of distinctness in terms of which it is defined. But evidently, that *very* notion is employed in the version of the exclusion principle that is at issue in this argument. So, if that notion is not sufficiently clear, the proponent of the argument has no business using it. Hence if you are inclined to reject emergentism as unclear, you must in consistency reject this argument against emergentism on the same ground.

Second, in view of the fact that it invokes a potentially unclear notion of distinctness, it is likewise unclear whether this version of the exclusion principle is true. An emergentist might agree that there are other versions of the principle that are plausible. For example, they might agree that the version that is used against the traditional dualist is very plausible. But he or she must insist that the version that invokes mereological distinctness is implausible. By contrast, the proponent of the exclusion argument against emergentism will deny this, saying that the exclusion principle that invokes mereological distinctness is plausible. Who is right? Of course the answer depends on whether we can make sense of the notion of mereological distinctness. And of course this in turn is just the question of whether we can make sense of emergentism. Can we make sense of emergentism? Well, there is no outright contradiction in it. But some positions just smell implausible even if they are not formally contradictory. So my conclusion is this. If it is coherent, the emergentist might be able to escape the exclusion problem. But it is unclear that it is coherent.

REFERENCES

Armstrong, D. M. 1997. *A World of States of Affairs*, Cambridge: Cambridge University Press.

Bennett, K. 2003. 'Why the Exclusion Problem Seems Intractable, and How, Just Maybe, To Tract it', *Noûs* 37/3 (Sept.): 471–97.

Broad, C. D. 1925. *The Mind and Its Place in Nature*, London: Routledge & Kegan Paul.

Crane, T. 2001. 'The Significance of Emergence', in Gillet and Loewer 2001.

Davidson, D. 1970. 'Mental Events', repr. in Davidson, *Essays on Actions and Events*, New York: Oxford University Press, 1980: 207–24

Fine, K. 1994. 'Essence and Modality', in J. Tomberlin, ed., *Philosophical Perspectives* 8: *Logic and Language*, Atascadero: Ridgeview Publishing Co., 1–16.

Fodor, J. A. 1974. 'Special Sciences (Or, The Disunity of Science as a Working Hypothesis)', *Synthèse*, 28: 97–115; repr. in N. Block (ed.), *Readings in the Philosophy of Psychology*, vol. i, Cambridge, MA: Harvard University Press, 1980, 120–33.

—— 1992. *A Theory of Content and Other Essays*, Cambridge, MA: MIT Press.

Gillet, C. and Loewer, B. (eds.) 2001. *Physicalism and Its Discontents*, Cambridge: Cambridge University Press.

Horgan, T. 1983. 'Supervenience and Microphysics', *Pacific Philosophical Quarterly* 63: 29–43.

—— 1993. 'From Supervenience to Superdupervenience: Meeting the Demands of a Material World', *Mind* 102: 555–86.

Kallestrup, J. 2006. 'The Causal Exclusion Argument', *Philosophical Studies* 131/2 (Nov.): 459–85.

Kim, J. 1993. *Mind and Supervenience*, Cambridge: Cambridge University Press.

—— 1998. *Mind in a Physical World*, Cambridge: Cambridge University Press.

—— 2005. *Physicalism or Something Near Enough*, Princeton: Princeton University Press.

Lewis, D. 1986. *On the Plurality of Worlds*, Oxford: Blackwell.

Pereboom, D. 2002. 'Robust Nonreductive Materialism', *Journal of Philosophy* 89 (Oct.): 499–531.

Sanford, David H. 2005. 'Distinctness and Non-Identity', *Analysis*, 65/4: 269–74.

Yablo, S. 1992. 'Mental Causation', *Philosophical Review*, 101: 245–80.

14

Exclusion Again

Karen Bennett

1. INTRODUCTION: TWO USES OF THE EXCLUSION PROBLEM

I am not moved by the exclusion problem. I am not alone in this; many others agree that the argument is not convincing. However, I think that there is more to be learned about what exactly is wrong with it. I therefore propose to say a few more words about why the exclusion problem is not really a problem after all—not, at least, for the nonreductive physicalist. The genuine *dualist* is still in trouble. Indeed, one of my main points will be that the nonreductive physicalist is in a rather different position vis-à-vis the exclusion problem than the dualist is. Properly understanding nonreductive physicalism—and clearly recognizing that it is, after all, a form of *physicalism*—goes a long way towards solving the exclusion problem. My goal in this paper is to further defend my preferred solution (2003), and to argue that it is not available to the dualist.

Let us begin by reminding ourselves how the exclusion problem is supposed to go. The basic idea is that if everything that happens can be accounted for in purely physical terms, then the mental seems to be left with nothing to do. More precisely, the problem is that the following five claims are incompatible with each other:

I intitally drafted a version of this chapter for a conference on mental causation put on by the NAMICONA group at Aarhus University. Many thanks to all the conference participants for very helpful discussion, particularly Helen Beebee, Frank Jackson, and Barry Loewer. Thanks also to the Corridor reading group, constituted on that occasion by Cheryl Chen, Adam Elga, Liz Harman, Sean Kelly, Jim Pryor, and Ted Sider. I presented a more recent version at the AAP meetings and at a workshop on mental causation at Macquarie University. Thanks especially to David Chalmers, Kit Fine, Peter Menzies, Adam Pautz, Denis Robinson, and Daniel Stoljar. Finally, thanks to Jesper Kallestrup and Jakob Hohwy for comments on the final version.

Distinctness: Mental properties (and perhaps events) are distinct from physical properties (or events).[1]

Completeness: Every physical occurrence has a sufficient physical cause.[2]

Efficacy: Mental events sometimes cause physical ones, and sometimes do so in virtue of their mental properties.

Nonoverdetermination: The effects of mental causes are not systematically overdetermined; they are not on a par with the deaths of firing squad victims.[3]

Exclusion: no effect has more than one sufficient cause unless it is overdetermined.

This way of presenting the problem is neutral about which claim should be rejected. It is not always presented that way—simply as a package of inconsistent claims, some one of which has to give, and any one of which will, in principle, do.

One virtue of presenting it this way is that doing so lays bare what solving the exclusion problem does and does not require. The question is simply how to avoid commitment to an apparently inconsistent set of propositions. That means that solving the exclusion problem requires, *and only requires*, doing one of two things—either arguing that one of the five incompatible claims is false, or else somehow arguing that they are not incompatible after all. Solving the exclusion problem decidedly does not require *defending* any of those premises. In particular, solving the exclusion problem does not require defending the causal efficacy of mental events and properties.

This makes it different from the various other problems about mental causation—such as concerns about whether Cartesian souls or second-order functional properties are the right sorts of things to cause anything—with which it can easily be entangled. The point of the exclusion problem is not that there is a special problem establishing the causal efficacy of the mental, but instead that the *assumption* that it is efficacious leads to trouble (see my 2003, 471–2).[4] My point

[1] Different versions of the exclusion problem arise depending upon whether it is type identity, token identity, or both that is denied. I shall be as neutral as possible on this question.

[2] Three quick points. First, not much is affected by weakening Completeness to the claim that every physical occurrence that *has a cause* has a sufficient physical cause. Second, not much is affected by weakening Completeness in a different direction, to the claim that every physical occurrence merely has its probability fixed by entirely physical antecedents. Third, notice that none of these versions says that everything that happens has *only* physical causes. That claim is stronger, and is not a good way to start out the exclusion argument (Kim flirts with using it in 2003, 162–4, but rightly decides not to).

[3] It is purely a terminological matter whether this is formulated as stating that the effects of mental causes are not overdetermined at all, or as stating that they are not overdetermined in some particularly *bad* way. The important point is the insistence on the disanalogy.

[4] The point here can also be made by virtue of the standard metaphor about how the physical 'does all the causal work'. The problem is not that the mental lacks the requisite skills; the problem is rather that there are no job openings. It is one thing to be fit for work, and quite another to

here is that responding to the exclusion problem requires less than is sometimes supposed. It does not require providing a positive story about how the mental manages to be causally efficacious. Telling such a story is of course required by a full defense of mental causation from all challengers, but not by a defense from the exclusion problem in particular.

As I have said, the exclusion problem is not always presented as a package of inconsistent claims. It is sometimes instead presented as an argument against Distinctness in particular. When it is framed like that, it is supposed to show that the mental is not distinct from the physical after all. But that conclusion is somewhat ambiguous, and so is the role of the exclusion argument in the philosophy of mind literature. The argument gets used for two rather different purposes. Sometimes it is used as an argument for physicalism, as against property or substance dualism (see, e.g., Papineau 1995, 2001).[5] Sometimes it is used as an argument for reductive physicalism, as against nonreductive physicalism (see, e.g., Kim 1989*b*, 1993*a* and *b*, 1998, 2005). That is, sometimes it is used to defend physicalism, and sometimes to defend a *version* of physicalism. These two uses can blur into each other, and it is not always obvious which a given author is doing. However, they need to be carefully distinguished. Doing so opens up the possibility of trying to preserve one while rejecting the other. As a proud card-carrying physicalist, that is what I would like to do.

The thought is that we physicalists should set our sights higher than we have in the past. We should not merely argue that we are not in trouble over the exclusion problem; we should argue that we are not in trouble *while the dualist still is*. That is, we should do our best to deny that we are in the same boat as emergentists vis-à-vis the exclusion problem and the commitment to so-called 'downward causation' (*pace* Crane 2001, Kim e.g. 1989*b*, 1993*a*). We should do our best to deny that the exclusion argument is a good argument for reduction, while nonetheless insisting that it *is* a good argument for the claim that the mental is nothing over and above the physical. At least, that would be the ideal conclusion. It would be better than the claim that the exclusion problem is so deeply flawed that it is not a genuine problem for anyone. After all, actual arguments for physicalism are rather hard to come by, and we should not throw the baby out with the bathwater.

I am going to argue for something slightly short of this ideal conclusion. The trouble is that it is not clear that dualists need to accept Completeness. Physicalists presumably do; physicalism itself arguably entails it. But it is not clear that dualists do. Many, notably Descartes, reject it, and those that do reject it do not contradict themselves in doing so. So perhaps dualists can escape the exclusion problem by claiming that some physical effects have purely mental

actually find a job. The exclusion problem comes in at the *second* stage; the other arguments enter at the first.

[5] That is, it is used to get from the completeness of physics to physicalism proper.

causes. Perhaps. But perhaps not. The question is not just whether dualists can *consistently* reject Completeness, but whether they can *plausibly* reject it. It is not clear that they need to endorse Completeness, but it is also not clear that they can happily deny it and walk away whistling. Many contemporary property dualists, including David Chalmers (1996, 150), *do* endorse Completeness. Indeed, the current Chalmers-inspired trend towards 'naturalistic', scientifically responsible forms of dualism would seem to be a trend towards forms of dualism that are much friendlier to Completeness. It is an interesting and important project, I think, to see whether even dualists have compelling reason to accept that physics is causally complete. Perhaps the best reasons to accept that claim do not presuppose physicalism. David Papineau comes close to showing this, with his illuminating discussion of the scientific history of Completeness (1995, 2001, 2002). However, it is not a project I am going to undertake here.

Since I am not going to argue that even dualists must accept Completeness, I cannot quite argue that the exclusion problem constitutes a successful argument against dualism. And since I cannot quite argue that the exclusion problem works against the dualist, I obviously cannot quite argue that it works against the dualist but does not work against the nonreductive physicalist. However, I am still going to do better than simply argue that it does not work against the nonreductive physicalist. I have already done that (2003). Here, I am going to argue for something in between that conclusion and what I now take to be the ideal conclusion. What I am going to argue is that the nonreductive physicalist's best strategy for avoiding the exclusion problem is not available to dualists. Defending nonreductive physicalism does not require defending full-blown dualism, too.

All physicalists have a well-motivated solution to the exclusion problem that no dualist has. Physicalists' best option is to deny Exclusion, and thereby endorse a strategy that I call 'compatibilism', and have defended in more detail elsewhere (2003). Dualists, I shall argue, must accept Exclusion. They therefore really do have to choose between denying Efficacy, denying Nonoverdetermination, and denying Completeness. That is, they must either endorse epiphenomenalism, claim that the effects of mental causes are systematically overdetermined in the standard firing squad way, or else claim, with Descartes, that the mental injects itself into the physical causal order. None of these options are particularly appealing. Indeed, I claim that if a case can be made that dualists should accept Completeness after all, the fact that they must also accept Exclusion would amount to an argument for the ideal conclusion. It would mean that the exclusion problem *is* a good argument against dualism, though it does not succeed against nonreductive physicalism.

My primary goal in this paper is to argue that only physicalists can be compatibilists. Here is the rough outline of the argument. There are two *prima facie* ways to motivate the central compatibilist claim that Exclusion is false. However, only one of them is successful, and it is not open to dualists. In arguing that one of the strategies does work, I will argue that, despite possible appearances, the force of the exclusion problem does not rest on any particular account of causation. In arguing that the successful version of compatibilism is only open to physicalists, I will rely upon the claim that the physicalist and the dualist mean rather different things when they endorse Distinctness. When nonreductive physicalists deny that mental properties are physical, they are saying something much weaker than dualists are. Physicalists have a clear argument for the falsity of Exclusion. But because dualists mean something rather different by Distinctness, they wind up with no argument against Exclusion at all.

As those last remarks make clear, however, pursuing this line of argument requires sorting out what the various positions are, and what the labels mean. Here, then, is the plan for the rest of the paper. In the next section, I will briefly clarify the relations between dualism and physicalism, both reductive and nonreductive. In sections 3 through 5, I will argue in detail that compatibilism requires physicalism. In section 6, I will turn to some objections and replies.

2. TAXONOMY: REDUCTIVE PHYSICALISM, NONREDUCTIVE PHYSICALISM, PROPERTY DUALISM

So what is physicalism, anyway? It is notoriously hard to define the view adequately, but I can at least offer up the same slogans as everyone else. Physicalists not only endorse the completeness of physics, but also think that all the facts are physical facts—that there is nothing 'over and above' the physical. Physicalists believe that everything globally supervenes[6] on the physical as a matter of metaphysical necessity. More precisely, physicalists typically endorse a thesis like the following:

> Any world which is a minimal physical duplicate of our world is a duplicate *simpliciter* (Jackson, 1998, 12),

where a minimal physical duplicate is what results from duplicating all the physical facts and "stopping right there". This allows the possibility of worlds physically like ours, but with ghostly 'extras', and thus does not require that physicalism be *necessarily* true. It is a contingent truth about the actual world. (See also Lewis 1983 and Chalmers 1996; see Hawthorne 2002 for interesting challenges to all three definitions.) Given the actual physical facts and physical laws—and no extras—everything else follows necessarily.

Crucially, note that physicalists deny that there are special psychophysical laws in addition to the physical ones—breakable laws that merely link or *tether* the mental to the physical. That is a dualist claim. Physicalists instead think that

[6] I invoke global supervenience because it is both standard and convenient. As I have argued elsewhere (2004), however, any claim made with global supervenience can also be formulated in terms of strong supervenience.

mental events and properties are not truly distinct existences that can be snipped away from their physical bases. There is no room for any wedge. That is why the metaphysical necessity of the supervenience claim—rather than the mere nomological necessity endorsed by some dualists (e.g. Chalmers 1996)—is of crucial importance to their view.

Now, many physicalists do endorse a claim that can sound vaguely dualist—namely, "mental properties are not identical to physical ones". These are nonreductive physicalists, and it is their endorsement of this claim that makes them appear vulnerable to the exclusion problem. It is, after all, the Distinctness premise. Both nonreductive physicalists and property dualists endorse Distinctness, although they have different motivations for doing so.

Property dualists typically endorse Distinctness for the same reason that they reject physicalism—namely, they do not think that consciousness can be explained in physical terms. Nonreductive physicalists, in contrast, typically endorse Distinctness for a combination of reasons having to do with the purported multiple realizability of mental state-types, and with the semantics of mental terms. They typically think that words like 'pain' rigidly designate a second-order functional property—the property of having some physical property or other that plays a particular causal role. Reductive physicalists, in contrast, do identify mental properties with first-order physical properties. The most plausible version, best articulated by David Lewis (especially 1978, 2000*b*), accommodates multiple realizability intuitions by taking terms for mental state-types to be nonrigid designators that can refer to different first-order physical properties in different contexts.[7]

Now, I myself think that there are many interesting complexities here, and suspect—somewhat heretically—that the distinction between reductive and nonreductive physicalism is probably not metaphysically very deep. However, I am not going to argue that here. What I *do* want to argue is that even if the line between reductive and nonreductive physicalism is indeed important, it is *less* important than the line between physicalism and non-physicalism. My claim is that the commonalities between reductive and nonreductive physicalists swamp their differences, at least as far as the exclusion problem is concerned.

One can picture nonreductive physicalism as occupying middle ground between reductive physicalism and property dualism. After all, there are two

[7] This position is sometimes called 'realizer functionalism.' It is more plausible than the position standardly attributed to early type-identity theorists like U. T. Place (1956) and J. J. C. Smart (1959), which simply takes a term like 'pain' to rigidly designate a first-order physical property like C-fiber stimulation. This view identifies *pain itself*, rather than a 'local' property like pain-in-humans, with C-fiber stimulation, and is consequently subject to the multiple realization objection (Putnam 1973).

However, it is at least debatable that these so-called 'identity theorists' actually had something closer to Lewis-style realizer functionalism in mind. Consider, for example, Smart's insistence that the identity between pain and C-fiber firings was merely contingent (1959, 147.) We could take this as an unfortunate pre-Kripkean failure to recognize the necessity of identity, but we could also take it as an indication that he was not using 'pain' as a rigid designator.

choice points here. One is the question of the Distinctness premise—are mental properties identical to physical ones? The other is the question of physicalism—does the mental, along with everything else, supervene with metaphysical necessity upon the physical? The reductive physicalist says 'yes' to both. The nonreductive physicalist says 'no' to the former and 'yes' to the latter. The property dualist says 'no' to both. (Terminological caveat: one can occasionally find the label 'nonreductive physicalism', or at least 'nonreductivism', used in the way that I use 'property dualism'. See Chalmers 1996, and, fascinatingly, Kim 2005, 49.[8]) However, this "middle ground" occupied by nonreductive physicalism does not lie halfway between the other two views. It lies closer to reductive physicalism, because the decision that matters is the one the reductive and nonreductive physicalist share—namely, that physicalism is true.

One way to put the basic upshot of this paper is that whether mental and physical properties are numerically distinct matters less than whether physicalism is true. Another way to put the same point is that the property dualist and the nonreductive physicalist have rather different claims in mind when they endorse Distinctness. The nonreductive physicalist is simply asserting that mental and physical properties are numerically distinct. The property dualist, in contrast, is asserting both that the properties are numerically distinct *and* denying that any dependence relation with modal strength holds between them. (See Stoljar, Chapter 13 in this volume, for more detail on the importance of the difference between various distinctness claims.)

Whichever way we put the point, what matters is that nonreductive physicalists endorse, and dualists reject, the claim that everything supervenes with metaphysical necessity on the physical facts and laws. In the next three sections, I will argue that this makes all the difference.

3. DENYING THE EXCLUSION PRINCIPLE: COMPATIBILISM

Exclusion, recall, says that no effect has more than one sufficient cause unless it is overdetermined. The idea behind the name is just that the existence of one sufficient cause somehow blocks or excludes all others, except in the presumably

[8] This passage appears to suggest that Kim always had property dualism in mind when he used the label 'nonreductive physicalism'—which, if true, changes the impact of many of his claims. Here is the passage:

> I think we can set aside the possibility that mind–body supervenience is logically or metaphysically necessary, since such a view is essentially a reductionist view, and we are here considering [mind-body supervenience] as a part of nonreductive physicalism (2005, 49).

He also says in a footnote that "there are independent reasons for thinking that mind–brain supervenience, if it holds, must be construed as nomological, not logical or metaphysical, supervenience" (49 n. 15).

rare case of overdetermination. To deny this claim is to insist that there is more to overdetermination than that—to claim that in certain circumstances effects can have several sufficient causes and nonetheless not count as overdetermined in the paradigmatic firing squad sort of way.[9] The resulting view is both popular and plausible. It is the view that I have called Compatibilism, and defended in more detail elsewhere (2003).

As I argued there, however, we cannot simply *proclaim* Exclusion false; we have to at least make a modicum of an effort to say *why* it is false. There are two strategies for doing so, based on two diagnoses of what overdetermination requires. To see this, think about some paradigm cases of overdetermination: firing squads, two children (presumably named Billy and Suzy) simultaneously throwing rocks at a window, your alarm clock sounding at just the same moment as a jackhammer starts up outside your window. Paradigm cases like these seem to involve a) two completely distinct b) transfers of energy. That is, there are two separable components in there—first, that there are *two* causes, and, second, that the causes are *oomphy* in some sense that I will try to say a bit more about later. A compatibilist can focus on the latter, and reject the oomphy notion of causation in favor of something along the lines of a pure counterfactual dependence notion. Or he can focus on the former, and claim that in the relevant cases the requirement of twoness is not quite met—i.e., he can claim that in the relevant cases the causes are tightly related in some way that defuses the threat of overdetermination.

So one strategy for denying the exclusion principle focuses on the notion of causation in play, and the other focuses on the relation between the causes. Only one of them works, and only one of them is available to a dualist. Unfortunately, it's not the same one. The one that works is the strategy that claims that certain kinds of tightly related causes can both be causally sufficient for the same effect without overdetermining it. In section 4, I will briefly sketch my own preferred version of this strategy, and argue that no dualist can avail herself of it. In section 5, I will argue that although the dualist certainly *can* move to a pure dependence notion of causation, doing so does not defeat the Exclusion principle. Doing so consequently cannot itself ground compatibilism.

4. MOTIVATING COMPATIBILISM I: TIGHT RELATIONS BETWEEN THE CAUSES

The thought that the mental and physical are so tightly related that they do not overdetermine their effects is a natural one, and I am not the only person

[9] Again, it does not matter whether I say that sometimes effects can have more than one sufficient cause without being overdetermined, or whether I say that sometimes effects can have more than one sufficient cause without being overdetermined in some particularly bad way (see n. 3). It is a purely terminological matter whether I say that not all double causing is overdetermination, or whether I say that all double causing *is* overdetermination, but not all overdetermination is on a par.

to have it (see in particular Yablo 1992, Shoemaker 2001, Pereboom 2002).[10] But unlike some people who push this line, I think that we both must and can say more about just *why* certain kinds of tight relation moot the threat of overdetermination. I think it is unsatisfactory to say, while emphasizing one's nonreductivism, that mental event or property *m* is not identical to physical event or property p, and then to say in practically the same breath that of course *m* and *p* do not causally compete in any way. If they are distinct, the threat of competition must be *argued against.* We cannot just assert that we can have it both ways. We nonreductive physicalists must properly shoulder the burden of proof and say *why* these intimately-related-but-*distinct* causes do not overdetermine their effects. This is what I tried to do in my earlier paper (2003).

What I claimed is that overdetermination requires the nonvacuous truth of certain counterfactuals. In order for two causes, *m* and *p*, to overdetermine some effect *e*, it must be nonvacuously true that

(O1) if *m* had happened without *p*, *e* would still have happened: $(m \,\&\, {\sim}p) \;\Box\!\!\rightarrow e$, and

(O2) if *p* had happened without *m*, *e* would still have happened: $(p \,\&\, {\sim}m) \;\Box\!\!\rightarrow e$.[11]

A couple of caveats here. First, this is only meant to be a necessary condition, not a sufficient one. In particular, overdetermination also requires that *m* and *p* both be causally sufficient for *e*.[12] Second, this is not meant to require a counterfactual analysis of causation; it is simply a test for overdetermination that reflects our everyday reasoning about causation and overdetermination. Take any case you like. If only one of the putative causes really was a cause, only one of the counterfactuals will be true. If they were joint causes, both of the counterfactuals will be false. If *m* and *p* are in fact the very same event, both counterfactuals will be vacuous. And if *e* really is overdetermined by *m* and *p*—think firing squads, Billy and Suzy throwing rocks at the window, etc.—both counterfactuals will be nonvacuously true.

[10] I take it that in trying to say more about *why* certain pairs of causes do not overdetermine their effects, I am addressing a question that Stephen Yablo (1992) does not address. I think he can more or less take my view on board if he likes. In contrast, both Derk Pereboom (2002) and Sydney Shoemaker (2001) *are* addressing the same question as me. However, both of their views are more metaphysically committal than mine. My approach is much more neutral on questions about the nature of properties, causal powers, the constitution relation and the like. Perhaps this is a weakness; perhaps it is a strength. Regardless, all four of us are compatibilists, with views in the same rough vicinity.

[11] This test is supposed to be fully general; I only name the causes *m* and *p* in order to streamline the ensuing discussion. Also, the counterfactuals can be tweaked in various ways to account for the fact that a version of the exclusion problem can be run on mental *properties*.

[12] It is perhaps worth emphasizing again that I am not arguing that mental events or properties *can* be causally sufficient for anything; I am arguing that the assumption that they can be does not lead to widespread overdetermination.

If I am right that the nonvacuous truth of these counterfactuals is necessary for overdetermination, the next step is clear.[13] The question is whether the dualist, the physicalist, or both, can deny the nonvacuous truth of at least one of the counterfactuals. I shall argue that although the physicalist can deny the nonvacuous truth of (O2), the dualist cannot deny the nonvacuous truth of either (O1) or (O2). I shall only take a quick look at the status of (O1) before turning to a more detailed discussion of the status of (O2).

First, (O1). The status of (O1) is complicated for the physicalist (see my 2003, 481–4). Luckily, however, I can dodge those complications here, because the status of (O1) is not particularly complicated for the dualist. She will not claim that it is either vacuous or false. She will not claim that it is vacuous, because she thinks that *m* can indeed happen without *p*. It can certainly happen without *p* in particular, and she will also think that it can happen without any physical realizer at all. Even physicalists, recall, usually think that physicalism is contingent. Cartesian souls are possible, just not actual; worlds where they exist are worlds in which physicalism is false, and mental properties can be instantiated without being physically realized. And the dualist will not want to say that (O1) is false, either. Doing so certainly appears to undermine the claim that *m* is causally efficacious with respect to *e*. To say that (O1) is false is to say that if *m* were to happen without *p*, *e* might not occur. But that suggests that *p* is required, that *m* is not in fact good enough to do the work. Thus there is a real tension here between saying that (O1) is false, and that *m* is causally sufficient for e.

Let us move on to (O2). I have argued elsewhere (2003) that the *physicalist* gets to say that (O2) will come out either false or vacuous in all cases of mental causation, depending on what sort of physical events or properties he takes to be causally sufficient for the effect in question. In the remainder of this section, I

[13] Martin Jones has raised the following counterexample to my claim that the nonvacuous truth of the counterfactuals is necessary for overdetermination. Suppose that there is a small firing squad of just two shooters, Billy and Suzy, with their weapons trained upon the victim. Suppose further that Billy is standing closer to the victim than Suzy is. Billy is a sensitive chap, however, and wants to avoid being the only person to shoot the victim. So he waits a split second to make sure that Suzy has fired her gun, and only then fires his. If Suzy does not fire when the command is given, Billy fires into the air. But if Suzy does fire, he aims properly and fires at the victim too. Although he fires later than Suzy, his bullet nonetheless strikes the victim at the same moment that Suzy's does. This certainly looks like a case of overdetermination—after all, the victim gets shot with two bullets! Yet one of the two counterfactuals is (non-backtrackingly) false. Had Billy fired his gun and Suzy not fired hers, the victim would not have died. So it looks like this is a counterexample to the claim that overdetermination requires that both counterfactuals be nonvacuously true.

There are several possible responses to this kind of 'staggered' overdetermination case. One is to insist that the relevant event here is Billy's firing *at the victim*, not his firing full stop. The overdetermination counterfactuals are nonvacuously true for that choice of cause. Another, which is more neutral about the individuation of events, is to grant that the death is not overdetermined by Billy and Suzy's firings, and to claim that it is instead overdetermined by some *intermediate* pair of events for which the counterfactuals are nonvacuously true. Billy and Suzy's firings count as overdetermining the death in a slightly derivative sense, because they cause events that nonderivatively overdetermine it.

would like to argue that the same is not true of the dualist. The dualist cannot claim that (O2) is either vacuous or false.

Let's start with the easy bit. It is clear that only the physicalist can say that (O2) ever comes out vacuous. The dualist cannot, because she does not think that there are any physical events or properties that metaphysically necessitate mental ones. She precisely thinks that there are—at best!—contingent psychophysical laws that link the two. So the dualist denies that there is any legitimate substitute for *p* that would make the antecedent metaphysically impossible. She at most thinks that there are choices of *p* that would make the antecedent *nomologically* impossible. So the dualist cannot claim that any instance of (O2) is vacuous.

The interesting and complicated question is whether the dualist can claim that (O2) is false, despite thinking that *p* is causally sufficient for the effect. I do not see how. Here, just as in the case of (O1), there is a real tension between the falsity of the counterfactual and the efficacy of the putative cause held constant. However, the *physicalist* can escape this tension, and say that (O2)'s falsity is consistent with *p*'s causal sufficiency for *e*. Let me sketch my story about how the physicalist can do that, and then explain why the dualist cannot say the same thing.

The first move the physicalist has to make towards establishing the falsity of (O2) is to convince us that he is not committed to thinking that all instances of (O2) are vacuous. He is not. If he holds a particular view about the nature of causal sufficiency, he can think that some physical event *p* is causally sufficient for effect *e*, that some mental event *m* is as well, and that *p* fails to necessitate *m*. After all, most of the events and properties that we talk about when we talk about the exclusion problem—things like patterns of neural activity, or properties like *being a C-fiber firing*—do not necessitate anything mental. These ordinary, everyday events and properties tend to be spatio-temporally localized, and they only guarantee the existence of the mental events and properties that they 'realize' *given certain background conditions*. For example, it is perfectly possible for C-fiber firings to occur without pain. They could be hooked up rather differently, or not hooked up to anything at all. Context matters. It is not an accident that physicalism is usually characterized by means of a *global* supervenience thesis rather than a local one.

There is, in short, an important mismatch between the sorts of physical properties and events that are typically invoked in instances of the exclusion problem, and those that constitute the supervenience base for the mental. It is only complicated extrinsic physical properties, and physical events with complicated extrinsic essences, that will metaphysically necessitate mental ones. Thus as long as it is legitimate to plug the more intrinsic, everyday physical events and properties into the counterfactual (O2), it will not come out vacuous. Whether it is legitimate to do so depends on whether such things ever count as causally sufficient for anything, which in turn depends upon one's views about the nature of causal sufficiency. If you think that causal sufficiency is a kind of strict sufficiency, according to which only big complicated sums of everyday events, background conditions, causal intermediaries and the like count as causally sufficient for anything, then the only physical occurrences that will ever be causally sufficient for action will be the complicated nonlocal occurrences. These do guarantee the mental ones, and thus all instances of (O2) come out vacuous. If, on the other hand, you think that causal sufficiency is mere sufficiency in the circumstances, then the more ordinary, localized physical events and properties will count as causally sufficient for action, and not all instances of (O2) will be vacuous.

So even the physicalist can indeed say that there are nonvacuous instances of (O2). These are claims like the following:

> had these C-fibers fired occurred without the pain, my hand would still have jerked back from the stove.

However, these claims are typically *false*—by physicalist lights, anyway. The idea here is simple. The context within which the physical event or property guarantees the mental one *is the same as the background conditions within which it brings about its effects.* So the C-fibers can perfectly well fire without the pain. They could be wired up differently, or perhaps twitching away in a Petri dish. But in such a situation, they will not at all cause the sorts of things they actually cause—they will not cause me to pull my hand away from the stove, and they will not cause me to jump around swearing like a sailor. For localized choices of p, then, p can indeed happen without m, but if it did, there is no reason to expect the occurrence of e. Those instances of (O2) are false. So says the physicalist, anyway.

Let's pause for a quick rundown: the physicalist says that if your notion of causal sufficiency requires you to plug in complicated extrinsic properties and events for p, then (O2) is vacuous. If, on the other hand, your notion of causal sufficiency allows you to plug in more ordinary sorts of events and properties, instances of (O2) will not be vacuous, but will typically be *false*. Now, we have already seen that the dualist cannot claim that any instance of (O2) is vacuous. So can she claim that all instances are false? Can she adopt this strategy, and say with me that if the physical cause had occurred without the mental one, it would not have caused the same effects?

Not without abandoning standard ways of evaluating counterfactuals. For the dualist, the closest world in which the C-fibers fire without pain is not a world in which various surrounding physical facts go differently. It is not a world in which the C-fiber stimulation takes place in a Petri dish, or otherwise without crucial background conditions that actually obtain. It is instead a world in which the psychophysical law that links appropriately situated patterns of C-fiber stimulation to pains is violated. It is not a full-blown *zombie* world, mind you—that would clearly involve the kinds of "big, widespread, diverse violations of law" that Lewis says it is of the first importance to avoid (1979, 47).

It is instead simply a world in which just that particular physical occurrence fails to give rise to the sort of mental one that usually accompanies it. That is merely a "small, localized, simple violation of law", that allows us to "maximize the spatio-temporal region throughout which perfect match of particular fact prevails" (1979, 47–8). This one tiny little violation of psychophysical law is a lot easier to accomplish—if it can be accomplished at all—than a big sweeping change in circumstances.

Crucially, of course, the nonreductive physicalist does not think it can be accomplished at all. As I have already emphasized, he thinks it is a mistake to think of psychophysical laws as contingent nomological connections between distinct things. The dualist and the nonreductive physicalist disagree about what is possible, about what worlds there are—and this forces them to disagree about which is the closest world in which the antecedent of (O2) is true. For the relevant choices of *p*, the closest *p* & ~*m* world that the nonreductive physicalist recognizes is *not* an *e* world. But for those same choices of *p*, the closest world that the *dualist* recognizes *is* still an *e* world. Nothing physical changes at all; given Completeness, *e* still occurs.[14]

Consequently, the dualist cannot say that (O2) is either false or vacuous, and therefore cannot motivate compatibilism in this way. For the dualist, cases of mental causation *do* meet the necessary condition on overdetermination. She thus has no argument for the claim that mental and physical events and properties are so intimately related that they can both be causally sufficient for the same effect without overdetermining it. She has given us no reason to think Exclusion is false of mental and physical causes. In short, it *matters* that the dualist does not think that the connection between physical facts and mental facts is as tight as the nonreductive physicalist does. A mere nomological connection does not fly.[15]

5. MOTIVATING COMPATIBILISM II: THE NOTION OF CAUSATION

Let us move on, then, to the other strategy for motivating compatibilism. Recall that I said there were two strategies—one that focuses on the intimate relation between the putatively competing causes, and one that focuses on the notion of causation in play. The latter strategy claims that the plausibility of the exclusion principle, and thus the force of the exclusion argument as a whole, turns upon

[14] Of course, the dualist may at the end of the day want to avoid the exclusion problem by denying Completeness. But the question at the moment is whether she can avoid the exclusion problem *without* doing so, by means of compatibilism.

[15] It turns out that Barry Loewer has given a very similar argument for a slightly different conclusion. In his case, it is for the claim that the dualist cannot say that ~*m* □→ ~*e* is true, rather than (as for me) for the claim that the dualist cannot say that *p* & ~*m* □→ *e* is false. See 2001, 51–2.

a mistaken view about the nature of causation—namely, that it involves some kind of *oomph* over and above mere counterfactual dependence.

I shall not say anything about whether this really *is* a mistaken view about the nature of causation, and I also shall not argue that the dualist faces any special difficulty claiming that it is mistaken. Presumably, she can wade into the causation literature and emerge with whatever view she likes. I certainly see nothing stopping her from adopting the sort of pure dependence view that is allegedly friendly to compatibilism. Instead, I will argue that this strategy simply does not work. Rejecting oomphy causation does not in fact provide any reason to think that the exclusion principle is false. The force of the exclusion problem does not turn upon any substantive view about the nature of causation.

The two views about causation I have in mind are those that Ned Hall has called 'dependence' and 'production' (2004).[16] The rough distinction is this. According to the production view, causation is a matter of the transfer of energy, or—to use the slang of its detractors—the transfer of 'causal juice', 'oomph', or 'biff'. This is the kind of view according to which causes generate their effects by means of a connecting process (Salmon 1984, Dowe 2000). It entails that there is no such thing as causation by omission or double prevention. According to the dependence view, in contrast, causation is *purely* a matter of counterfactual dependence (or probability-raising, or something of the sort). Patterns of counterfactual dependence do not indicate underlying oomphy causes, but fully constitute causal reality.

People sometimes suggest, both in conversation and (to some extent) in print, that the exclusion problem does not get off the ground on the pure dependence notion of causation.[17] But while I certainly agree that the production view is often in the background of discussions of the exclusion problem—Kim admits as much (2002, 675)[18]—I do not agree that the exclusion problem itself actually *requires* it. I do not agree that rejecting it makes the problem go away.

My claim here is ripe for misinterpretation, so let me be clear about what it is that I am disputing. I am not denying that a dependence notion of causation might be handy in establishing the causal efficacy of the mental in the first place. That is, it might well help block the worries about the causal relevance of mental properties that arose around Davidson's anomalous monism (see Lepore and Loewer 1987), and it will quite likely also help block Princess Elisabeth's worries

[16] Hall himself thinks that our causal intuitions are not univocal, and that we actually have two concepts of causation.

[17] Loewer 2002 is a possible example, though he does not in the end endorse the strong claim in the main text above (personal communication).

[18] Kim says that "Loewer is right . . . in saying that my thinking about causation and mental causation involves a conception of causation as 'production' or 'generation' " (2002, 675). He goes on to try to defend the production model against Loewer's claim that contemporary physics has no place for such a notion. I think Kim is right to admit this, but wrong to assume that the pure dependence notion alone would dissolve the problem completely.

about the causal powers of Cartesian souls.[19] Whether it can or not depends on whether it is good enough as an account of causation full stop. However, those questions are not currently on the table (see section 1). The only question that *is* on the table is whether a pure dependence notion of causation can defuse the threat of overdetermination by falsifying the exclusion principle. The question on the table is whether thinking that the presence of one cause excludes others requires thinking of causation like causal juice of which some effects get a double dose. Is it true that if we reject that in favor of dependency, the exclusion principle will fall away, bringing the exclusion problem with it like a house of cards?

No. This second strategy for defending compatibilism does not work. Moving to a pure dependency notion of causation is not sufficient to establish that allegedly competing mental and physical causes do not overdetermine their effects. I actually do not think that it is necessary, either—as long as one believes that mental and physical causes are appropriately intimately related, I suspect that one can think that causation is as 'oomphy' as one likes and nonetheless claim that mental and physical causes do not overdetermine their effects—but I will set that aside for now.[20] All I will argue is that moving to a pure dependence notion is not by itself enough. The real work must be done by an appeal to the relation between the causes, à la first strategy.

To see this, note that most believers in a pure dependence theory *also believe that genuine overdetermination occasionally happens*. They think that classic firing squad cases do happen, and that they are importantly different from cases of mental causation. Consider, for example, the familiar point that simple counterfactual theories, according to which c is a cause of e just in case e would not have happened if c had not happened (Lewis 1973), do not allow overdetermining causes to count as causes at all. Such views are forced to say that all apparent cases of overdetermination are really cases of joint causation. They are forced into what Jonathan Schaffer calls the 'collectivist' view of overdetermination rather than the 'individualist' view (2003). But—and this is the crucial point—everyone thinks that this is a *problem*, and starts looking for a less simple counterfactual

[19] While it is very hard to see how nonphysical, nonextended souls could actually *transfer energy* to physical things like neurons, it would not be very hard to argue that there are counterfactual connections between, say, acts of will and the contraction of muscle fibers. See my 2007, section 2.

[20] The trick would be to claim that mental property instances (or events, etc.) and their physical realizers *only provide one injection of oomph*. Events, properties, and the like are individuated differently than are transfers of oomph. Two events, one dose of oomph. To see the idea, imagine two events, one a proper part of the other, such that the part constitutes what might be called an 'efficacious core': the other parts of the larger event are wholly inert. One might well want to say that both the larger and the smaller event are causally sufficient for some effect, but do not overdetermine it. And in such a case, surely one could say that even if causation was literally the transfer of a magic pellet from one event to the other. That was all by way of cartoon analogy, but do note that Sydney Shoemaker can probably think of causation as being as oomphy as he likes, while nonetheless maintaining his compatibilist solution to the exclusion problem (2001, 2007). Thus while I myself do not actually endorse the metaphysics of realization that adopting this strategy for the mental/physical case would require, I nonetheless think it is worth mentioning.

theory. Lewis did, for example (cf. 1986, 2000*a*). Everyone agrees that the right version of a dependence theory must accommodate genuine overdetermination.

But that means that the dependence theory alone cannot dismiss the charge that some particular effect is overdetermined. It says that sometimes effects have two causes and are overdetermined, and that sometimes effects have two causes and are not overdetermined. *No* theory of causation that allows both cases can *all by itself* distinguish between them. Only information about the two causes—and, in particular, how they are related—can do so. A mere insistence that causation is not oomphy cannot do the job; it cannot distinguish cases of mental causation from cases in which a person is simultaneously hit with two bullets from two independent shooters. So the mere appeal to a pure dependence theory of causation cannot itself establish that the exclusion principle is false and compatibilism is true. It cannot show that mental and physical causes do not overdetermine their effects.

Indeed, I am inclined to suspect that the only way in which the dependence view of causation can help is because anyone who endorses it will be amenable to my counterfactual test for overdetermination, and will consequently be amenable to my own version of the *first* strategy for motivating compatibilism. Be that as it may, the fact is that the only way to properly motivate compatibilism is by appeal to the tight relation between mental and physical causes. And once we go beyond simply asserting that tightly related causes cannot overdetermine their effects, and provide an actual *test* for overdetermination that some pairs of causes pass and others fail, we can see that *compatibilism requires physicalism.* The dualist cannot avail herself of the nonreductive physicalist's solution to the exclusion problem.

6. OBJECTIONS AND REPLIES

Some readers will object to my claim that my version of compatibilism works for physicalists. Other readers will object to my claim that it does not work for dualists. That is, some will protest that not even physicalists can dodge the exclusion problem in the way I have suggested. Some will agree that physicalists have a viable answer, but will insist that dualists can in fact help themselves to it too. Although the former sort of complaint is really more targeted against my 2003 than against my claims in this paper in particular, I will consider two of each sort of complaint, in reverse order.

6.1. Your claim that dualists cannot endorse your compatibilist solution seems to rest on a rather small point. The Lewis–Stalnaker semantics for counterfactuals has to bear a lot of weight here. Can't I just reject it?

If the dualist rejects the standard semantics for counterfactuals, she can disagree with the physicalist about which worlds there are without disagreeing with him about which is the closest world in which the antecedent of (O2) is true. That is correct. The only question is whether that is an acceptable price to pay. It is not.

Bear in mind that not just any quibble with the Lewis story will help the dualist. The dualist's goal here, recall, is to insist that (O2)—(p & $\sim m$) $\Box\!\!\rightarrow e$—is false despite the fact that she thinks there are metaphysically possible worlds in which p happens without m and without any change in surrounding circumstances or preceding occurrences. Consequently, what she needs to do is reject Lewis's way of reckoning the relative similarity of possible worlds. In particular, what she needs to do is insist that worlds with quite different matters of particular fact but perfect nomological match are closer to the actual world than are worlds with localized nomic violations but perfect match of particular fact.

But this similarity metric gets other counterfactuals wrong—and, indeed, gets other *causal* counterfactuals wrong. The dualist who opts for the modified similarity metric will be committed to backtracking evaluations being the norm rather than the exception. Consequently, any such dualist who is also tempted towards a counterfactual analysis of causation will have to work out a different response to the problems of effects and epiphenomena than that which Lewis offers. I simply direct the reader to Lewis's own defense of his similarity metric (especially 1973, 170–1; 1979, 43–8); I have nothing of substance to add. The dualist should listen to Lewis, and should not jettison that metric in order to count (O2) false. The cost is too high.

6.2. Suppose you're right that motivating compatibilism requires endorsing the claim that the mental supervenes upon the physical with metaphysical necessity. That's not to say that compatibilism requires *physicalism*.

The objection here is an objection to the definition of physicalism upon which I am relying. Although there is widespread agreement that physicalism does require the claim that everything supervenes upon the physical with metaphysical necessity, a number of people think it also requires more. They think that the definition I have provided, though necessary, is not sufficient for physicalism. If this is correct, it would follow that supervenience with metaphysical necessity is compatible with dualism, and thus that dualists who are willing to endorse it can be compatibilists after all.

Now, if worst comes to worst, I am willing to downplay my claim. If a version of dualism that accepts that the mental supervenes on the physical with metaphysical necessity is both coherent and well motivated, I will allow its proponents to help themselves to my solution to the exclusion problem. After all, it is the metaphysically necessary supervenience claim, and not any further requirements on physicalism, that is doing the work. If necessary, then, I am willing to downgrade my claim from

- compatibilism requires physicalism.

to

- compatibilism requires the metaphysically necessary supervenience claim.

But I am only willing to do this if it is necessary, and I am not convinced that it is. I do not think that there is any real reason to deny that the metaphysically necessary supervenience claim is sufficient for physicalism, and some reason to think that it indeed is sufficient.

Why would anybody think that it is not sufficient for physicalism? Let me quickly canvass a variety of reasons, some of which can be found elsewhere and some of which cannot. First, Jessica Wilson (2005) argues against the sufficiency claim in two stages. She begins by arguing that physicalists should be necessitarians about the laws of nature (with Shoemaker 1980, Swoyer 1982), and then argues that necessitarianism collapses the distinction between nomological and metaphysical necessity. But even assuming both the controversial necessitarian premise and the ensuing merging of the two grades of necessity, it is not clear why it would follow that supervenience with metaphysical necessity is not sufficient for physicalism. The mere claim that there is no real distinction between nomological and metaphysical necessity can only show that there cannot be any nomologically-but-not-metaphysically-necessary supervenience relations—and thus that Chalmers' version of property dualism (1996) is not coherent. It cannot itself show that a position that endorses a nomological-*and*-metaphysically-necessary supervenience claim can legitimately count as dualist. In fact, perhaps the proper upshot of Wilson's premises is that genuine dualists have to think that all connections between physical properties and mental ones have to be *completely*—even nomologically—contingent. Thus I do not think that Wilson has provided reason to believe that the metaphysically necessary supervenience claim is consistent with dualism.

Second, one might argue that metaphysically necessary supervenience cannot be sufficient for physicalism by appeal to a variety of technical features of supervenience itself. All of these are reasons to think that supervenience does not guarantee that everything that happens genuinely *depends* upon what happens at the most basic physical level, as physicalism surely requires. For example, supervenience can hold symmetrically, but dependence is usually thought to be asymmetric. Further, there are various odd versions of global supervenience that are too weak to count as genuine dependence relations, *even if* they hold with metaphysical necessity (see my 2004). Neither of these are real concerns, however. At worst, we would simply need to specify which version of global supervenience is used to characterize physicalism, and add 'and not *vice versa*'—e.g. it is metaphysically necessary that everything strongly globally supervenes upon the physical, and not *vice versa*.

A more important threat to supervenience's ability to capture dependence claims is posed by necessary existents. Anything that exists necessarily exists regardless of what else exists, or what properties other things have. It follows that necessary existents supervene on anything whatsoever. For example, every two worlds that are just alike vis-à-vis the distribution of rutabagas will be just alike vis-à-vis whatever necessary existents you wish to countenance—perhaps God, or the number three. So God and the number three supervene on the distribution of rutabagas. But surely they do not in any intuitive sense *depend* on the rutabagas—we are assuming that they exist no matter what.

This is a real issue. I am not sure what best to say about it. I simply note two points. First, the very fact that there is no sense in which God or platonic numbers or what-have-you depend upon the physical means that physicalists should view them with suspicion, and arguably should repudiate them altogether (see Jackson 1998, 22–3). Second, even if the case does show that one set of properties can supervene upon another without depending on it, it does not obviously show that the *mental* can supervene on the physical without depending upon it. After all, no one thinks that mental properties or particular mental states exist necessarily. So this line of thought is not obviously relevant here.

A third argument derives from the idea that there are more informative characterizations of physicalism to be had. A variety of people have suggested that if everything supervenes with metaphysical necessity on the physical, there must be some explanation of why it does. Supervenience itself is simply a relation of property covariation, and it is not in general plausible to say that it is just a brute fact that two sets of properties covary with each other (see Blackburn 1984, 186; Horgan 1993; Kim 1993*c*, 167–8; Melnyk 2003). Andrew Melnyk, for example, thinks that the supervenience of the mental on the physical is best explained by the fact that each instance of a mental property either is or is realized by an instance of a physical property. He consequently thinks that physicalism is best characterized in terms of realization.

Now, that is all well and good. I agree that supervenience claims typically require explanation, and am happy to grant for the sake of argument that realization provides the best explanation of the physicalist's claim that the mental supervenes on the physical with metaphysical necessity. But it is important to see that what this sort of argument at best shows is that the metaphysically necessary supervenience claim is not a sufficiently informative *characterization* of physicalism. It cannot show that the metaphysically necessary supervenience claim is not sufficient for the *truth* of physicalism. After all, it might be the case that metaphysically necessary supervenience guarantees that realization holds, which in turn means that physicalism is true.

Melnyk himself denies that metaphysically necessary supervenience guarantees that realization holds. He suggests, as does Frank Jackson, that the metaphysically necessary supervenience claim is consistent with dualism (Melnyk 2003, 58; Jackson 2006, 243). However, neither really argues for this. They both seem to take it to be obvious that a dualist could endorse that rather strong claim.

However, I don't think it *is* obvious. Indeed, I find it quite hard to make sense of a version of dualism according to which the mental is both genuinely distinct from and metaphysically necessitated by the physical. I cannot understand what makes such a view properly *dualist*, because I cannot understand how genuinely distinct mental properties (let alone full blown souls!) could be metaphysically necessitated by the physical. I realize that this is not really an argument, of course. Settling the dispute in favor of either party probably requires settling the status of the Humean dictum that there cannot be necessary connections between completely distinct existences, and I do not intend to do that here. I simply note that I am not convinced that the view is coherent.

Further, it is not clear why anyone would endorse it even if it is coherent. Note, in particular, that this sort of dualist cannot appeal to the conceivability of zombies to help motivate their view. In fact, they would need to respond to the argument just as much as a physicalist does! Zombies are *not* metaphysically possible on this view. So the dualist would have to explain why they seem possible. Presumably, she would either claim that they will not seem possible upon properly informed reflection, or else that although they will always continue to seem possible, this indicates something about the structure of our concepts rather than about the structure of reality. These are familiar options; they are the same options that the *physicalist* has. Indeed, we can borrow Chalmers' labels for types of physicalism (2002), and call these type A and type B metaphysical-necessitation-dualism, respectively.

So I am not convinced by any of the arguments in favor of requiring more from physicalism; I do not think that dualism is consistent with the metaphysically necessary supervenience of everything on the physical. I consequently do not see any compelling reason to backpedal from my claim that compatibilism requires physicalism.

6.3. Haven't you been paying attention? Kim's latest version of the problem is the 'supervenience argument'. His claim is that not only does the supervenience of the mental on the physical not *help*, it actively *hurts*—it only makes the problem worse.

It is true that I have focused upon the original exclusion problem, which Kim (1989*a*) extracted from Norman Malcolm (1968), and refined and ingeniously defended through the 1980s and 1990s. It is also true that Kim has recently shifted his attention to what he calls the 'supervenience argument' (1998, 38–47; 2005, ch. 2), and has been quite explicit that he does not expect supervenience to do the nonreductive physicalist any good.[21]

[21] The supervenience argument does not affect dualism, with the possible exception of the unmotivated and possibly incoherent 'metaphysical-necessitation-dualism' discussed in Section 6.2.

However, the supervenience argument is best understood as a further twist on the exclusion problem. The exclusion problem proper only challenges the idea that mental causes sometimes have physical effects. The supervenience argument extends the reach of the exclusion problem to also challenge the claim that mental causes sometimes have *mental* effects. I am going to skim over the details, but here is the basic idea. Suppose some mental occurrence M_2 has a mental cause M_1. Either M_1 causes M_2 directly, or it does so by causing M_2's physical supervenience base P_2 to be instantiated. If it causes M_2 directly, we have a tension between the two 'determiners' of M_2. The competition between M_1 and P_2 is not exactly *causal*, and would only be ruled out by a modified version of the exclusion principle, but the point seems clear. P_2 itself guarantees M_2, so what need of M_1?[22] Alternatively, M_1 could cause M_2 by causing its supervenience base P_2 to be instantiated. Even aside from the appeal to some non-causal exclusion principle, it seems plausible to require this (see Kim 1998, 42–3). But the causal completeness of physics tells us that P_2 must also have a sufficient physical cause . . . and we are back at the original exclusion problem.

However exactly it is fleshed out, then, the supervenience argument rests upon the exclusion problem. The point of the supervenience argument is simply that physicalists must think that mental-to-mental causation requires mental-to-physical causation. Since the exclusion problem challenges the possibility of mental-to-physical causation, it gives rise to a challenge to the possibility of mental-mental causation as well. But if the exclusion problem can be solved, the supervenience argument does not get off the ground. More precisely, if the exclusion problem can be solved in a way that does not presuppose the possibility of mental-to-mental causation, the supervenience argument does not get off the ground. (In my view, one important lesson of the supervenience argument is that 'dual explanandum' responses to the exclusion argument are in trouble (see my 2007).) I have argued for a solution to the exclusion problem that does not presuppose the possibility of mental-to-mental causation. The supervenience argument poses no additional threat.[23]

[22] In the latest version of this argument, Kim explicitly refuses to formulate any exclusion-like principle here (2005, 41 n. 8).

[23] Another way to put a similar point might be this. The supervenience of the mental on the physical only makes the original exclusion problem worse if the original exclusion problem works in the first place. I claim that the original exclusion problem only works if it is not the case that the mental supervenes upon the physical with metaphysical necessity. It follows that only views according to which the mental *does* supervene upon the physical, but *not* with metaphysical necessity, face an additional challenge from the supervenience argument. In short: the supervenience argument makes matters worse for Chalmers-style property dualists. It does not make matters worse for me.

6.4. You're only getting out of the problem—if you are—by giving up on mental causation. You haven't said anything about how the mental can really be causally efficacious, and it is starting to feel as though its efficacy is only derivative. Isn't this at best a Pyrrhic victory?

Two points. First, recall my remarks in the first few pages to the effect that solving the exclusion problem does not require providing a positive account of the efficacy of mental events and properties. Second, the objector's underlying thought is correct: no one can say that mental and physical causes are completely independent of each other, and yet do not overdetermine their mutual effects. That is the truth at the heart of the exclusion problem.

Thus I am happy to acknowledge that the dualist has something the nonreductive physicalist does not have—namely, the claim that the mental is *independently* causally efficacious. Perhaps doing without independent efficacy is a disturbing thought. But the fact is that it is a mistake to think that a *physicalist* can say anything else. Physicalists need to bite this bullet for reasons having nothing to do with the exclusion problem. It is a direct consequence of their physicalism. Kim is surely right that physicalists need to accept something like his 'causal inheritance principle' (e.g. 1992, 326; 1998, 54).[24] That is, he is right to emphasize that physicalists cannot believe in causal powers that "magically emerge at a higher level and of which there is no accounting in terms of lower-level properties and their causal powers and nomic connections" (1992, 326). That is part of what it is to be a physicalist.

So the objector here needs to either stop deluding himself about the consequences of his physicalism, or else decide that he prefers dualism, all things considered. But if he prefers dualism because he thinks it is the only way to avoid epiphenomenalism, he must either deny the completeness of physics, or accept rampant overdetermination. That is the lesson of the exclusion problem. Compatibilism is not an option for him.

7. CONCLUSION

I have argued that the exclusion problem does not exert the kind of force on a physicalist that it does on a dualist. Dualists really do need to choose between systematic overdetermination, epiphenomenalism, and the incompleteness of physics. Nonreductive physicalists do not. Thus although the argument does

[24] The physicalist is only committed to the 'subset' version of the causal inheritance principle proposed in 1998, not the stronger 'identity' version of 1992.

M1 → M2

↑ ↑

P1 → P2

Fig. 14.1

provide pressure towards physicalism, it does not provide pressure towards reductive physicalism. A proper understanding of nonreductive physicalism—an understanding that puts the right emphasis on the 'physicalism', and does not get distracted by the 'nonreductive'—makes the exclusion problem look a lot less threatening.

One lesson to be drawn, then, is that these familiar diagrams are dangerous (see Fig. 14.1). They blur the line between emergentism and nonreductive physicalism, and mislead us into thinking that both views are in the same boat vis-à-vis the exclusion problem—which they are not. They obscure the fact that the upward arrows that symbolize Distinctness come to something rather different for those who endorse physicalism than for those who deny it. The dualist really does need to choose between denying Efficacy, Nonoverdetermination, and Completeness. The physicalist does not. And if, as seems likely, the dualist does have reason to endorse Completeness, I can get even closer to the ideal conclusion I discussed back in section 1. The exclusion argument is an enormous problem for the dualist; not for those who say—and mean it—that the mental is nothing over and above the physical.

REFERENCES

Bennett, Karen. 2003. Why the exclusion problem seems intractable, and how, just maybe, to tract it. *Noûs* 37: 471–97.

—— 2004. Global supervenience and dependence. *Philosophy and Phenomenological Research* 68: 501–29.

—— 2007. Mental causation. *Philosophy Compass* 2: 316–37.

Blackburn, Simon. 1984. *Spreading the Word.* Oxford: Oxford University Press.

Boyd, Richard. 1980. Materialism without reductionism: what physicalism does not entail. In Ned Block (ed.), *Readings in the Philosophy of Psychology*, I. Cambridge, MA: Harvard University Press.

Burge, Tyler. 1979. Individualism and the mental. *Midwest Studies in Philosophy* 4: 73–121.

Chalmers, David. 1996. *The Conscious Mind: In Search of a Fundamental Theory.* Oxford: Oxford University Press.

—— 2002. Consciousness and its place in nature. Repr. (2002) in Chalmers (ed.), *Philosophy of Mind: Classical and Contemporary Readings*. New York: Oxford University Press, 247–72.

Crane, Tim. 2001. The significance of emergence. In Carl Gillett and Barry Loewer (eds.), *Physicalism and its Discontents*. Cambridge: Cambridge University Press, 207–24.

—— and Mellor, Hugh. 1990. There is no question of physicalism. *Mind* 99: 185–206.

Crisp, Thomas, and Warfield, Ted. 2001. Kim's master argument. *Noûs* 35: 304–16.

Dowe, Phil. 2000. *Physical Causation*. Cambridge: Cambridge University Press.

Hall, Ned. 2004. Two concepts of causation. In J. Collins, N. Hall, and L. A. Paul (eds.), *Counterfactuals and Causation*. Cambridge, MA: MIT Press.

Hawthorne, John. 2002. Blocking definitions of materialism. *Philosophical Studies* 110: 103–13.

Hempel, Carl. 1980. Comments on Goodman's *Ways of Worldmaking*. *Synthese* 45: 193–9.

Horgan, Terence. 1993. From supervenience to superdupervenience: meeting the demands of a material world. *Mind* 102: 555–86.

Jackson, Frank. 1998. *From Metaphysics to Ethics: A Defence of Conceptual Analysis*. Oxford: Clarendon.

—— 2006. On ensuring that physicalism is not a dual attribute theory in sheep's clothing. *Philosophical Studies* 131: 227–49.

—— and Pettit, Phillip. 1990. Program explanation: a general perspective. *Analysis* 50: 107–17.

Kim, Jaegwon. 1989*a*. Mechanism, purpose, and explanatory exclusion. Repr. (1993) in *Supervenience and Mind*. Cambridge: Cambridge University Press, 237–64.

—— 1989*b*. The myth of nonreductive physicalism. Repr. (1993) in *Supervenience and Mind*. Cambridge: Cambridge University Press, 265–84.

—— 1992. Multiple realization and the metaphysics of reduction. Repr. (1993) in *Supervenience and Mind*. Cambridge: Cambridge University Press, 309–35.

—— 1993*a*. The nonreductivist's troubles with mental causation. Repr. (1993) in *Supervenience and Mind*. Cambridge: Cambridge University Press, 336–57.

—— 1993*b*. Postscripts on mental causation. In *Supervenience and Mind*. Cambridge: Cambridge University Press, 358–67.

—— 1993*c*. Postscripts on supervenience. In *Supervenience and Mind*. Cambridge: Cambridge University Press, 161–71.

—— 1998. *Mind in a Physical World*. Cambridge, MA: Bradford.

—— 2002. Responses. *Philosophy and Phenomenological Research* 65: 671–80.

—— 2003. Blocking causal drainage and other maintenance chores with mental causation. *Philosophy and Phenomenological Research* 67/1: 151–76.

—— 2005. *Physicalism, or Something Near Enough*. Princeton: Princeton University Press.

Lepore, Ernest, and Loewer, Barry. 1987. Mind Matters. *Journal of Philosophy* 84: 630–42.

Lewis, David. 1966. An argument for the identity theory. *Journal of Philosophy* 63: 17–25.

—— 1973. Causation. Repr. (1986) in *Philosophical Papers*, ii. NY: Oxford University Press, pp. 159–172.

Lewis, David. 1978. Review of Putnam. In Ned Block (ed.), *Readings in the Philosophy of Psychology*, i. Minneapolis: University of Minnesota Press, 232–3.

—— 1979. Counterfactual dependence and time's arrow. Repr. in *Philosophical Papers*, ii, New York: Oxford University Press, 32–66.

—— 1983. New work for a theory of universals. *Australasian Journal of Philosophy* 61: 343–77.

—— 1986. Postscripts to "Causation." In *Philosophical Papers*, ii, New York: Oxford University Press, 172–213.

—— 2000*a*. Causation as influence. *Journal of Philosophy* 97: 182–97.

—— 2000*b*. Reduction of mind. In S. Guttenplan (ed.), *A Companion to the Philosophy of Mind*. Oxford: Basil Blackwell, 412–31.

Loewer, Barry. 2001. From physics to physicalism. In Carl Gillett and Barry Loewer (eds.), *Physicalism and its Discontents*. Cambridge: Cambridge University Press, 37–56.

—— 2002. Comments on Jaegwon Kim's *Mind in a Physical World. Philosophy and Phenomenological Research* 65/3: 655–63.

Malcolm, Norman. 1968. The compatibility of mechanism and purpose. *Philosophical Review* 78: 468–82.

Melnyk, Andrew. 2003. *A Physicalist Manifesto: Thoroughly Modern Materialism*. Cambridge: Cambridge University Press.

Merricks, Trenton. 2001. *Objects and Persons.* Oxford: Clarendon Press.

Papineau, David. 1995. Arguments for supervenience and physical realization. In Savellos and Yalçin, eds., *Supervenience: New Essays.* Cambridge: Cambridge University Press, 226–43.

—— 2001. The rise of physicalism. In Carl Gillett and Barry Loewer, eds., *Physicalism and its Discontents*. Cambridge: Cambridge University Press, 3–36.

—— 2002. *Thinking About Consciousness*. Oxford: Oxford University Press.

Pereboom, Derk. 2002. Robust nonreductive materialism. *Journal of Philosophy* 99: 499–531.

—— and Kornblith, Hilary. 1991. The metaphysics of irreducibility. *Philosophical Studies* 63: 125–45.

Place, U. T. 1956. Is consciousness a brain process? *British Journal of Psychology* 47: 44–50.

Putnam, Hilary. 1973. The nature of mental states. Repr. (2002) in David Chalmers, ed., *Philosophy of Mind: Classical and Contemporary Readings*. New York: Oxford University Press, 73–9.

Salmon, Wesley. 1984. *Scientific Explanation and the Causal Structure of the World.* Princeton: Princeton University Press.

Schaffer, Jonathan. 2003. Overdetermining causes. *Philosophical Studies* 114: 23–45.

Shoemaker, Sydney. 1980. Causality and Properties. In *Time and Cause*, ed. Peter van Inwagen, Dordrecht: D. Reidel: 109–35.

—— 2001. Realization and mental causation. In Carl Gillett and Barry Loewer (eds.), *Physicalism and its Discontents*. Cambridge: Cambridge University Press, 74–98.

Smart, J. J. C. 1959. Sensations and brain processes. *Philosophical Review* 68: 141–56.

Sturgeon, Scott. 1998. Physicalism and overdetermination. *Mind* 107: 411–32.

Swoyer, Christopher. 1982. The nature of natural laws. *Australasian Journal of Philosophy* 60: 203–23.

Unger, Peter. 1979. There are no ordinary things. *Synthese* 4: 117–54.
Van Inwagen, Peter. 1990. *Material Beings*. Ithaca, NY: Cornell University Press.
Wilson, Jessica. 2005 Supervenience-based characterizations of physicalism. *Noûs* 39: 426–59.
Yablo, Stephen. 1992. Mental causation. *Philosophical Review* 101: 245–80.

Index